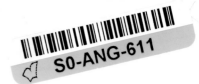

Disclaimer

Healing the Symptoms Known as Autism is not intended as medical advice. This book is for informational and educational purposes only. Please consult a medical professional when the need for one is indicated. For obvious reasons neither the author, co-authors, contributing authors, the publisher, nor their associates can take medical or legal responsibility for having the contents herein considered as a prescription for everyone or anyone. You are ultimately responsible for the uses made of this book.

All content, including text, graphics, images, and information, contained in this book or our website, is for general information purposes only. We take no responsibility for the accuracy of information contained herein, and such information is subject to change without notice.

Healing
the symptoms known as
Autism
Second Edition

by Kerri Rivera
with Kimberly McDaniel & Daniel Bender

Healing the Symptoms Known as Autism
Second Edition

by Kerri Rivera
with Kimberly McDaniel & Daniel Bender

ISBN: 978-0-9892890-4-7
Library of Congress Control Number: 2013945511

1st Edition released May 2013
2nd Edition released January 2014
Printed in the United States of America

Mailing Address:
AutismO2
PO Box 10334
Chicago, IL 60611

Feedback Email: kim@cdautism.org

For further information:
    www.cdautism.org
    www.HealingTheSymptomsKnownAsAutism.com

The Kalcker Parasite Protocol as integrated into Chapter 8 has portions Copyright ©2013 by Dr. Andreas L. Kalcker & Miriam Carrasco Maceda. Original English Translation by Mercy Acevedo
Edited & revised by Michael Harrah, Kimberly McDaniel & Daniel Bender

Original Cover Design: Eduardo A. Davad
http://edudes.weebly.com/

Back cover photo of Kerri Rivera by PaulVanVleckPhotography.com

I would like to dedicate this book to the families
of children on the spectrum the world over.

May all of our children
find the healing that they need.

~ Kerri

This book is dedicated to my Dominick.
I love you forever; thank you for being our angel.

~ Kim

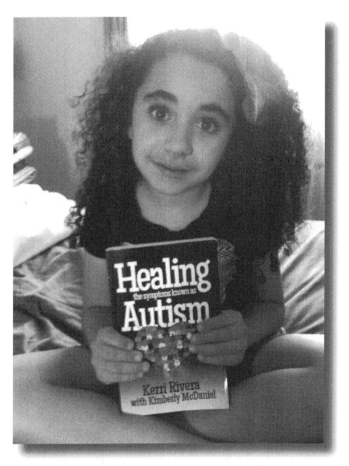

One of our fans currently working towards recovery thanks to the protocol.

Table of Contents

Foreword

Autism, not the one described by Kanner in 1943, but the one that we see today diagnosed in 1 of 50 kids is a combination of immune disorders that need to be treated biomedically. There is a lot that we still need to understand about why and how these immune dysfunctions affect our kids' development, causing near complete impairment of their social interaction and communication.

There is a long, hard road ahead to fully comprehend the integrated system that comprises "autism," but our kids cannot wait. It takes more than just medical, professional, or even scientific interests working hard day and night to find a suitable and effective solution to help our kids. It takes drive, passion, and guts to do the right thing; to hear and read the overwhelming stories of parents from all over the world and not turn our backs, but help. It takes an eternal and extreme will to help, even when your own child is on the spectrum.

Kerri's protocols have been indispensible to the full recovery of many of the kids in our Curando el Autismo (CEA) Foundation. These protocols represent a readily available and effective solution to alleviate most of the pathogenic insults to the immune system. Years from now, when "autism" diagnoses do not exist, when we find ourselves fully knowledgeable about the now mysterious immune-brain-behavior connection, I will remember Kerri not only as a friend but as one of the first courageous leaders that dared to change the path for our ill kids. She goes against all odds, sharing knowledge, experience and simply making it happen.

~ Lorna B. Ortiz, PhD.
President of Curando el Autismo, CEA

"Based on parent reports, the prevalence of diagnosed ASD in 2011–2012 was estimated to be 2.00% for children aged 6–17. This prevalence estimate (1 in 50) is significantly higher than the estimate (1.16%, or 1 in 86) for children in that age group in 2007."

US Department of Health & Human Services
National Health Statistics Reports
Number 65, Pg. 2 - March 20, 2013
www.cdc.gov/nchs/data/nhsr/nhsr065.pdf

Preface

by Kimberly McDaniel

Darkness cannot drive out darkness; only light can do that.
Hate cannot drive out hate; only love can do that.
~ Martin Luther King, Jr.

Welcome to the Second Edition of *Healing the Symptoms Known as Autism!* We are absolutely thrilled to share with you the latest protocol updates and everything else that has happened since May, 2013.

You may be thinking: Why a second edition so soon? Our first edition gave us the structure to explain the protocol, and a foundation to build on. This book has already helped many families around the world, and in fact some parents read it and recovered their children without even contacting us until afterwards! Keep in mind that when it was released in May, 2013 it was absolutely up to the minute, but as we mentioned, this protocol will continue to evolve until we have something that is consistently recovering people on the spectrum of all ages. As of January 2014, we again are sharing the latest updates, as well as a whole lot more information that we hope will be as interesting and beneficial to you as it was to us.

Here are some of the exciting new additions:

- Olive Kaiser of www.GlutenSyndrome.net has written a section on gluten and its role in molecular mimicry and autoimmunity. Since many of you are not new to the autism community, a gluten free diet for your children is nothing new. However, you may be interested to find out just how damaging gluten can be for folks who are off the spectrum as well.

- Scott McRae has contributed a chapter on CDH (Chlorine Dioxide Holding [Solution]). A new method of preparing chlorine dioxide that many families are now using with success. This gives us an even wider variety of preparations available to accommodate the needs of our families.

- The Kalcker Parasite Protocol chapter now has some beautiful charts that spell out the timing of all the components for the 18 days a month that a child will be on the parasite protocol. Thanks to Dan Bender, a lot of the confusion surrounding how to make it all fit will be cleared up. You will also find years of lunar calendars to make it easy to see when the protocol is active. You won't have to check Google again to see when the full or new moon is coming.

- The "Worm Whisperer" Robin Goffe shares with us part of her journey towards healing for her 19-year-old son. Her advice is for the Extreme Cases—Self Injurious behavior, aggression, violence, etc. If you are the parent of an older child on the spectrum, or a child who displays these behaviors, or you know someone who is living with a child like this, you owe it to yourself to read Robin's suggestions. They are full of hope and wisdom.

- The one and only Marco Ruggiero, lead researcher on GcMAF, (Gc Macrophage Activating Factor—an immune system supplement) has written an entire chapter on GcMAF and its applications for autism. A must read.

- Last but not least, a whole new crop of testimonials that will make you cry. If after reading this book you still have doubts about giving this protocol a chance, I highly recommend you revisit these testimonials. If I had to pick one part of the book that was absolute favorite, this would be it. It may be because I collect a lot of them, and usually have a little correspondence with the families to get their permission, and genuinely get to feel their excitement, their sense of accomplishment when they see their child start to heal, and not to mention their endless gratitude for being able heal their own children.

I pray that all of these testimonials find their way to the people who need them and as a result children stop suffering because their parents see them reflected in those words and understand that if other children can heal, their children can as well.

To me, there is nothing more real than hearing from someone that has walked a mile in your shoes. There is nothing more inspiring that to hear someone say, "I know it's possible, because I did it, I lived it, and I am here to tell you about it."

The families that courageously walked this path and then took the time to share their stories are pioneers and heroes to their own families and to our entire community and beyond. They are blazing a trail for others to follow and countless lives will benefit from their diligence, fortitude and dedication. The stories of healing come from all over the world... from children and adults of all ages. We hope that they move you as much as they moved us. We are eternally grateful for the service these families have provided to humanity and thankful that they were generous enough to take the time out of their lives to pay it forward and share.

- The book now as an extensive index making it much easier to use as a reference.

As of this printing, families are healing their children with autism using this protocol in over 58 countries! Our Facebook groups have over 3,500 members in many of these countries. CD officially knows no borders. It is absolutely thrilling to us that people are coming together with the common goal of healing their children themselves, and to help others do the same! It fills our hearts with joy to be a part of this and to be able to see and feel the love that is shared every single day.

The development of this protocol has been a growing grass roots effort, in sharp contrast to how modern medicine usually works. The reason for this is clear: Modern medicine has not really helped to heal autism and may very well be part of its cause. While we don't have any double blind studies to rest on, we do have a slew of anecdotal evidence, which may not mean much to those in the arena of modern medicine or modern science, that doesn't make it any less real. Time and time again, our *results*—children dropping ATEC points—are being duplicated by families all over the world. For a family who is using this protocol, there is absolutely nothing more real than watching their child come back to them. Ask any autism parent what they would rather have... a long-term double-blind study published in a peer reviewed journal... or a healthy child. My money's on the latter.

As exciting as it is to be a part of this, and as wonderful as it is to hear about gains and read uplifting testimonials, we know there are still families working to heal children that are very sick, and our groups share the highs as well as the lows. Kerri will tell you that some months are better than others and the gains ebb and flow. I urge you to read and reread the testimonials. These are real stories of real healing and if you haven't already I invite you to believe that your child can be one of the success stories in those testimonial pages.

All of our families are proving what many were told was impossible: Children with the symptoms known as autism can heal! This grass roots movement is creating a paradigm shift in the way the world views healing from autism. The second edition of this book will be translated into at least 13 languages including Spanish, Portuguese, French, Flemish, German, Czech, Norwegian, Arabic, Polish, Italian, Hungarian, Bulgarian and Serbian. This is exciting. This is real. And, this is a living protocol. Every family that uses it every single day is helping to shape the future and heal the children who are affected today, and quite possibly prevent children from becoming affected tomorrow. For this we are eternally grateful.

Here's to you and the continued healing of humanity,

Terminology & Units of Measure

Throughout this book we talk about "CD," which is an abbreviation for *chlorine dioxide*, a well-established oxidizer. Chlorine dioxide is also often referred to as MMS, which is the common name given to it by Jim Humble, the man who discovered various applications of chlorine dioxide. There are many books, videos, blogs and articles using the name, "MMS," which is surrounded by a fair amount of controversy. We choose to not get tangled into that debate since our focus is on helping our children recover from autism. For us, our only concern is that (1) it is safe for our children, and (2) that it works. Based on extensive use of CD on thousands of children with autism, we can confidently say that both those statements are true. If this were not so, this book would not exist.

Units of Measure

Throughout this book we talk about various measured treatment components and containers using fluid volumes and weights. Since this book primarily addresses a US audience, we sometimes talk about measures in the US system of pounds and fluid ounces; while also using the internationally recognized metric system, which is frankly... easier to use.

The common abbreviations of measure you will see throughout this book include:

l	=	liter (volume)
mg	=	milligram (weight)
ml	=	milliliter (volume)
lb	=	pound (weight)
lbs	=	pounds (weight)
ppm	=	parts per million (concentration)
fl. oz.	=	fluid ounce (volume)
net. wt. oz.	=	net weight ounce (weight)

For easily measuring small amounts, syringes (without needles) are a great tool. Don't bother going to a chain store pharmacy... they won't sell them to you without a prescription. Instead, check your local medical supply store, animal supply store, private pharmacy or protocolsupplies.com. Cost: Surprisingly dirt cheap. The complete set of five below cost about $1.00 in Mexico—less than most candy bars—and not much more in the US. Note: Some brands of syringes have printed on scales that easily rub off, especially if your hands are a little oily. To prevent from losing the markings, cover the scale with some clear tape or clear nail polish.

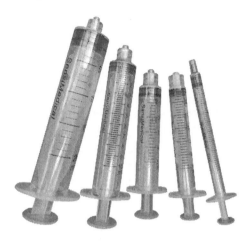

When it comes to accurately measuring larger volumes, you can buy a set of 7 Polypropylene Graduated Cylinders. Of course this is not a requirement. You can use common kitchen measuring utensils, but these are more accurate and easier to read. If you decide to get them, avoid those with printed on lettering (it rubs off). Raised lettering is best, although sometimes a bit difficult to read. Typical cost on ebay™ or Amazon® for a set is around $25USD. The sizes range from 10ml to 1000ml. You can also buy individual cylinder sizes made of plastic or glass.

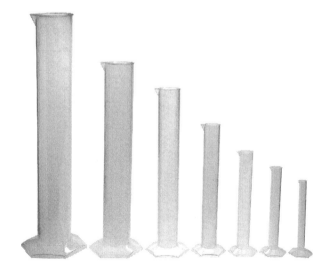

Acknowledgements

Gratitude makes sense of our past,
brings peace for today,
and creates a vision for tomorrow.

~ Melody Beattie

Thank you to my Mother who taught me by example the value of volunteerism and to help others who are less fortunate. Thank you for always telling me that I am the best and that I could do anything. I believed you :)

Thank you to my husband of nineteen years for supporting me on this journey. As challenging as it is, you have always stood by me. You are the love of my life, and father of the sweetest boys on the planet. Thank you for giving me the strength to be strong enough to do a mammoth job. It would not be possible without a pillar of your magnitude.

Thank you to Alex, the best big brother in the world who supports and enjoys what we do as a family and who sees the big picture. I couldn't be prouder than I am of you. I am so grateful you chose me as your Mom, and you chose to be on this journey with me, the road less traveled. I love you forever!

Thank you to Patrick for bringing to our family a higher good. You are an angel. You have brought light to all who meet and know you. Thank you for choosing me to be your mother. You and your brother have taught me more about myself and about life than I could have ever dreamed. I am grateful to you and I Love You more than words can say. Through me, you have given people their lives back. You have forever changed the face of autism.

Thank you to Linda for giving me my sister and one of my greatest friends.

Thank you Slimmie for your support, love and dedication, you are my BFF and we speak the same languages. Thank you for the support of my projects and always having me look prepared.

Lorna, thank you for supporting me, believing in me, trusting me, being faithful to your heart, and for being one of the most honest people I have ever known. You are my sister of the heart and I love you very much.

Susan Wiseman, thank you for offering your connection on that day when I most needed it. That one act of humility changed the future forever. I will never forget what you did for me.

Norrah Whitney, thank you for pointing me toward the direction of recovery, and explaining to me what I needed to do. You are without a doubt my first angel on this journey.

Ana Meckes, thank you for being another much needed angel and teaching me how to advocate for my son. I have not stopped ever since.

Anju, thank you for being my friend, for sharing with me, and for believing in me. You are a unique treasure.

Pina, thank you for helping and supporting me, we will be friends forever. I will always remember what you did for me, the clinic, and the kids.

Kenny, thank you for you excellent books full of sage advice and making biomed user friendly. Most of all, thank you for sharing fever therapy with us.

Carolina, Yamileth y El Jefe... gracias por apoyarme, defenderme y creer en mi. Son amigos en todo el sentido de la palabra. Estoy orgullosa de ustedes, moviendo montañas con el amor que solo una familia puede tener por un hijo....y ustedes lo han hecho por un pais. Les quiero mucho.

Bob Sands, thank you for seeing something special in me, thank you for taking me to meet Bernie and Mrs. Rimland. That day changed my life forever. Thank you for giving us the best hyperbaric chamber in the world. With that chamber we have seen so many miracles.

Jim, you have brought light to many and hope to all who have had the fortune to know the miracle that is CD (Chlorine Dioxide). I am grateful to you every day of my life. I have witnessed first-hand the miracle that is autism recovery. Thank you for staying the path that has never been easy. But it is as you say, "The right thing to do..." I love you.

Andreas, my dear friend, thank you for your dedication, your research and for your willingness to help. You are the science, the reason and the truth that is chlorine dioxide, the molecule that has the power to save humanity. Thank you to you and Miriam for your unfailing support over the years. Your contributions to the world of autism are changing the way the world views autism forever. And the lives of so many children are now recovered thanks to your contribution to The Protocol. Without you both, these recoveries would not have been so abundant.

Dan Bender, thank you for seeing the big picture and for giving so generously of yourself to help us help children with autism. Your selflessness has allowed this protocol to reach more families all over the world. Thank you for making the second edition of this book a reality, we never would have gotten it off the ground without you.

Thank you Michael Harrah for standing by me and working tirelessly to share the information that has had such a positive effect on so many families all over the world. Your wisdom and know-how have been invaluable to me in this book, our website and forums. You were a friend when I most needed one. I am grateful that you are in my life.

Dr. Bernard Rimland, even though you have left us all too soon, you moved mountains while you were here. Thank you for letting me train as a DAN! Clinician, and for allowing us to translate the protocol to Spanish. Thank you for giving us Infantile Autism in 1964, changing forever the thinking that autism was caused by the refrigerator mother. And setting into motion biomedical interventions for healing our children I wish we had more like you. I try to think "What would Bernie do?" and I usually get the answer. Always helping and always available. Humility. You set the standard for humanitarian.

Thank you to all the families on our forums for blazing a trail for others to follow and fighting for the health of your children every single day. You are an inspiration.

To all the Mods; Ginette, Caryn, Joy, Alison, Heidi, Michael, Pam, Katya, Carolina, Nilesh, Mirena, Robin, Debbie, Sue, Susan A., Brandi, Don, Clint, Maggie, Claire, Amber, Dawn, Naomi, Maryann, Susan R., Stacey, Jessi, Lina, Boris and Susanne, Olive, Dana, and Pat, for being the best mods in the world. Your help changes lives for the better each and every day. This is for you:

> It's in our interest to take care of others. Self-centredness is opposed to basic human nature. In our own interest as human beings we need to pay attention to our inner values. Sometimes people think compassion is only of help to others, while we get no benefit. This is a mistake. When you concern yourself with others, you naturally develop a sense of self-confidence. To help others takes courage and inner strength.
>
> ~ The Dalai Lama

Thank you Joy for sharing with Alison that you had heard about CD for autism through the seminar that Jim had in the Dominican Republic. That gesture opened the gates to the north and from there to everywhere. You are a special healer.

Teri and Ed Arranga, thank you for the platform and for helping so many families find what they need for their children, and never blinking, even when it gets really scary.

Thank you Doll, for a much-needed distraction from autism when I really need it most. BFFs are good at doing that.

Thank you to the Mansours, for believing in my projects and me. Your support made this book and our website possible.

Thank you to the various proof readers who helped with that fun process, including Michael Harrah, Pam Gotcher, Joy Whitcomb, Charlotte Lackney, Don Kalland, James Beyor, Cathy Fuss, Jeremy Horne, Ph.D., Luane Beck, Candace, Andreas Schreiber, Olive Kaiser, Susan, and Clint Melanchuk.

Thank you Mads, for your website magic and our beautiful logo.

Thank you Carolyn Unck for helping get this book into shape and all your support and advice.

Thank you Marco and Stefania for thinking out of the box and preserving the truth because it works.

Thank you so much Pam Gotcher for going above and beyond everyday to make sure our readers get their books!

Thank you Scott McRae, Brenda McRae, and Charlotte Lackney for contributing the CDH chapter. This new method of preparation has already been beneficial to many of our families, and is an exciting new addition to this book.

The purpose of life is to contribute
in some way to making things better.

~ Robert F. Kennedy

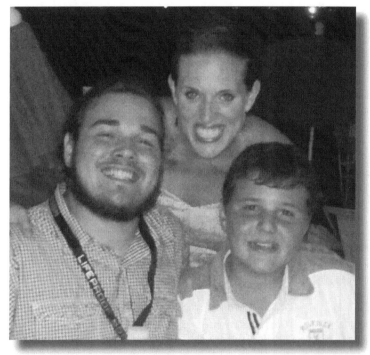

Alex Rivera, Kim McDaniel (Kerri's sister), & Patrick Rivera

Introduction

Autism is Avoidable, Treatable and Curable

*Your body's ability to heal is greater
than anyone has permitted you to believe.*
~ *Anonymous*

Congratulations on finding this book, and welcome to the world of autism recovery. This book comes to life as more and more children with an autism diagnosis respond and recover in more than 58 countries around the globe. This book gives families a do-it-yourself guide to an *Autism Spectrum Disorder* (ASD) recovery program with answers all in one place.

I have, on my ASD recovery journey with my son Patrick, personally been frustrated with the lack of information and answers leading to lost time and money. For example, when I first knew that Patrick was no longer developing "normally" (in 2003), I was unable to get a diagnosis. Seven years, dozens of interventions and hundreds of thousands of dollars later I was still searching for pieces to Patrick's autism puzzle.

I learned over the years of many people recovering their children using various protocols and interventions, and I looked into all of them. Some gave us improvements but not recovery (most specifically for Patrick, diet). Some gave us nothing.

My goal with this book is to alleviate that frustration and loss of time and money for other parents.

I became interested in chlorine dioxide (CD) in 2010 but I was unable to find any information about using it with autism on the Internet. Since I knew that almost every child with autism suffers from similar pathogens (viruses, bacteria, candida, and parasites), heavy metal toxicity, inflammation and allergies I researched those conditions in combination with chlorine dioxide—removing "autism" from my vocabulary.

I realized with further research that CD would be excellent for curing the symptoms collectively known as autism. When Patrick was first diagnosed in 2004, his *Autism Treatment Evaluation Checklist* (ATEC) score was 147 and after six years of biomed he was at a 63. (The diets made the biggest difference in those initial dropped ATEC points). 2½ years of CD later he is at a 21. CD has made all the difference in his life, in my life, and in so many lives around the world.

I brought CD to my *Defeat Autism Now!* style Clinic in Puerto Vallarta in 2010. Today more than 115 children globally have lost their diagnosis of autism (meaning an ATEC score of under 10 points). Additionally, thousands of children around the globe have dropped points on their ATEC and are moving towards recovery. 27 children in less than 1 year in Venezuela alone lost their diagnosis of autism with a combination of diet, CD, and ocean water to the surprise of the doctors who diagnosed them in the first place. Many of those same doctors are now looking at CD for other patients.

It is my dream that every family of a child with autism be given this information so that they can decide for themselves whether they want to give it a try.

This book is a protocol for all of us. Some of you may be completely new to autism recovery; some of you may be a veteran like me and/or parents of older children and adults on the spectrum. This protocol works for even the classic "non-responders" and for those who are so close to recovery yet can't seem to get through the door. This book is for you. CD helps the body heal the symptoms we call "autism" across the board—it is an equal opportunity healer.

I know from experience that an autism diagnosis is devastating on many levels. The initial regression of a neurotypically developing baby takes away eye contact, speech, and the emotional connection between parent and child. Then, when strange new behaviors such as flapping, squealing, rocking, spinning or even self-injurious behaviors appear, you know in your deepest mommy (or daddy)-gut that your child was not born like this. It seems to take forever to get the truth about what happened to your happy, healthy baby. It takes even longer and is more confusing when you have to figure out how to heal that sick child. Far too many "health" providers in the autism field are focused on making money so we can't blindly trust anyone. We must do our own homework. The journey itself is a lot of trial and error coupled with misinformation.

Many supposed "autism experts" don't know much about recovery, or the effective order of treatments and end up costing our children time and the parents money. The less time a child spends chronically ill, the easier and faster it is to recover them. Not to mention the child spends less of their lifetime suffering the physical, emotional and mental effects of autism.

I feel that all parents who begin this protocol should expect a full recovery from autism because this protocol treats what causes this diagnosis. Our research indicates that every person with a diagnosis of regressive autism has virus, bacteria, candida, parasites, heavy metals (biofilm), inflammation and allergies. This protocol handles every one of these issues, and that's why it has been so successful. Some recover faster than others. But, every day we are one step closer to the end of autism.

How do you know if the protocol is working and how long does it take to see results?

The *Autism Treatment Evaluation Checklist* (ATEC) is our measure. The ATEC is an online survey that evaluates the severity of a child on the spectrum. For more information see Appendix 4, page 447. Many families notice changes from day one, while others take longer. You will get results when you correctly apply the interventions in this book in the proper order and without breaks.

What are the results you can expect from the protocols in this book?

I would love to say that everyone who follows the protocol will get their child down to an ATEC of 10 or less—what we call a recovery—and we have 115 of those already. The majority of those I'm in contact with report substantially significant improvements, even if they have not reached recovery. In the case of my son Patrick, he started at 147 in 2004 and has come down to 26. I'm optimistic as I continue to search for further answers, and will continue to share what I find.

If you are not getting results and have gone through this book including the Frequently Asked Questions (FAQs) and troubleshooting, please contact me through the forum at...

www.cdautism.org

...there are always tweaks we can make to keep moving towards recovery.

I recommend you read this book straight through in the order that it is written as that is the order in which it is to be applied. Jumping around the interventions can lose time for your child and waste money for you. Doing interventions in the correct order, when your child is ready for them, is the best to way to achieve recovery. Diligence and perseverance win the race every time.

My mission is to share with whoever is interested, the blessings that I have received. If the information presented here feels right and resonates with you, then please, give it a try. It might just be what your child needs.

This book in a nutshell:

If you want the best chance at recovery, here's the overview of how to do it:

1. The Diet: Eliminating gluten, dairy, soy, sugar, and toxins, to stop inflammation and reduce the overall toxic burden.

2. The CD Protocol to kill pathogens while using a multimineral like ocean water.

3. The Kalcker Parasite Protocol.

4. Explore and implement other potentially synergistic supplements to aid in speech facilitation, neurotypical behavior and/or seizure reduction.

5. Consider gentle chelators.

6. After 3 parasite protocols and consideration of all above steps, find a hyperbaric chamber (1.75ata).

7. Consider adding in GcMAF.

It is important to consider all of the pieces of information in Chapter 14, *Miscellaneous Information You Should Know* (page 323) and apply them from the beginning when they make sense for your child. You also may find the *Summary of Protocols* in Appendix 12 a good resource when you do not have time to reread a chapter to find something specific.

On the right is what we call the *Stairway to Recovery*. Joy Whitcomb, one of our amazing moms, came up with this so you can see just how each step rests on the previous steps, and without them you would not reach the top step… RECOVERY!

Author's Note: It is never my intention to "change someone's personality" or take away their character by healing autism. I see it quite the opposite. When children start to recover, their personality starts to shine through. The behaviors that we saw before (spinning, flapping, squealing, smearing feces, auto aggression, lining things up, tantrumming, etc.) are not personality traits but symptoms of a sick body. These symptoms start to disappear once the body begins to heal and our children can express who they really are through smiles, eye contact, words, gestures, etc. They can show us what they need and want and play an active role in their own lives. It is my dream that every child has the opportunity to mature and choose the life they want for themselves, and be responsible for making their own decisions. I truly believe this is possible for all of our children and adults on the spectrum, and I want families to have the opportunity to offer healing to their children.

Throughout this book we have used the pronoun "he" when referring in general to "a child on the spectrum." This is not to alienate families with girls or women on the spectrum. It is simply a question of fluidity. To use *he/she* or *his/hers* every time we chose to use a pronoun seemed cumbersome, so therefore we are using "he" or "his" throughout the book. We chose "he" rather than "she" because autism is five times more common among boys than among girls. As of March 2013 the CDC revealed the results of a new study conducted during 2011 and 2012 which surveyed 95,000 families and estimated the prevalence of autism at 1 in 50 children.

The acronym DAN! is no longer applicable to *Defeat Autism Now!*, as it belongs to *Divers Alert Network*. The acronym has been used in several places in this book as several of the personal anecdotes are from a time when its use was still appropriate. Today, a "DAN! Doctor" could be defined as a practitioner who received training through the network formerly known as *Defeat Autism Now!*.

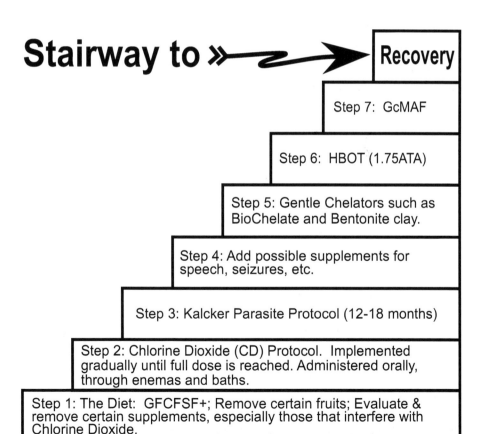

Stairway to ≫ ⟶ Recovery

Step 7: GcMAF

Step 6: HBOT (1.75ATA)

Step 5: Gentle Chelators such as BioChelate and Bentonite clay.

Step 4: Add possible supplements for speech, seizures, etc.

Step 3: Kalcker Parasite Protocol (12-18 months)

Step 2: Chlorine Dioxide (CD) Protocol. Implemented gradually until full dose is reached. Administered orally, through enemas and baths.

Step 1: The Diet: GFCFSF+; Remove certain fruits; Evaluate & remove certain supplements, especially those that interfere with Chlorine Dioxide.

Concept by Joy Whitcomb.

Everything yields to diligence.

~ Antiphanes

IMPORTANT NOTICE

Please keep in mind that the protocols in this book are still evolving, and will continue to be improved as new discoveries are made. We will release new editions to incorporate those new discoveries. The topics of CDS & CDH are particularly new and rapidly evolving. This book is current as of January 2014. Please be sure to check this book's website for important corrections and updated information beyond this and subsequent editions:

HealingTheSymptomsKnownAsAutism.com

Chapter 1

Kerri's Story

*"The impossible is now declared possible as soon as you agree to it.
It's just a flip of the mind, letting go really, nothing more."*
~ *Stuart Wilde*

"What happened, what did you do to Patrick?" That was the first thing my husband asked me when he first saw our son, after returning from a weeklong trip. This was just five days after our youngest son Patrick received his last vaccine—the DPT (diphtheria-pertussis-tetanus) + Hepatitis B + Influenza B (what is known in Mexico as the *Pentavalente*) on the 13th of August 2002 at two years and one day old.

That question was the first of many to propel us down our path paved with autism. I told Memo (my husband) that we shouldn't worry. The nurse mentioned that we could expect a fever, or he could be listless. These were completely normal reactions. Contrary to what she said, what we observed during those first days and weeks were loss of eye contact, flapping, toe walking, high-pitched marine noises along with excessive drooling—drooling that would soak the front of his clothing.

Patrick had also lost all of the speech he had acquired; Mama, Pa, *agua* (*water* in Spanish), letters of the alphabet, numbers... all of it. The only thing he wanted to do was watch videos while running back and forth in his bedroom squealing the "ambulance sound," flapping and banging his gut, and drooling through all his clothes.

Not being well versed at the time in these problematic symptoms, we chalked it up to a case of the terrible twos. But these particular terrible twos led to loss of sleep for Patrick as well as the rest of the family, antibiotic use for green nose and eye mucous, and raging diarrhea that was so acidic it would burn his skin upon contact. This would be the story for the rest of the third year of his life.

The first of many to associate Patrick's behavior with autism would be my great aunt. She mentioned to me that she believed Patrick had autism after observing him at a family get together in April of 2003 while we were visiting relatives in Chicago. It was the most ridiculous thing I had ever heard.

Nevertheless, I went home that evening and immediately Googled the symptoms of autism. Laid out on the website were symptoms like spinning objects, lining up objects, self-injurious behavior, lack of socialization, and several other factors that I felt in no way described my son. I dismissed the comment, and continued to watch my son display strange behaviors, without understanding why.

I was back in Chicago a few months later in July. While going out for a run, I saw a girlfriend of mine who has a child the same age as Patrick. We stopped to chat and she asked me how he was doing. I said, "fine." She asked me if he was talking yet. I told her he had developed language, but since March he had lost all the vocabulary that he had previously acquired. My girlfriend looked at me and said "Oh…" with a look of concern on her face. I asked her, "What's wrong? What does that mean?" Now I was extremely nervous. "Well," she said reluctantly, "loss of language is a red flag for autism." There was that word again. I told her that we had already gone through all that, because by then I had taken Patrick to a neuro-pediatrician in Guadalajara, a psychologist with a huge center in Guadalajara, and a local psychologist in Puerto Vallarta. All three of these experts had told me that he was fine; they didn't see any problems with his development.

I started on my jog, and about halfway through, it hit me that Patrick did have autism, so I sprinted home, sat down at the computer and went to the *Autism Society of America*'s website and found a checklist of 16 symptoms of autism. The directions said if your child had 12 or more than most likely he has autism, Patrick had exactly 12. Looking back, he most likely had 14 or more, but I wasn't ready to see those just yet.

That same day I called his pediatrician in Puerto Vallarta and I told her I thought my son had autism, and she told me, "No, I have never seen anything like that in your son, but bring him and I will take another look." When we went in she observed him. She said that he didn't line things up, he didn't hit his head, he would still come to me, he was 'playing' with some toys in the waiting room, so therefore my son didn't have autism.

The pediatrician told me to go home that day to wait for him to straighten out. All the experts told me he was the way he was because he was the baby of a bilingual family that—according to them—traditionally produces late talkers; his parents and brother were all late talkers. He was spoiled. He had a nanny. And, he's a boy—boys are late talkers, etc., etc. The pediatrician successfully talked me out of the diagnosis once again.

As nothing was wrong, that fall we put Patrick into a kindergarten. His teacher would tell me Patrick isn't doing this activity or that, and I replied that we had taken him to see all the specialists, and he was just a late talker. She was super sweet about it and every few months she would make a comment to me because she saw him drastically different from his classmates.

Then one day it happened, I got a call from the director of the school saying that her friend, a neuropsychologist was in town from the United States, and she would like her to see my kids. At 6pm on March 12, 2004 I had an appointment with this neuropsychologist. I had already figured that this woman wanted to see Alex, my older son because he hadn't been doing well at school. He hadn't been sleeping well since Patrick hadn't been sleeping, which led to some poor performance in school. I had already gotten the news that Patrick was fine, so when she started focusing on him and his behaviors I was slightly confused. We sat down in his classroom, and she started asking me if he always... runs in circles, flaps, drools excessively, squeals like a dolphin, etc., (we actually used to joke that his mother must have been a dolphin). After that, I told her how we had already gone to all of these specialists and they said he was fine.

I was tired of getting the run around, and then everybody asking me what was wrong with my kid when he was just taking some extra time getting going. That's when she said to me, "I can't believe they didn't tell you your son has autism."

These words changed my life forever. Of course I asked her if she could be wrong, and she said, sure there exists a possibility, but she had done her post grad in autism, had seen hundreds of cases and this diagnosis was her professional opinion. That opened the floodgates for a river of tears that didn't end for years to come.

Being a positive person, I asked her what I should do. She said, "I would like to introduce you to a group of psychologists that are in town." The next day I went with her to a hopeless place, with hopeless people and I asked her if this is something that we can cure, and she said, "No, you can do therapy with these psychologists, and that's it." Children are born with autism and they will die with it, was the basic sentiment. I knew for sure that my son was NOT born with autism. He was the smartest, bright-eyed baby ever, and we had the photos and the videos to prove it. He was not born the ghost of a child that we had now. I knew that I would keep searching until I found something else for Patrick. I became proactive and never returned to that place.

The very next day I saw another girlfriend and she mentioned that she had a book on ADD and autism, so I immediately picked up the book and it was all about diet. Gluten-free, casein-free to be specific, and I decided to start it right away. Truth be told, Patrick's diet was horrible, he had self-restricted to only dairy and wheat. Bread products and cheese were his staple foods, but the good news was he still ate potatoes. Even as an autism novice, I knew I couldn't take him to a fast food chain because those fries were coated in gluten. We started off with just homemade fries with sea salt, because that was the only thing left on his diet that he would eat. After three days of being on the diet he said three words, the first three words he had said in over a year. I knew we were onto something.

The next week I ran into a friend from tennis, I really didn't want to say hi, because I was really depressed, but I heard a voice saying to me "It's not about the road but about smelling the flowers along the way." So, I forced a smile on my face, and went to say hi to her in my great depression. Well, she started to complain about her week, so I listened patiently, and then I told her about my week; Thursday my identity was stolen on the Internet, Friday my son was diagnosed with autism, and Saturday my dog of 14 years had to be put to sleep.

When she heard all this she turned off her car and told me how sorry she was. She said that she would put me in touch with her friend that had opened the *Early Autism Center* in Toronto, Canada. When I woke up the very next morning, I had a long email from Norah Whitney waiting in my inbox. She would turn out to be the first of many autism angels in my life.

I received a lot of precious information from that email, but what was maybe the most important detail for me was that what had happened to my son was an effect of all the vaccines he had received, he wasn't born with autism, as I knew. I also hadn't caused this, and I needed to start letting go of some of my guilt. Norah also told me that we can treat autism and I needed to immediately contact a DAN! Doctor, and Dr. Bobby Newman, Board Certified Behavior Analyst and Licensed Psychologist. Norah said that they were the best, and that this group of DAN! Doctors were curing autism.

I got in touch with everybody and that same month we started our own *Applied Behavior Analysis* (ABA) program. I also took Patrick to the States to see his first DAN! Doctor. When I got back home from that trip I had bought nearly $5,000 (US) of supplements and injectables. That didn't mean I knew how to use them, and by no means was I watching my son improving before my eyes. This was June of 2004, and we went through the rest of that summer with some supplements, other biomedical interventions, and 40 hours a week of ABA therapy.

That fall, some friends mentioned to me that their father was receiving chelation in San Diego, and I had just heard someone else saying that chelation was working for kids with autism, due to their extreme metal toxicity. By the end of the evening I had the phone number for the clinic that was providing his chelation. When I called for information, they told me that they referred all of the children's chelations to Dr. Woeller in Temecula California, so I made Patrick an appointment. In March of 2005, I took the whole family to Temecula to see Dr. Woeller, because basically nothing was happening with the supplements I had been giving to Patrick. I knew I needed to keep exploring other avenues.

Several thousand miles and various tantrums later, we arrived at Dr. Woeller's office. I told the receptionist that we had come to see Dr. Woeller. To my chagrin she said, "No, you have an appointment with some other doctor, Dr. Woeller isn't even in town right now." My husband was sure I had messed up the appointment and was extremely upset with me. Meanwhile, Patrick was screaming, crying and taking his clothes off in the waiting room. They finally let us through to speak with the other doctor and after going through Patrick's autism we explained that we wanted to chelate. We had the understanding at that point that his autism was coming from the mercury in the vaccines. She told us point blank that we couldn't do everything at once, and before we could chelate we would have to clean up his gut. I flew home with my family totally deflated. We started on the impossible journey of cleaning the gut.

My first ever autism conference turned out to be *AutismOne* in late May of 2005. I met a lady who was a rescue angel for *Generation Rescue*, and I told her I wanted to chelate my son with those DMPS drops, which were fashionable at the time. She told me that when it came to my son's recovery I shouldn't take no for an answer. I had to advocate for my son, and not let myself get pushed around. With that wisdom, I called Dr. Woeller's office again and told them I wanted my appointment with Dr. Woeller himself, and I would not be given the run around. The manager listened to me and said that she would put me through to him. After a long c'onversation, Dr. Woeller agreed to take Patrick's case and that he would help me chelate my son. He agreed with me that it was silly to think that we could have the gut completely under control before beginning chelation. Eventually I got the DMPS drops for Patrick that I had so coveted, and I felt we were back on track. However, after about six months of using the drops we still saw no change.

Flashback to that same *AutismOne* conference, where I had attended a lecture about the *Specific Carbohydrate Diet* and the removal of all grains from the diet—a diet that helped Patrick inch forward minimal improvement by minimal improvement.

In November of 2005, I had a phone consult with Dr Woeller, and having been disappointed with the transdermal DMPS I decided to ask if there was anything new in the world of autism. The answer that would end up changing all of our lives was hyperbarics or HBOT (hyperbaric oxygen therapy).

I learned that there was a really nice man by the name of Bob Sands in San Diego who owned a corporation that manufactured hospital grade hyperbaric chambers. I phoned Bob's office because Patrick was going to need 40 sessions right away, and I wanted to check prices and see if there was a package discount for hyperbarics. The answer was yes, in fact there was a discount. I scheduled Patrick's HBOT, and took both of my kids to San Diego, where we stayed for 20 really long days to get Patrick his first 40 sessions of hyperbarics—two a day—everyday, morning and night.

During that time, my husband and mom would call and ask me if Patrick was better, but he was still naked in front of the TV, jumping up and down, flapping and squealing. It wasn't until we got back home that he began to pronounce the first syllables of all of the words for things he wanted, like "ap" for apple. We considered hyperbarics a great success, but like I said that wasn't until a couple of weeks after we finished the 40 sessions. That's when we really began to see the changes in Patrick. Bob always says that HBOT is the gift that keeps on giving; you can see benefits for up to two months after you finish your sessions.

Meanwhile, Bob and I hit it off right away. He had a real jovial and family-oriented atmosphere in the clinic. I told him my story and how I wanted to help people know that autism is avoidable, treatable and curable. I shared with him that there was no information, much less Biomed or autism recovery in Mexico (and most of Latin America). I wanted to help people and to share with people that there is a lot we can do to help our children heal.

The very next day he walked into the office and changed the course of my life forever. He told me that he was in fact friends with Dr. Bernard Rimland, "Bernie," the Grand Godfather of Biomedical treatment for autism, and the author of *Infantile Autism, Dislogic Syndrome*, and the founder of the *Autism Research Institute*. I told Bob that meeting Bernie today, would be akin to having met Mick Jagger when I was 15. He then announced that we would be having lunch with none other than Bernie himself and Mrs. Rimland. For the first time in my life, I admitted to Bob that I was so excited that I didn't know what to say. Bob told me that when it was my turn to say something that I should ask Bernie "What can I do for DAN!?"

In a tizzy I ran over to Marshall's, the discount retailer; bought a new suit, hose, and even a pair of high heels. The next afternoon, I put on my new ridiculous clothes, ditched my kids with my friend's maid, and hopped in Bob's Jag to meet Bernie and Gloria (Dr. and Mrs. Rimland)—an absolute dream come true. When we arrived at their favorite restaurant, I was completely overdressed. Gloria ordered a salad, and the guys had tilapia because Bernie didn't really like vegetables. The conversation ranged from Kinotakara patches, to the difference between soft-sided hyperbaric chambers and hard hyperbaric chambers.

I waited until there was a lull in the conversation and I went for it, I asked him what could I do for DAN!, and he said I should translate the DAN! Protocol and take it to all of Latin America. His words left me totally dumbfounded. Had I heard right? Latin America? I was thinking my town of Puerto Vallarta, or maybe Jalisco, (the state we lived in) and maybe in my wildest dreams all of Mexico, but this was much bigger than I had imagined. At this point, though there was no stopping the momentum that we had started. Within months we translated the Protocol to Spanish, and donated it to the Autism Research Institute, for dissemination throughout Latin America. Much later I would find out that one of my dear friends, Yeroline, would heal her son from autism using the translation of the DAN! Protocol, as well as others.

During that same trip my husband and I spoke to Bob about buying one of his chambers for the not-for-profit autism clinic we were planning on opening in Puerto Vallarta. The plan was to run the clinic on a non-profit basis, but anchor the clinic by charging the public for their sessions in the chamber, allowing all the profits to pay for children with autism to go for free in the chamber.

It was a green light all the way. We deposited the money for the chamber in March of 2006, and it arrived on October 31, 2006. AutismO2—Hyperbaric Clinic officially opened its doors on Dec 1, 2006. We threw a party for the inauguration, invited friends, family, Patrick's therapists, and our local priest came to Bless This House. We all wore white, and in honor of Patrick, who was our motivation for opening the clinic, we all had on nametags that said Kerri—Patrick's Mom, Memo—Patrick's Dad, etc. It was a special evening for all of us, but me especially, as it solidified what would be the path that I would still be walking as I write this book seven years later.

The clinic had a Sand's Hyperbaric Chamber, an allopathic physician with a specialty in Hyperbarics, 2 psychologists, 2 hyperbaric technicians, and me, to initially meet with the parents. As for the chamber, we always knew that it was going to help a lot of kids with autism, but it has helped a lot of others as well. The chamber was what gave language back to Patrick in 2006.

Later that same year we sent our allopathic doctor with our naturopathic hippie doctor to Ixtapa, Mexico for a hyperbaric conference, where they serendipitously met Dr. Giuseppina Feingold, (Dr. Jo) a DAN! doctor using hyperbarics for children with autism. As soon as our guys got back to Puerto Vallarta they started insisting that I had to contact her because she is curing kids with a protocol that included hyperbarics. Never one to waste time, I emailed her immediately, but at the time I didn't know she wasn't an email person and, because I am just not a phone person, we didn't connect.

Fast forward to January 2007, my husband, Memo, was buying a 1951 Desoto on eBay. We had to pay for the Desoto with a check, and therefore started to talk to Bryan, the seller of the car. During their conversation, Memo, my husband, said to Bryan "If you don't want to sell, because it's worth more than your selling price I will understand." Bryan had already decided to let it go, but at the same time he was interested in where the car was going, what Memo did for a living, etc. Memo told him about our life in Puerto Vallarta, and the classified ad magazine business that he owns. That's when Bryan stopped him and said, "I've heard of that magazine!"

It turned out that this Bryan was a nurse who works with a doctor who does hyperbarics and heals kids with autism. Well, that piqued Memo's interest, so he told Bryan about Patrick's autism and then Bryan says you must call Dr. Jo, yes, the very same Dr. Jo that our clinic doctor had met months earlier at the Hyperbaric Conference in Ixtapa. So, I called her immediately and when she answered I said who I was, and I told her Bryan told me I had to call her. I asked her if she believed in God and she said yes. I went on to tell her that in September she had met with my clinic's doctor and how I had emailed, but never heard back. At the time, Dr. Jo had been receiving so many emails that sometimes she couldn't get to all of them.

Finally we had connected, and we hit it off right away. I immediately told her all about the clinic and Patrick, hoping that she could come to Vallarta. She told me that I had to go see her in New York first, and we would get Patrick some treatment. So off we went to freezing cold New York in March of 2007.

We immediately started treating Patrick with IV chelation. The theory at the time was the main factor causing autism were heavy metals coming from vaccines that were damaging the methylation pathways. During my daily treks to Dr. Jo's office I finally met Bryan, the owner of the Desoto that my husband bought on eBay. We started talking about my clinic and what we could do collaboratively if Bryan were to move there. Bryan had already been in nursing for almost 30 years and was an expert in ozone and other alternative therapies. He told me he was ready for some changes, and we were very interested to have someone of Bryan's caliber and relaxed personality to join us at the clinic.

Within a week of my return to Puerto Vallarta Bryan came for his first visit, to see if he could call Vallarta home. Two months later he came back with all of his equipment to set up his office. We were a great fit, and Dr. Jo would fly down from time to time to help out with patients.

From 2007 to 2008 we were treating Patrick with IV chelation on top of his regular GF/CF/SF, diet, supplements, and hyperbarics. In May of 2008, I met a mom who had recovered her autism spectrum child with homeopathy. Almost immediately I started working with a world class homeopath from June 2008 to May 2009, but I didn't see anything to make me feel that the cure to autism was down that path. That same year I met a doctor doing the Yasko protocol, and she had some ideas, so we gave it a try from August 2009 until the end of May 2010. At that point, Patrick honestly looked worse than before we had started giving him 80 supplements a day.

By now I had become disenchanted with *Defeat Autism Now!* based megavitamin protocols. A precious few of the families that we helped recovered their children with diet, supplements, chelation and hyperbarics. However, the overwhelming majority still had an autism diagnosis after tons of work by their parents, and usually a lot of money spent on supplements and treatments. I started feeling like it was a fraud, telling people to follow this protocol, which I knew wasn't going to be enough to recover most of the kids. That's not to say that we weren't seeing vast improvements, but counting all of the children that we worked with, only two children recovered.

By July of 2010, I was totally disillusioned and befuddled and I didn't want to continue doing what I was doing the way I was doing it. So, I asked the Universe/God/Angels—whoever was listening, for help. If my mission truly was to help families recover their children from autism then I was going to need a tool to work with. One that was available on every continent and that was affordable to everyone, because what we had just wasn't doing the job.

No magic voice came, thank God! Because that would have really freaked me out. However, I started to remember these colorful little bottles of chlorine dioxide that I never used. I decided to research their use on Google. Disappointingly, there was absolutely nothing on the Internet about autism and Miracle Mineral Solution (MMS) aka chlorine dioxide (CD). So I started thinking about what autism is made up of. So, I Googled chlorine dioxide with virus, bacteria, candida, heavy metals, blood brain barrier, allergies, and inflammation. The evidence was overwhelmingly positive, which showed me that CD could treat all of the components that make up autism. I had hope once again.

I was especially interested because at the clinic, we specialize in oxidative therapies such as hyperbarics and ozone. As chlorine dioxide is more benign than what we were already using, I decided to investigate further.

No side effects except a possible Herxheimer reaction; which is not a side effect of chlorine dioxide itself, but can happen with any detoxification protocol. I decided to speak to my husband and son Alex, who were also excited. The next day at the clinic, my husband's best friend's cousin and his wife were getting out of the chamber. I said, "Hi!" and she immediately said to me, "I'm taking CD." She didn't say "Hi!" or "Kerri!" just, "I'm taking CD." That was the definitive moment for me—my Aha! moment. I told her I had been researching it for weeks, and I was extremely interested. She was having great results, so my husband said he would try it first. If after three days on the drops he was still alive then we would start Patrick on them.

I contacted Jim Humble, discoverer of CD. I was hoping he would help me to better understand how to dose CD for children with autism. I explained to him that there was nothing on the Internet for kids. He helped me do just that. He gave the following recommendations: 1 drop 8x a day for children under 25lbs, 2 drops 8x a day for children under 50lbs, and 3 drops 8x a day for children under 100 lbs. He told me that the more doses that we can get in one day the better, 8 doses are the minimum.

That first week Patrick vomited (classic Herxheimer reaction), because I went too fast with the dosing. On the Internet, the only protocols I found gave high doses a few times a day, and as I found that week low and slow doses all day was the way to go. However, despite the Herxheimer reaction I caused Patrick (through lack of a low and slow dosing protocol) he was still noticeably better. Seven days later my son had improved eye contact and was asking for things that he had never requested in his life. At 9pm he looked me straight in the eye and said, "I want bed." With my jaw hanging open in disbelief, I followed him upstairs to his room. When we got there he turned to me and looked me straight in the eye again and said, "I want take bath." I knew I was not dreaming, and I had really just heard that. After his bath he looked me straight in the eye and said "I want brush teeth" and the whole time we brushed his teeth he was giggling... so I asked him what he wanted and he said, "I want 'kanket'" so I said, "blanket" and he repeated, "blanket, yes" and ran to the bed, and jumped on it to enjoy the blanket. He had never jumped into the bed in his life before that. This was the first seven days on CD. I was blown away.

By September of 2010, every person that was previously only using herbs or medications to kill viruses, bacteria, candida and other pathogens was about to hear about CD. That's when things really started to happen.

Back in 2007, I learned how Dr. Anju Usman was having great success with her biofilm protocol. She concluded that virus, bacteria, candida, parasites, and heavy metals are all joined together in the biofilm (more on this in Chapter 5, starting on page 117). And when I saw that CD killed pathogens and neutralized heavy metals and so many other things that make up the core of autism, I knew we would kill a lot of birds with one stone. I was also hoping to sidestep a few pharmaceutical pieces of the biofilm protocol, i.e. antifungals, antibiotics, antivirals and be able to use something with no side effects (a Herxheimer reaction is different than a side effect).

I was in the process of discovering how we could use this extremely inexpensive oxidizer that is available all over the world to help the body heal from autism. The other important part of CD is that you don't need to take your child somewhere for treatment, as in the cases of hyperbarics, ozone or IV chelation... there is no doctor needed, or trips to visit doctors in other countries. It's as simple as taking a supplement and you modify your dose depending on what you feel and see. Basically, any family with access to the internet, diet, CD and a few choice supplements can heal their child with autism.

After having limited success with my son on different biomedical treatments, even with the best doctors in the world, it was time for a change. With CD we are attacking the biofilm all day as CD destroys the electron shells of the different molecules making up pathogens, therefore releasing toxins into the bloodstream. This release of toxins is the principal reason one must go slow and build up the dose, to avoid a Herxheimer reaction as so many of these children are very toxic. If we kill too many pathogens at once, too many toxins enter the bloodstream. The body will immediately look to eliminate them, most notably through diarrhea and vomiting. This is unpleasant and totally avoidable.

CD is so benign you can use it on your skin, hair, ears, eyes, orally, rectally, vaginally, inhaled, etc. At the doses we use CD in aqueous solutions; it is not detrimental to healthy cells. It specifically targets pathogens due to their negative charges. Once I understood the basics, and Patrick was still improving, I started to share with others to understand how to use CD. Very quickly we were having success that many other clinicians weren't having. Kids on the spectrum were improving, some started recovering, and we had to sit up and take notice. I was blown away again.

In November, a child recovered and then in December another child recovered. Their families took them to psychiatrists and their doctors to have their diagnosis removed. These were the very important first steps that convinced me that this is something that we must continue to do. We started to spread the word that this was an inexpensive treatment modality available in every continent of the world.

With my background in biomed I learned that you watch for reactions while you load the dose. *Low and slow* is the rule. We arrived at the one-drop at a time dose and as kids recovered, parents shared their stories with other parents and more and more people started using it. It was very grass roots.

This is when the explosion happened. I started to think that this might be the missing piece of the puzzle that we had been looking for. In all seriousness, there is no one cure for all kids with autism, which is why each child's protocol and path to recovery is different. While we have seen great success with CD today I keep working to discover new modalities that help these children heal as non-invasively as possible. Now that we had had success in the Spanish-speaking world, I needed to share these treatments with families of children with autism all over the world.

Around this time something very interesting started happening with the CD enemas... parasites; more specifically roundworms were coming out with the CD enemas of the parents and their children using the Protocol. Today I have hundreds of photos, which were sent to me from parents all over the world (first world and third world nations) who have seen worms passed in stools.

At the moment laboratory testing is woefully inadequate, but a keen veterinarian can easily check for the presence of parasites in a stool sample using a high-powered microscope. The children who have had stool samples reviewed by microscopy have come back positive. Pinworms, roundworms, tapeworms and hookworms are the most common findings. Stool analysis done by laboratories have consistently come back negative even when worms have clearly been seen and photographed and seen under the microscope. In fact, one mother I know sent in a live, moving worm that her child had passed. The result? Negative for parasites! At this point it is simply not enough to trust a coprological analysis when looking for parasites.

Dr. Andreas Kalcker and Miriam Carrasco have been instrumental in this piece of the puzzle and have designed an amazing parasite protocol that has already helped many children including Patrick. In October of 2011, Andreas gave me the first parasite protocol and families in Spain, Mexico, Venezuela and others throughout Latin America began to use it. We'll talk about it in depth in Chapter 8, page 165 and how it has affected my life as well as the lives of so many other families with children on the spectrum.

In January of 2012, I got in touch with Teri Arranga and I was invited to speak at *AutismOne* in May of 2012. This would be the first time I would present at *AutismOne* in English, and obviously the first ever presentation on CD. After eight years of biomed and six years of helping families in Latin America I would be flying above the radar, knowing full well there would be a tradeoff. While I would reach families all over the US, for the first time I would end up taking a lot of flak in the blogosphere. We survived!

When I first came across CD in 2010 and began to watch it work it's miracles with autism, I expected parents, doctors and professionals who dealt with autism to be excited. I assumed they would begin to do research as to how and why the chlorine dioxide molecule was healing/curing autism. Much to my chagrin, many people were disinterested. Some even went so far as to say that what I had seen was impossible or that CD was toxic. Well, to that I would say that healing/curing autism with a toxic substance is impossible. Since then a handful of some of the best doctors in the world have become interested (that number is growing) and quite a few parents are taking note. Hundreds in fact went to my presentation at *AutismOne*. Several told me in hindsight that they had thought about not attending because the title of the presentation sounded too good to be true... *40 Children Recovered in 21 Months*.

The people who did attend were pleased with the information and many began the Protocol. However, what was to happen the days and weeks after my presentation blew my mind and was absolutely beyond my wildest nightmares. Some parents attacked me in print and on the Internet. I received threatening and accusatory emails filled with hate speech and foul language.

In most cases these emails and blogs were from anti-biomed parents. Others in the biomed movement told me not to worry, that these people were notorious for doing this sort of thing to others. They jump on the newest and brightest intervention in order to get their time in the limelight. Stealing attention away from the treatment, altering the truth, and in some cases lying to people about what is happening just to get other parents up in arms. Never could I have imagined anything like what transpired. However, as time passed, so did the threats, negative blog posts, etc.

Update for 2014

One of my favorite quotes states:

> *"All truth passes through three stages. First, it is ridiculed. Second, it is violently opposed. Third, it is accepted as being self-evident."*

Fortunately, the 2013 *AutismOne* conference was a totally different experience—which may indicate we are slipping into that third stage. In May of 2013, we were at 93 recoveries, and during my presentation at *AutismOne*, some courageous parents took the stage with me to share their children's stories of healing and recovery. There were no attacks. As the first edition of this book launched at the conference, many of our wonderful moderators were on hand to answer questions, and assist parents who were interested in getting started. I had a book signing along with the pleasure of meeting many parents I had up until then only known through email or Facebook. By January 2014, the first edition had already sold thousands of copies. If you searched for "autism" in the category of "books" on Amazon, it was showing up in various positions of the first two pages of over 10,000+ results, with the majority being five-star reviews. If you changed the order to "Average Customer Review," it was in the top 10, sometimes in position #1.

This has always been a grassroots parent driven movement, and today help is available in 7 languages online to answer questions and offer support. As with anything, if you attract enough attention, you will also attract some "haters," however CD has already earned itself a place in the treatment modalities that are healing the symptoms known as autism.

CDS (chlorine dioxide solution) was introduced in the first edition, as we were still hoping that it was something better than it turned out to be. It was a better tasting and more tolerated form of CD, and still remains an excellent preparation choice for those who are extremely sensitive, and have trouble tolerating even one drop of classic CD. However, we found that over the long haul, only one child so far has recovered with strict CDS use—the other 114 were with classic CD.

In this edition we are introducing *Chlorine Dioxide Holding [Solution]* (CDH). When this preparation technique was introduced it was touted as something similar to CDS... having a better taste, is better tolerated, along with less Herxheimer reactions. However, there is one big difference; CDH still contains a small amount of the raw materials required for the preparation of CD (sodium chlorite and citric/hydrochloric acid). On the other hand,

CDS was chlorine dioxide gas ONLY dissolved in water. That small amount of raw materials in the CDH preparation may be what makes the difference. After 90 days of CDH use with over 70 families, it has not failed. Gains have not plateaued, and parents seem to be having an easier time increasing their children's dose, without any Herxheimer reactions. Another amazing thing about CDH is that the natural sweetener *Stevia* can be added to improve the flavor, while the potency of the dose does not change. This can be a game changer for kids that have taste aversion to classic CD. It should be noted that not all brands of Stevia are created equal and there may be some that can't be used. We are still testing various brands.

CDS and CDH have both earned their place in methods of chlorine dioxide preparation, thus allowing more people to benefit from the healing properties of CD who might not have otherwise been able to tolerate it.

People are always interested to know how my son Patrick is doing, and I am happy to share a little bit about what has been going on in his life lately. This past August 2013, Patrick turned 13. I had expected him to be recovered by now; however, we are still working towards a full recovery. He is better every month and his current ATEC is somewhere between 22 and 24. Patrick is very social, he loves a party. This Halloween, my sister threw a party and it was 11:30pm before he was finally ready to go home. He also loves spending time with his family. Every night he tells me, "I love you Mommy, gimme kissy." That is not only his way of telling me he wants a kiss, but that he wants me to come spend time with him before we go to sleep.

He has been preparing his own food in the kitchen, and while he has always liked to help chop, his being able to place his selection in the toaster oven and heat it himself is new. We didn't show him how to do this. He decided on his own that he would heat and serve himself his dinner one day. Another major advancement is that he is now able to clean himself after toileting, which is something he always asked for help with before. He will even wear headphones when listening to YouTube videos or watching DVDs if someone has to make a phone call.

We don't have any conduct issues, and if no one told you I had a son with autism, and you saw us out, you would never know. Apraxia remains the biggest factor delaying Patrick's recovery. That said, Patrick does communicate more than ever, and attempts more language than ever before.

As far as where I see this movement heading in the future, I believe that if truth does pass through 3 stages then we have finally entered the third stage of "self-evidence." The CD Protocol has now recovered 115 children (as of

December 2013); is used in 58 countries; and has already helped over 5,000 people on the spectrum, with more and more being added every day. The power of social media allows for parents to share with other parents their successes with the protocol, thus forming a stronger bond. Parents in the autism community trust other parents above doctors, and rightfully so.

At this point we are breaking many stereotypes associated with healing autism. For example, we now know that after the age of 9, recovery is still very possible (a 31 year old man is nearing recovery as I write these words). You do not have to be rich to recover your child from autism. You do not have to speak English—there are Facebook groups in 7 languages and this book will be translated into at least 13 languages. We now know that autism is not a psychological disorder. It is biomedical... viruses, bacteria, candida, parasites, and heavy metals cause the behaviors that lead to an autism diagnosis. Once you remove what is causing the symptoms, you can remove the diagnosis.

I witness on a daily basis what was not supposed to be possible: the healing of autism.

The future is bright, and it is up to us to share it!

Best in health,

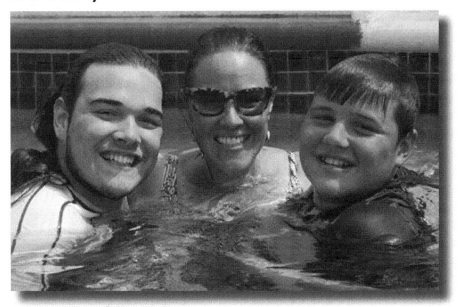

Alex, Kerri & Patrick Rivera

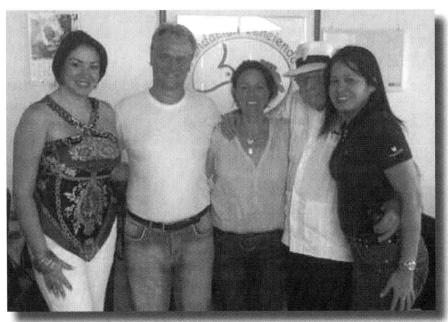

Jim, Andreas and myself in Venezuela where 2 of the most amazing women in the world have a foundation to help Venezuela heal from the autism epidemic. I am so grateful to Yamileth Paduani and Carolina Moreno for their foundation and hard work. 28 recovered children from their foundation with this protocol in their first year of service. Thank you ladies. I am so proud to be your sister of the heart.

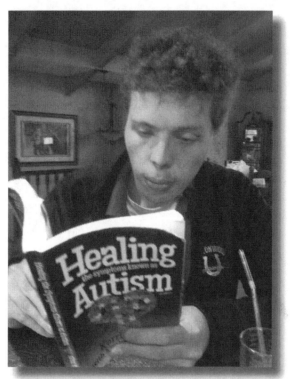

Ty reading and healing

Chapter 2

<u>Yes We Can!!!</u>

Without faith, nothing is possible. With it, nothing is impossible.
*~ **Mary McLeod Bethune***

Before we embark on the path of healing autism, it may provide you some comfort and encouragement to hear from those who have gone before you.

Some of the parents of the children who lost their diagnosis through this Protocol were generous enough to share a photo of their children along with a "thank you note." You will see that a couple of the older children wanted to write their own notes and share their success with the world.

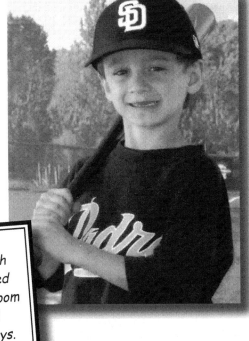

1 My son gets to play little League!

Thanks to ATEC of 4, autism IS treatable!

THANK YOU KERRI!

2 OMG! I'm still rubbing my eyes. Nathan just played with cars appropriately! He pushed them along while saying, "vroom vroom!" Until now, he would simply mouth, spin or tap toys.
-Week 5 of MMS

③ Today in my son's school they had an "I Can Run" day for good health and to collect food for families in our community. Last year he couldn't make it 1 mile - they run / walk around a track. This year he ran 2 miles... Whhaattt? 7 months on mms and 6 months treating parasites.

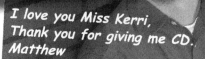

④

I love you Miss Kerri, Thank you for giving me CD. Matthew

⑤ Wow! Here is something to be grateful for! It was time to do my son's one year ATEC doing MMS (7 months detoxing parasites) and his score was...drum roll please...15! You read it right, a 15! I am tearing up right now writing this. My son is 14 years, 4 months old. He was at a 27 when we started, then went up to a 34 when we started treating parasites (behaviors worsened), then down to 21 three months ago, and now a 15! Thank you so much Kerri! Without you, who knows where he'd be.

⑥ Before MMS we were able to get my sons atec score down to a 24. Although he mainly functioned as a "neurotypical" child, he still would have behavioral problems. He was easily agitated and would struggle with some anxiety and OCD. We were constantly battling yeast, constipation, metals and come to find out, parasites! We began MMS very slowly. We noticed his moods were improving. He was smiling more and over all just really pleasant to be around. We decided to retake his atec after only 1 month. It was a shocking 4!!! It dropped 20 points in 1 month!!! We have our boy back and will forever be grateful! We will be starting the parasite protocol this month and looking forward to an atec of 0!!!

I just wanted to share that today my daughter said a full sentence!

She normally only makes two word sentences and often stutters and stammers, with a lot of articulation problems.

My husband came home after a week away for work and she walked up to him as he sat at the computer and she said: "I want... to sit with daddy."

And in the bathtub (I'm doing the MMS steambath as both my kids are coughing right now), she turned to her brother and said "Look brother, cup." and she held the plastic cup in front of him. She has never been this coordinated and 'present', nor articulate. I am so grateful.

Even though we still have a long way to go, I feel like a huge weight has been lifted off my shoulders.

Thank you for your hard work.

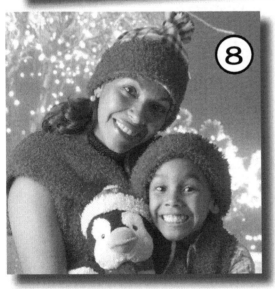

Thank you for helping me to rescue my son. God bless you Kerri Rivera!

My son is at a three-day camp with 100 NT 5th graders! We have provided all his food, and go up to give supplements twice a day... other than that, he is on his own sleeping with friends for the first time in his life! I have no words other than Praise The Lord for bringing me Kerri Rivera and also for giving me and my family the strength to never give up! Our little bird had taken flight... thanks be to God!

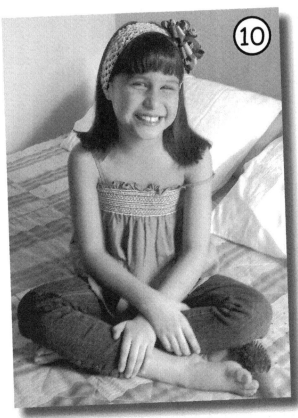

(10) *Thank you God for your fidelity, thank you my beautiful girl for giving me your gaze and your smile every day, thank you Kerri McDaniel de Rivera for walking with me.*

(11) Hello, I'm Silvia, Alejandro's mom, we live in Spain. I was giving MMS to my son for 10 months without seeing any changes. Kerri told me that I wasn't doing something right... and that was correct. Being the warrior she is, she made me tell her everything I was giving Alejandro and she got it, Alejandro drank pineapple juice all day long, he would take more than a liter a day and that made the MMS not work, I stopped giving him pineapple juice 2 months ago, and he is a new child... He pays attention, his comprehension is almost 100% I must say my baby did not speak, but with this he started saying: "Come on, mom!" "My mommy" All this because I started giving him the MMS as I should. I want to say NO juice near MMS because it anulls its effectiveness. I thank God for putting Kerri in my path. My son improves everyday, slowly but you can see that he is saying goodbye to his little world. Thank you Kerri for being in our lives and for making us see the light. Also thank you JIM HUMBLE for giving hope to our lives.

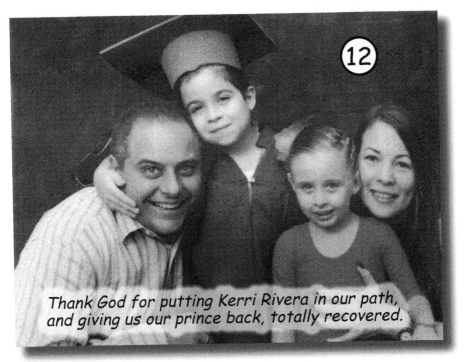

Thank God for putting Kerri Rivera in our path, and giving us our prince back, totally recovered.

(13)

My son turned 12 today - hooray!! This is truly the very first time since his 1st birthday that my heart didn't shatter into a million pieces because it's another year down the road, and still so far away from recovery!! He decided that he was staying at home today to play with his birthday toys, he told his teacher (several times over), and when she asked if she could take the day off too, he said "nooooo!!. When his grandpa called from Holland to sing Happy Birthday, he sat quietly listening with a smile on his face - the usual is "no singing!" Besides that - here's my brag for the day - his teacher told me that she had to move him and his best class buddy away from each other because they were copying each other's work!!! YAHOO - we were SO excited - yes I know, we're crazy, but hey - if it's typical, I don't care what it looks like, I WILL TAKE IT!!! If you think this is weird, you should've seen me when he bit a child when he was 3!! I want to encourage you all today, look for the small things, check in with the people who are in contact with your kids and keep a journal of the changes. You will be amazed at how much we miss, because we spend every waking moment watching over them! I feel SO blessed!!

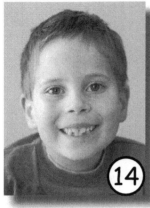

Dear Kerri,

Thank you so much for bringing our son's smile to life. The happiness you see in these eyes comes from listening to you and your amazing protocol.

We were stunned when his ATEC dropped 18 points in 3 weeks, and has now reached a staggering 1 from the original 36 in less than one year.

(14) I thank God every day for having me in that AutismOne lecture in 2012 where you opened my eyes to what else we could do to help him. I want every parent out there to know this is a real Protocol with real results.

Thank you again and God Bless everything you do for our Children.

You Rock! Love Maryann

(15) Greetings from Monterrey.

Just to let you know, we went to visit you in Puerto Vallarta on June 21st, and my child started treatment in July with MMS. As of today my son eats almost all on his own, and wipes his mouth whenever he needs to. For about a month now he has been doing funny things; like covering up his cards when we play as if to hide them, if he sees me squatting on the floor he runs over and jumps on me. He shows expectation on his face when he knows that I am coming to tickle him. He hides behind a wall when we play hide-and-seek.

In both of the institutes where he goes they have told me he is able to pay attention for longer periods of time, his way of being has changed, and they have also said that his eye contact is much better. According to his therapist he is now a candidate for speech therapy because he is able to pay attention.

For us, Kerri, this is a miracle come true, to see our son waking up little by little and to see him eat all on his own. Thank you so much for sharing all of this with us.

Since starting MMS my daughter's play skills improved, (16) she actually looks into my eyes and gives me eye contact which means a lot. She started answering questions, more engaging and now I started to feel as if the end of the tunnel is not too far. I am so grateful to Kerri for showing me a way to recover my child. GOD BLESS.

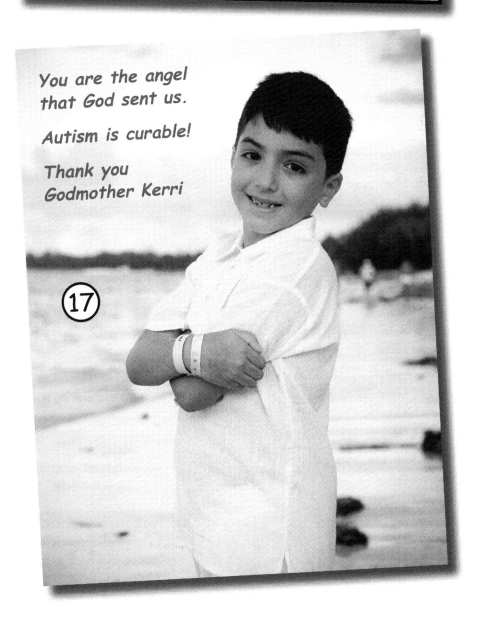

You are the angel that God sent us.

Autism is curable!

Thank you Godmother Kerri

Hi Kerri,   (18)

I cannot believe it has been 5 weeks since we spoke on the phone.

My son turned 22 yesterday. He actually opened each birthday card, and read the inside. We always knew he could read, but he Never showed an interest in opening cards or gifts. He had some interest in his gifts last night. He has been wearing only light grey shirts for 5 years. This week he wore a blue one and a charcoal grey shirt.

Looking straight at me, and asking for what he wants. No real bad effects yet. We are on 22 drops as of today. 2 enemas a day 300ml - 8 drops - ocean water in the morning.

I have attached 2 pictures from this week, I think these are worms.

Can I hope that he can get better?... After all the treatments we have been through?... well I am. I think, what will I do with my time when he is better (possibly recovered)?... I will yell from the roof tops and dedicate myself to helping other families. Is this what I was meant to do? My purpose? I would love it!

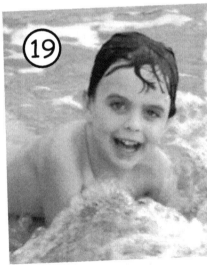

(19)

Thank you for this look. I share this look with you, the same look that you have given back to my Mom, this photo would not be, if it hadn't been for you. I love you very much, your Godson Gabriel

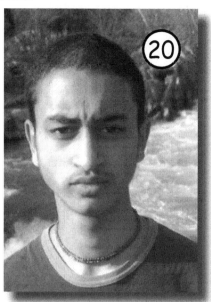

My family and I are very grateful to Kerri Rivera for making available the CD protocol to treat ASD which has recovered myself and made a huge difference to thousands of kids and families all over the world.

CD can recover even a teenager like me whom others had given up on. Of all the bio-medical interventions, CD cost the least and made the biggest difference.

Muchas Gracias por salvar mi vida Kerri.

This is Benjamin. 4 years 5 months old, current atec of 4 and dropping weekly :) Diagnosis atec at 3 years 2 months was 134. Atec when starting CD protocol was 18 and was stagnant after full on bio-med/ diet intervention. Dropped all supps except melatonin when starting protocol and obviously can't be happier with that decision. Thank you to Kerri Rivera of course for giving me a way to save my baby boy... We will continue with protocol until atec = 0 :)

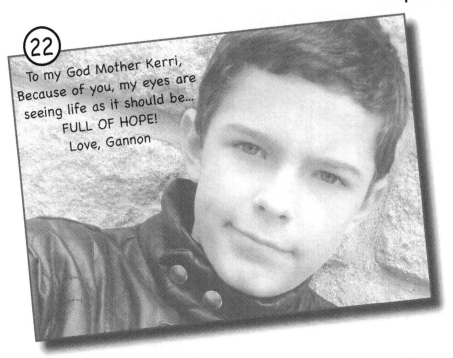

To my God Mother Kerri,
Because of you, my eyes are
seeing life as it should be...
FULL OF HOPE!
Love, Gannon

My sons started using MMS exactly 2 and a half months
ago and we saw improvements almost immediately, my twins
attention got better just days after we started the treatment
and at 10 days after starting my son Juan Pablo started calling
me mom! He has never done that before. (Neither of my twins
were verbal, meaning they were not able to speak a single
word.) A few days later Jesus Alejandro said "Mom, water"
while pointing to the fridge, it was shocking for me.

My two sons can now say 4 or 5 words and their communication
skills have gotten a lot better, even if it's not verbal they
are very good at expressing what they want. There is a
lot of improvement in comprehension, following orders and
accomplishing small tasks, they react when you say their
names, they are controlling their bowel movements, and in
general their whole quality of life has gotten so much better
since they started with MMS.

I know we have a long road to go but we are on the right track
and I trust that thanks to the science that discovered the
great effects of this wonderful formula for our children with
autism we will recover them, as it truly does detoxify!

Ing. Artebys Cedeño
Mother of Jesus Alejandro and Juan Pablo

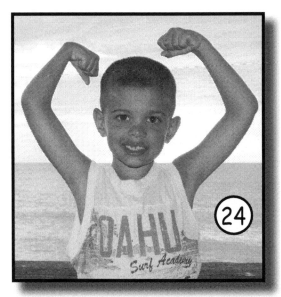

Dear Godmother Kerri,

How can we ever thank you enough for crushing autism out of TJ's life? We now have a smart, happy, helathy boy that has great confidence in himself!

We are forever grateful to you!!!

25

We started using MMS a month ago. We are not even at the full dose yet but have been seeing some amazing gains.

I took my son to the mall about a week ago because it is one of his favorite things to do. When we got home he did something he has NEVER done before. He came up to me, hugged me and said "Thanks". Wow.

Two days ago my husband had to go to the local farm supply store because something broke in the barn. So we asked my son if he wanted to go and he literally jumped off the couch and excitedly came with us. While he was there he picked out a couple of books he was interested in and a couple of small vehicle toys. When we got home I was helping him with his coat and boots he said "you're great mom". Never have I ever had spontaneous comments like this and the only thing I can attribute it to is the MMS because we stopped everything else. This gives me inspiration to continue the protocol and I look forward to what the future holds for my son and our family.

Thank you Kerri!

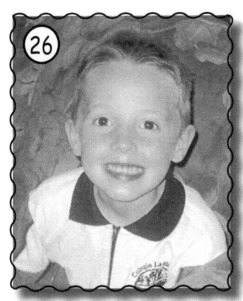

If it were not for you Kerri, my mother would still be worried about my future.

You are my Guardian Angel!!!!

Autism is curable!

Thank you Kerri Gracias Kerri!

27 His speech therapist told me today that his sentences are so much better, more organized, also his ability to converse back and forth and also his concentration have improved!! Soooooooo..... Yay!
Oh, before we went to see his speech therapist he said: Mummy, my speech is getting so much better!
Yup, he said that! He knows!

28 I can't believe it! I just did my daughter's ATEC and in one month it dropped from 72 to 48!!! I am so shocked! Is this a dream? We revised the scores over and over with my husband and accepting that some of our answers could be just very positive feelings, still the improvement is huge!! I am so thankful Kerri Rivera! I have no words!! I am praying this is not a dream!! THANK YOU SO MUCH!!!! I believe there is more to come but right now I am so much in shock!

(29)

I have to post our Sunday gain, my daughter is and always has been on sensory overload, those of you who deal with this know that teeth brushing, hair combing and showers can be torturous for child AND parent. I literally dread washing her hair. She screams so loud she could break the windows. She smacks her wet thighs so hard that they've been bruised for years. This morning she gets in the tub, sits down and sees me roll my sleeves up (which is usually the moment she loses her mind because she knows I'm about to grab the shower head), she stood up, looked me dead in the eye, smiled at me and said "R. shower". I began to wet her hair down, still convinced that the screaming was about to begin any minute. I started shampooing and she said "well done", I smiled and said "VERY we'll done baby". My husband peeked in to see why it was so quiet and she looked at him and said "Daddy shower", smiling from ear to ear as to say 'I'm taking a shower Daddy'..... what a great way to start our Sunday. HUGE, HUGE deal for her and for us. I feel like I finally exhaled today. MMS rocks and so do all of you!!! Happy Sunday ;-))))

Dear Kerri,

(30)

Thank you SO MUCH for helping us with our daughter's complicated health issues. The CD/PP protocol allowed my daughter to sleep through the night, for the FIRST time in 7 years! One month on the parasite meds, she began sleeping perfectly and has slept perfectly ever since!

We are FOREVER grateful! Also, the more her pathogen load decreased on the protocol, the more foods she would eat and LIKE!

My daughter eats SALAD now! AND will try any food I give her. I thank you from the bottom of my heart and will be forever grateful!

With love,

The WHOLE Clark Family!

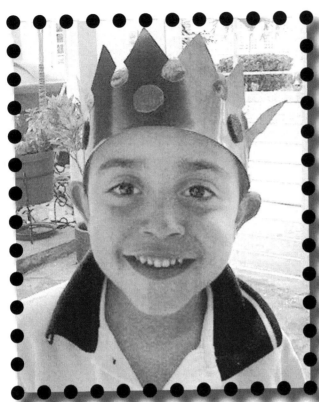

31

*I was cured,
Yes we can.*

*I love you
very much
Godmother
Kerri!*

32

My son had a great week - yesterday we went bowling as a
family. It's difficult with him to notice gains sometimes because
he is really close - his ATEC was a 7 last time I did it and the
changes in him may be subtle and harder to notice. While we
were bowling he was calm (despite the loud music, lights and
commotion) he sat in between his turn watching everyone, (and
the music videos playing) knew when it was his turn and cheered
for me (I was beating my husband at the time - lol). He carried
his ball down the lane and swung it with one arm - omg!! It was
the most NT I have seem him! He now is a brown belt in Tae
Kwon Do and this was the first time he was able to swing the ball
- I used to have to carry the ball to the ramp, help him lift it
and count to 3 for him to push the ball. He was diagnosed
hypotonic at 3.5 years, MMS and PP are what helped him get
some strength, energy and endurance. I increased his MMS by
a drop about 2 weeks ago and we are also ramping up on GcMaf.

Great FUA moment today. My son took his first
ever lesson.... swim lessons. He did amazing!!!
Followed all instructions, waited in line, smiled,
talked, and let the instructors help him.
Amazing.... I cried almost the entire time. At
one point he smiled, waved, and said "hi mommy."

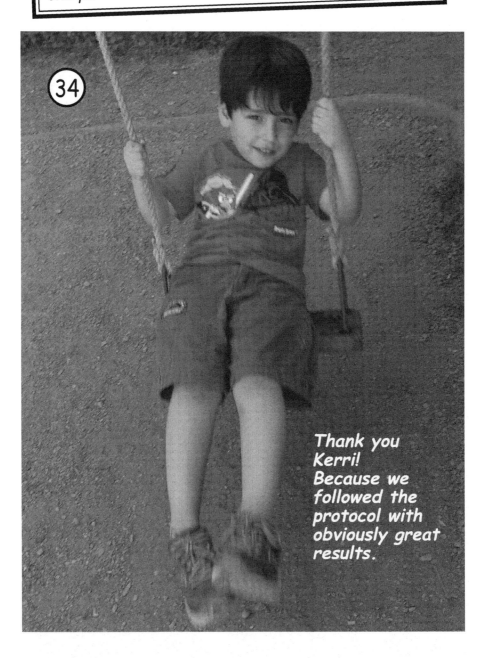

Thank you
Kerri!
Because we
followed the
protocol with
obviously great
results.

(35)

My son has continued to improve on his handwriting and his anger has melted away. We had an IEP today and we lost 2.5 hours of services because he has done so well he does not need those services. They were surprised at how well he is doing. And he fed his little brother soup tonight to get him to eat his dinner.

Thank you Kerri for
helping us to recover our son!

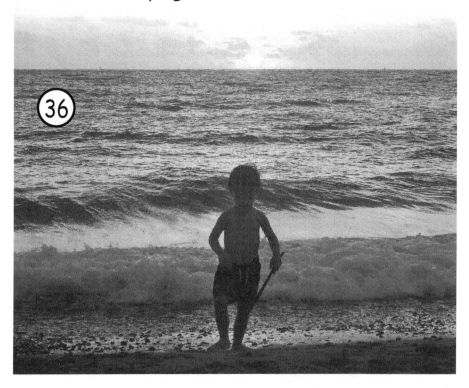

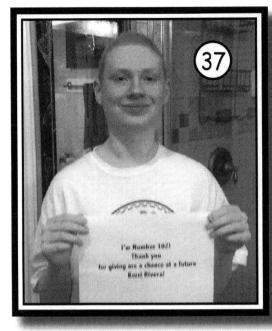

I'm Number 102!
Thank you for giving
me a chance at a
future
Kerri Rivera!

On any given day, I probably rattle out the words I LOVE YOU, directed at my boys at least a dozen times. My NT boy almost always will reply back. My ASD boy usually says, YES YOU DO as his answer. And I have completely accepted that that is his way of receiving my I love yous.

On very rare occasion he will say I love you to me...

Well, by now you know where this is going.

This morning I was walking past him and he said to me.... I LOVE YOU!

I wasn't at first sure what he said as he didn't shout it, So I asked him, what was that?

He repeated, I love you.

I said thank you son, I love you too!!!

Wait for it...

Bammity bam bam BAM!!!

Celebrating every little big thing. Appreciating my 3 favorite words. Loving every minute of every day. Even loving those big red lips this morning knowing he is detoxing...

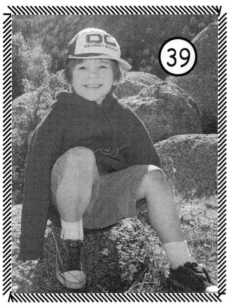

Our son was quickly slipping away from us. We were lost. This protocol gave us direction and ultimately brought our son back to us. He looks at us with smiling eyes and tells us he loves us. He has a full childhood now. Words could never convey the magnitude of our gratitude for Kerri and all who support her efforts to make a future for our kids. See Gunnar's full testimonial on page 378.

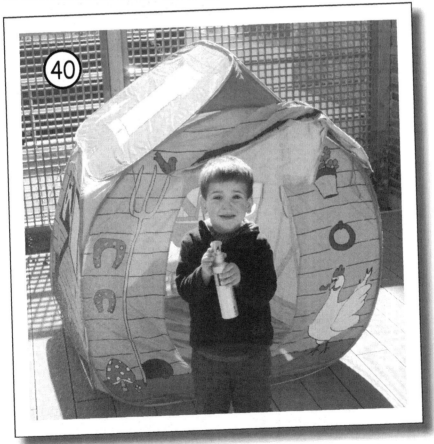

Gracias Madrina Kerri!! I now have an ATEC of 10!

We started the DAN protocol when our 10 year old daughter was 18 months old and remained on it for 9 years. Before starting CD, our daughter appeared neurotypical, but she was heavily dependent on supplements and her progress had stagnated for a few years. She had a distended belly, poor growth, severe constipation, anxiety, a touch of OCD, and focus/concentration/fogginess issues.

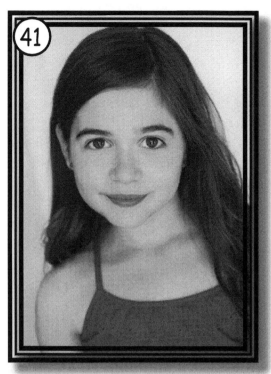

Her ATEC before starting CD was 24. Just 26 days later, her ATEC is 7. A 17 point drop in 26 days! We haven't even had time to do a parasite protocol or a 72/2 weekend yet! Her belly is much flatter and her anxiety, minor OCD, and focus issues are greatly improved! We're going to keep her on CD and I plan on starting the protocol myself this week. As a friend said, "DAN got her to third base and CD brought her home!"

My son just saw me reading this page, and asked what CD Autism was. I told him it was the medicine he's taking. He said, "I think my autism is gone. How do you know someone has it still?" Soon, baby, soon!

Spiro and Peter (9 year old twins)

After years of doing many interventions for our twin boys, and having moderate success at best, we learned about CD. It took about a year before we felt comfortable enough to try it. I can honestly say that, it is the BEST intervention that we've used. We started CDS in mid July 2013. In the 4 short months that we've been using CDS and now CD, we have had more gains in every area, than in the last 6 years of doing so many different treatments. What I love about this protocol, is the simplicity of it, less is more, and that was a huge change in thinking for me.

Just to give you an idea on how well our boys are doing, here are their ATEC scores so far:

Spiro: He was number 100 to recover on the "Healing Train" and the 1st child to recover using CDS.

ATEC prior to starting CDS - 22.

ATEC one month after starting CDS - 16.

ATEC two months after starting CDS - 9.

Peter: He was pre verbal prior to CDS and now uses single words and the odd 2 word combination to communicate. Well on his way to healing.

ATEC prior to starting CDS - 69.

ATEC one month after starting CDS - 55.

ATEC two months after starting CDS - 46.

We finally know, deep in our hearts, that our boys are well on their way towards "true healing". We don't have that stress and anxiety about what the future holds anymore. We finally feel like we can breathe easier, and that day by day, the gains keep coming consistently. The gains stay, and that feels better than anything.

Thank you, to my FB friends who introduced me to MMS and to Kerri Rivera who we have such admiration and respect for. I thank GOD everyday that we were fortunate enough to find out about this treatment. Our boys are coming back to us and their beautiful personalities are emerging. We now look to the future with such HOPE. Kerri, we will forever be grateful to you.

xoxoxoxoxoxoxoxoxoxoxo

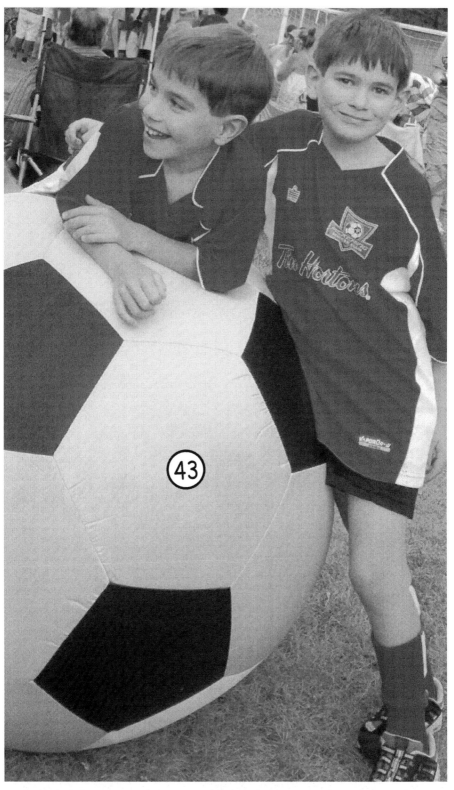

(44)

Whoa... My severe kid walked in the door and wrapped his arms around my neck and gave me a normal hug for the first time in his life (6.5 years). Umm... This is crazy. He wiped his butt for the first time EVER... no prompting, no asking! I wasn't even in the room with him! When I got excited and asked, "Did you wipe???" I swear to GOD... I heard "Yeah, Mom!" Kid's never said a word ever. Could be dreaming, but WOW!!! What a day!!!

Please share your experiences!

Testimonials are one of the best ways to share your experiences with this protocol. Perhaps you learned about it by reading or watching a video testimonial?

If you don't tell us your experiences, we can't share them or take action on issues that need improving or correcting...

Send your testimonials to:

testimonials@cdautism.org

Also, let us know if we are free to publish your testimonial, with or without your name.

More miracles & testimonials starting on page 358.

Chapter 3

<u>Step 1 – The Diet</u>

"Let food be thy medicine and medicine be thy food."

~ *Hippocrates*

If I could choose the one part of *The Protocol* that would be the single most important piece of the recovery puzzle it would be—*The Diet*. By *The Diet*, I mean the dietary plan that I recommend to all of the families that want to start *The Protocol*. It is a combination of the classic gluten-free, casein-free, and soy-free diet along with the elimination of sugar, corn syrup, coloring, preservatives, and other harmful foods. *The Diet* is the basis for the rest of The Protocol; similar to laying the foundation of a house that the rest of the structure will rest on. Adhering to *The Diet* is critical to the effectiveness of the rest of *The Protocol*.

When a family of a child with autism comes to see me, the first thing they want to know is:

What can I do to help my child?

I always, always start with *The Diet*. In fact, I send them away after that first meeting with hope that they will be able to recover their child, but only if they commit to *The Diet* 100%. I explain to the families that they must think about food the same way their great grandparents thought about food. In generations past, food came directly from the Earth, with little processing. Fruits, vegetables, nuts, and meats were dietary staples for our great grandparents and they should be for our children as well. We must think <u>whole foods</u> and not ~~processed foods~~. There is no point in going from regular junk food to gluten-free/casein-free junk food!

After my first meeting with a family, they leave with the list of permitted foods and I have them email me when they have a week straight with zero exceptions or "errors" in *The Diet*. That is where the parents who are truly hungry for recovery are separated from those who are interested in having someone else "fix" their child for them.

One of two things generally happens during that first week. In the first scenario, I get an email from an ecstatic mother or father saying, "I can barely believe it, Johnny slept through the night for the first time in years," or "Johnny had a normal bowel movement," or "Johnny said two new words yesterday!" That's what I hope for.

The second scenario is... I never hear from the family again. There may have been tantrums, or an adjustment period related to *The Diet* that proved too much for them, and they decided to pursue another avenue. That's not to say that everyone sees a miracle, or that there's no middle ground. Some of the results are less obvious, such as more eye contact or less redness in the face, but generally speaking, we see positive changes. Any change is a good sign. *The Diet* is only the first piece of the puzzle. We must continue from here, layering in interventions until we get the desired, end result.

> Kerri... Bless you! When my son was 3 years old he was prescribed Ritalin®, Risperdol® and Clonazepam... can you believe it? Obviously I never gave them to him, it hurt me to see my child "drugged." 2 days after starting the diet he slept through the night, the sparkle is back in his eyes... I can't wait to start with MMS, I am so happy!!!

Throughout this book "miracles," which are actual emails and forum posts from parents about their children's improvements, have been set in text boxes (like the one above) and placed in the chapters that they accent. Please note that as many of these miracles were collected some time ago the contributors have used the term MMS instead of CD. Due to time constraints it was impossible to request permission from these contributors to change the acronym of MMS to CD in their testimonials. MMS and CD are the same substance. Where the acronym MMS is used please know that chlorine dioxide is the substance being discussed and is responsible for the healing.

Author's note: I'm not against all prescription drugs, especially those necessary to bring about healing. However, I don't condone medicating a child with drugs, masking the symptoms known as autism. So, when I see an email like this, I know we've got a great chance to heal that child because we have a parent who has committed herself to healing her child, and who is excited to see what changes the next tool will bring.

Your child's doctor may not have heard of *The Diet* or may be misinformed of its benefits. The references section at the end of the book lists several studies and articles discussing dietary intervention for ASD's. You can use them as a jumping off point for your own study. If you are consulting with a doctor, it is important to choose someone who is familiar with autism and the recovery of autism.

Many doctors do not have time to study up on what's new in autism recovery and if they have zero recoveries then they are in dire need of overhauling their protocols. Another major problem in the mainstream medical community is gigantic egos. If what we are doing is not working to recover our children, then we need to look at what we are doing and why we are doing it. Let's check our egos, update our protocols, and look at what has worked for families who have recovered their children.

Researchers at the New Jersey Medical School's Autism Center found that "children with autism were more likely to have abnormal immune responses to milk, soy, and wheat than typically developing children," which is published in a chapter of Cutting-Edge Therapies for Autism 2011-2012, by Siri and Lyons.[1] In addition, interest is growing in the study of the link between autism and gastrointestinal (GI) ailments. Siri and Lyons also relate a study by the University of California, Davis Health System, where they found that children with autism born in the 1990s were more likely to have gastrointestinal problems, including constipation, diarrhea, and vomiting than children with autism who were born in the early 1980s.

If your doctor is uninformed, or tells you there is no evidence to prove that The Diet will help your child, do the research for yourself since only you are in charge of your child's diet. Heck, why not do The Diet? It doesn't cost you any money and it just might help your child heal. Whether he eats cheesy puffs or fruits and vegetables will ultimately come down to you. You are the one with the money in your pocket. The only way to know for sure if your child is going to be one of the individuals who recovers with The Diet, is to try. It can take gluten six months or more to be removed from the microvilli or "shag carpeting" of the small intestine. As I mentioned previously, some children have obvious changes in two to three days, but even if your child's evolution is taking a little longer than most, DO NOT GIVE UP! At the writing of this book, I have helped about 5,000 or more families of children with autism; all of the children who have lost their diagnosis, as well as those coming close to recovery, have used varied protocols depending on their symptoms. The one thing that they all—unequivocally—have in common is: **The Diet!**

In my opinion, it makes little difference what other interventions you apply to your child if you can't manage The Diet 24/7/365. Hyperbarics, chelation, ABA, etc., simply will not have the desired effects if you are still feeding "drugs" (aka garbage foods) to your child.

Why do I say drugs? Because that is what gluten and casein become in the bodies of our children on the spectrum; more specifically, gluteomorphin (also called gliadorphin) and casomorphin, which are similar to morphine. Gluteomorphin and casomorphin are produced in the gut due to improper digestion of peptides (as we will explain more in detail later). In a person with "leaky gut syndrome" (increased intestinal permeability), they are able to leave the intestine and cross the blood-brain barrier where they act exactly like morphine or heroin. Would you purposely give your child street drugs? NO!

Once we have this information and understand the severity of this issue, we have a responsibility to our children to do better. We must take away the foods that are keeping them ill. Invite your family and your child's school to help heal your child's ailing body. Explain that they can no longer give your child these items, and that if they do, it's like giving them a dose of morphine. If it sounds drastic... that's because it is!

Researchers have found an abnormal amount of these undigested peptides (gluteomorphin/casomorphin) in the urine of children with autism, proving their existence in the body. Among others, Dr. Knivsberg and colleagues in Norway have found that urine samples from people with autism, PDD, celiac disease, and schizophrenia contained high amounts of the casomorphin peptide.[2] Similarly, Gliadorphin (gluteomorphin) has been verified by mass spectrometry techniques to be present in unusual quantities in urine samples of children with autism.[3]

Do *The Diet*!

There are still plenty of food options that are permitted. I promise you—your child won't starve! We have included some recipes in Appendix 15 on page 513 to get you started. *The Diet* is absolutely the most important piece of the puzzle. If we can't remove what is directly linked to brain and gut inflammation, as well as immune-allergic reactions to offending foods, it is nearly impossible to heal a child on the spectrum. I have personally never seen a family recover a child without dietary intervention. That's not to say it hasn't happened, but I have never seen or heard of it.

Like I said before, when we started with my son Patrick, his only legal food was homemade French fries. So that's what he ate. Little by little he began to accept more foods. I assure you, the adjustment period will fade and they do eat. Stop the cycle of inflammation and addiction. Only then will your child begin to heal, and once your child starts to feel better he will accept more foods.

In the case of my own son, his acidic diarrhea and sleepless nights stopped the week we started *The Diet*. From that moment on I was hooked, not only on *The Diet*, but also on biomedical treatments for curing autism. I have never looked back. I strongly encourage you to experience *The Diet* for your child, or even as a family. It is an amazing thing.

I thought the following might encourage some of you who have recently made big dietary changes for your kids and are struggling with all that involves. I put my son on a GF/CF/SF... well, basically, EVERYTHING-free diet when he was 11 months old, following a major vaccine-induced crash. My choice to put him on a diet was criticized by nearly everyone in my life, beginning with his pediatrician who told me I was "just imagining" that he'd regressed and that he "probably wasn't allergic" to what I had taken out; she called a week later with the test results and an apology, and a long list of other things he was allergic to! He's now just a little over seven and doing GREAT. I just delivered a GF/CF muffin to him, and he said, "You know what I love best about you, Mommy? I love that you are so nice to us, and that you always make sure we have food that doesn't make us sick." So, don't feel bad about not giving your kid that ice cream cone when Mr. Softee comes by or not loading their Easter basket up with food dye this weekend. It may take years, but they will see that you loved them enough to NOT give them these things.

Some other tips include the following:

Review Your Child's Supplement List

Is your child taking 30+ supplements a day? We will talk more about this throughout the book, but this protocol is geared towards eliminating excesses and not about supplementing deficiencies. It's important to carefully review your child's supplements. In order to maximize the benefits from

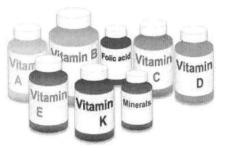

this protocol consider removing any antioxidants, (they kill CD—more on that in Chapter 5, page 88), calcium, magnesium (which feeds the biofilm), as well as iron and B_{12} (which are favorite foods of parasites). Supplements for increasing speech, reducing seizures, enzymes, and probiotics obviously have their place in individual protocols. B$_{12}$, while known to feed parasites, has also been known to greatly boost speech in some children. If your child saw benefits in speech from B$_{12}$, it may be worth keeping in. As always, these are decisions that each family has to make for their child on an individual basis.

If a certain supplement proved beneficial to your child, then don't remove it (the exception being antioxidants and the other aforementioned supplements). The goal of this step is to remove <u>unnecessary</u> supplements as they are most likely feeding parasites and creating "excess noise" in the body. Anything that is not serving a purpose needs to be eliminated.

Keep a Journal

Keep a record of the foods you have removed and those you have added in. Then, take note of the types of reactions you observe: rash, more or less hyper, more or less stimmy (self-stimulatory behavior), sleep patterns, frequency and consistency of bowel movements, tantrums, acceptance of

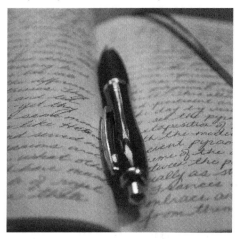

new foods, eye contact, language, etc. Write everything down so that you can follow any relationships or patterns that will allow you to identify when something is working, or when it is not. Record these observations in a notebook because it helps guide us, especially those of us who are stressed, frazzled, and sleep deprived.

Don't Stress About Raw Foods or Perfectly Balanced Meals...Yet!

When you are first transitioning, feed your child whatever legal foods he/she will eat. We are taking baby steps. Once your child is on *The Diet* 100%, you can start adding in new foods, bite by bite, if necessary.

Do the ATEC

Keep track of your progress with the ATEC checklist (see page 447), which you can find at...

www.autism.com/index.php/ind_atec

This is an excellent way to see how you are doing. Every time that you begin a new intervention, it's a good idea to do the ATEC, and then repeat it every three months or so to see how your child is evolving. Sometimes our children are recovering right before our very eyes and we don't even know it. The ATEC can be used to measure the effects of all new interventions, not just *The Diet*.

Using the ATEC is a great way to measure improvement. Many of us are tired, burned out, or don't have the best memory. A formal questionnaire can help us to discern when an intervention is working or not, and it only takes about seven minutes to fill out. See Appendix 4, page 447 for a sample survey and more information about ATEC.

Always Read Labels

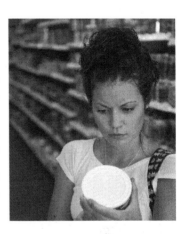

Read the label on the back of all packages—not just the one on the front that says "gluten-free." Many times they have sugar, yeast, carrageenan, or other items that are not allowed. We must know what we are putting into our children's bodies. If you can't pronounce it... you don't want to put it into your child. Be careful of hidden offenders like malt, natural flavors, artificial flavors, whey, and numbers (red 40, E-441), etc.

Have a Support System

It doesn't matter whether it is a friend, family member, rescue angel, or neighbor. Have a shoulder to lean on. Autism recovery is a marathon not a sprint, and no one should have to go it alone. There are so many amazing parents out there who have walked this path and are willing to help newbies! As of this writing we have several public forums open, including...

www.cdautism.org

and

www.facebook.com/groups/AutismCD

This is an excellent resource for finding the latest info, protocol changes, and share hope and/or frustration with parents all over the world who are walking the same path. Don't forget to sign up for our newsletter as well by visiting the home page at www.cdautism.org!

Take it One Day at a Time

Defeatist thinking will only harm your resolve to help your child "I can't do this for the rest of Johnny's life!" or "How will I get through this year?" are defeatist thoughts. Go hour-by-hour or minute-by-minute, and know there are victories every day in the world of autism. We must draw strength from those

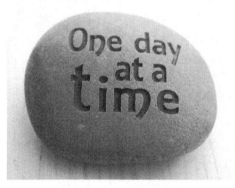

victories, even when they aren't our own. Both this book and my website have a section of miracles and testimonials (see Chapter 2, page 19 and Appendix 1, page 357), which are real correspondence I have received from parents describing the advances their children have made as a result of doing *The Protocol*. We receive these miracle emails and forum posts every day, but we had to pick and choose which ones to share in the book. You will also see them sprinkled throughout the chapters of this book. Take some time to read them, know that children are recovering every day, and believe your child can be next. If something doesn't go as planned, wake up the next day and know that, *THIS IS the first day of autism recovery.*

Why Does My Child on the Spectrum Need to Go on a Gluten-Free/Casein-Free/Soy-Free Diet?

As I said before I have never seen a child recover without *The Diet*. The following information comes from *www.gfcfdiet.com* and explains why *The Diet* is so important for people with autism.

Scientific studies have shown the presence of high levels of peptides derived from casein and gluten proteins.[4,5] The digestion process is considered "normal" in terms of protein digestion for most people, as they make smaller particles called peptides that are further broken down into amino acids. However, in people diagnosed with autism it is more difficult to properly digest some of these proteins, thus allowing them to enter the blood directly as peptides. This often happens due to a lack of enzymes that help with the optimal assimilation of food and can be a factor in causing exaggerated bowel permeability (aka, leaky gut syndrome). This results in poor digestion, which facilitates the entry of these harmful proteins directly into the bloodstream, where they can cross the blood-brain barrier.

Leaky gut syndrome has been attributed to many causes including viruses; Candida; gluten, which produces zonulin, a protein thought to cause leaky gut; amongst other things.[6]

Gluten-containing foods may destroy the digestive system if they are consumed excessively or are introduced too early into a child's diet. Wheat is hybridized through artificial processing, resulting in inadequately prepared grains. Casein-containing foods may also destroy the digestive system because they are pasteurized and/or homogenized. These processes may result in damage to the enzymes that break down gluten or casein, thus causing incomplete digestion of these proteins.

Recently, Dr. Andreas Kalcker introduced us to the theory that the inability to properly digest these proteins may stem directly from parasites in the intestinal tract. These parasites may contribute to a leaky gut and thereby play a role in the development of allergies towards gluten, casein, soy, etc.

Gluten is found primarily in wheat, rye, barley, oats, spelt, malt, most breads, cakes, muffins, cereals, flour tortillas, pizzas, pastries, and donuts, etc. Gluten is also found in food starches, semolina, couscous, malt, some vinegars, soy sauce, teriyaki sauce, flavorings, artificial colors, and hydrolyzed vegetable proteins. Casein is contained in milk from cows, sheep, goats and any or their derivatives such as yogurt, butter, ice cream, or cheese. No form of cow's milk may be consumed as it causes inflammation and mucous. Even if the product claims to be lactose free, cream free, or casein free—it is not allowed.

Improperly digested gluten and casein fragments can both enter the bloodstream and cross the blood-brain barrier. Because of their opioid properties, these peptides can react with opiate receptors in the brain to cause effects similar to those of an opiate drug such as heroin or morphine.[7] These opiates are called gluteomorphin (or gliadorphin) and casomorphin, and can react with some parts of the brain, for example, the temporal lobes, which are actively involved in the process of the integration of language and hearing. Interestingly, these are two of the areas most affected by autism.

Besides their effects on the brain, opioid-forbidden foods cause inflammation in the gut and brain. When a child has an allergy to a food—in this case gluten, casein, and/or soy, etc.—as it enters the body the immune system sees it as an invader and reacts by trying to protect the body from the substance.

The first time the body is exposed to a food allergen, the immune system makes antibody-specific immunoglobulin E (IgE) against the allergen. IgE antibodies circulate in the blood and adhere to types of immune cells called mast cells and basophils. Mast cells are found in all body tissues, especially in the nose, throat, lungs, skin, and gastrointestinal tract (GI). Basophils are found in the blood and in tissues that have been swollen due to an allergic reaction.

The next time the body is exposed to the same food allergens, the allergen binds to IgE antibodies that bind to mast cells and basophils. These connections between allergens and antibodies direct the cells to release large amounts of chemicals, one of which are histamines. After the liberation of a histamine by an activated mast cell, the permeability of the vessels near the site increases. Therefore, the blood fluids (including leukocytes, which are also involved in immune response) enter the area causing inflammation. Histamine release also causes the release of cytokines and inflammatory mediators by leukocytes. These chemicals, in turn increase the inflammatory response.

Welcome to The Diet!

Now that we've covered the science behind *The Diet*, it's time to get started. First, make sure you complete an ATEC and save the results so you have a baseline score. Next, prepare a shopping list based on the following allowed items.

Author's Note: Organic products are better but not required.

Permitted Foods List

Proteins:
- Beef
- Chicken
- Eggs
- Fish (small not large size)
- Pork
- Turkey
- No processed meats or cold cuts (hot dogs, bologna, etc.)
- No shellfish (preferably—full of toxins)

Fruits:
- Most fresh fruits are permitted (except citrus, mango, pineapple, kiwi and limit berries).
- Frozen fruit without added cream or sugar.
- NO canned fruit (nothing canned ever).
- Be careful of dried fruit as it may contain sugar.

Author's Notes:

Juice is not permitted on this protocol as it has proven time and time again to annul CD and cost families precious time and money. The amount of fruit necessary to make a glass of juice also causes it to be high in sugars, albeit natural, and they can still affect the immune system. Children on this protocol need to drink water and generally speaking most former juice drinkers transition from drinking flavored beverages to water without much issue. If your child must drink a flavored beverage it would be acceptable to blend and strain or juice one apple, for example, and add it to some water and if you choose you can sweeten it with stevia (SweetLeaf® or KAL® brands are ok).

Fruit should not be consumed after a meal as a dessert due to its rapid digestion. If it is eaten after other more slowly digested foods (i.e. meat, grains, etc.), it can ferment in the stomach, causing bloating, gas, or discomfort. Fruit is best eaten before a meal or separate from meals.

Vegetables:
- All vegetables!!!
- Including French fries, however, not frozen fries or fries from fast food chains; these are often coated in flour.

Author's Note: I don't condone the prolonged use of potatoes, as they convert to sugar in the body. However, it was the only "legal" food my son would eat when we began the GF/CF/SF diet.

Nuts:
- Almonds
- Cashews
- Coconut
- Hazelnuts
- Walnuts
- Plus, they all make great milks!

Grains:
- Amaranth
- Buckwheat
- Corn
- Millet
- Quinoa
- Rice
- Sorghum
- Tapioca
- Xanthan gum

Author's Note: I prefer a grain free diet for autism recovery, especially if your child suffers from "grain brain" (addiction to grains, undesireable behaviors and/or inability to concentrate after eating grains). If your child seems to be addicted to carbs, i.e. fruits and starches, you may want to consider the Ketogenic diet or the Rosedale diet.

Even though these grains are allowed, they can be difficult to break down, and can easily ferment in the intestinal tract due to excessive Candida overgrowth, bacteria, and parasites.

Beans:

- All beans—EXCEPT soy
- Garbanzo
- Lentils
- Navy
- Peanuts

Sweeteners:

- Stevia (This is the best of all the sweeteners, but make sure it does not contain erythritol—a sugar alcohol!)
- Agave syrup
- Honey
- Maple syrup (natural/real—not made from corn syrup)
- Xylitol
- NO piloncillo (unrefined sugar)
- NO sugar

Author's Note: Honey is allowed, however, it can create insulin spikes.

Prohibited Foods List

After working with thousands of families, and conducting independent research, it is my personal opinion that the products on the following list should be avoided if your intention is to heal autism:

- Acetic acid (E260)
- Artificial flavoring
- Artificial sweeteners
- Bouillon cubes
- Bread
- Cacao/Cocoa
- Candy
- Cane sugar
- Carrageenan
- Catsup
- Chocolate milk
- Coloring
- Corn flakes
- Corn syrup
- Cow's milk in any form (even lactose-free milk products)
- Flour tortillas
- Gelatin
- Malt
- Margarine

- Mayonnaise
- Microwave popcorn
- MSG (Monosodium Glutamate)

  (MSG goes by many names—too numerous to mention here. A detailed
  list is available at www.truthinlabeling.org/hiddensources.html)

- Natural flavoring
- Noodle soup
- Oatmeal (except for Bob's Red Mill GF oats)
- Pasta
- Children´s nutritional shakes
- Play-Doh™

  (Contains gluten—Gluten-Free Dough is available at
  www.discountschoolsupply.com)

- Preservatives
- Processed meats (hotdogs, ham, sausage, cold cuts)
- Sodas
- Soy/fruit beverages
- Soy milk
- Soy sauce
- Sports drinks
- Sugar
- Yeast

NO Cow's Milk:

- Not casein free
- Not lactose free
- Not organic
- Not raw
- Not evaporated
- No No No cow's milk!
- Sorry, no goat's milk either! It too has casein.
- All cow's milk, regardless of what is removed from it, causes mucous production in the body. This, in turn, provides an ideal environment for pathogens.

If you're thinking that once you go GF/CF/SF + that your child will starve, trust me they won't! The list of foods they eat may get shorter, but they will keep eating. As I mentioned earlier, my son Patrick ate homemade French fries for the first three weeks of *The Diet* until he began accepting different fruits, nuts, and chicken again, but we did it... we transitioned. What I have seen in my own son, and in other children, is that when they begin to get healthier in the weeks and months after starting *The Diet*, they become more open to accepting new "legal" foods.

> Wow... quite amazing Kerri...
>
> I have always believed that "you are what you eat" and have been very careful with what I give to my kids, so their diet has been quite healthy, except for the occasional ice cream, etc. My son even spits out candies when someone offers him one because he really doesn't like them. He is not into sweets at all, thank God.
>
> But I must say this diet is just what he needed! Yay!

There are a few loopholes to the above list. If you make your own catsup, mayonnaise, etc. with items from the permitted foods list, then your child can obviously eat those foods. The list refers to those items that come from the grocery store that contain white sugar, preservatives, and other problematic ingredients.

There are many items on the forbidden foods list that don't contain gluten, casein, or soy. Here is the explanation behind a few of those items:

White refined sugar: Refined sugar has been found to reduce immune system function as well as contribute directly to obesity and Type II diabetes.

The following list is excerpted from *Suicide by Sugar.*[8]

- Sugar can suppress your immune system.
- Sugar upsets the mineral relationships in the body.
- Sugar can cause juvenile delinquency in children.
- Sugar eaten during pregnancy and lactation can influence muscle force production in offspring, which can affect an individual's ability to exercise.
- Sugar can cause hyperactivity, anxiety, inability to concentrate and crankiness in children.

MSG: An excitotoxin that can literally "excite neurons to death." We need all of our neurons!

Yeast: Feeds Candida and other fungi.

Carrageenan: Contributes to inflammation in the body and studies have linked it to colon cancer in rats.[9]

Artificial sweeteners containing sucralose: In making sucralose, the chlorine in the sweetener bonds to carbon, producing a chemical known as a chlorocarbon. "According to physician and biochemist, Dr. James Bowen, chlorocarbons are never nutritionally compatible with our metabolic processes and are wholly incompatible with normal human metabolic functioning."[10]

Processed Meats (hot dogs, ham, cold cuts, and sausages): The fats found in these meats may contain high amounts of toxins such as heavy metals, pesticides, and herbicides. In addition, processed meats contain sodium nitrite, which can harm the liver and pancreas. They may also contain corn syrup and flavoring.

Natural Flavoring: The exact definition of natural flavorings & flavors from Title 21, Section 101, part 22 of the Code of Federal Regulations is as follows:

The term natural flavor or natural flavoring means the essential oil, oleoresin, essence or extractive, protein hydrolysate, distillate, or any product of roasting, heating or enzymolysis, which contains the flavoring constituents derived from a spice, fruit or fruit juice, vegetable or vegetable juice, edible yeast, herb, bark, bud, root, leaf or similar plant material, meat, seafood, poultry, eggs, dairy products, or fermentation products thereof, whose significant function in food is flavoring rather than nutritional.[11]

Basically if you start with a natural ingredient, you can process or manipulate it any way you choose. No matter how many chemicals or solvents are added it will be labeled as a "natural flavor."

Notice they can come from meat, seafood, dairy, and wheat, etc., can also contain MSG.

Coloring: Food dyes have been linked to allergic reactions, hyperactivity in children, and even cancer. Red No. 2, for example, was banned in 1976 after it was suspected to be carcinogenic. Red No. 40, in a number of tests, was shown to damage DNA in mice.

When we are dealing with children on the spectrum, their immune systems are already compromised, and their detox pathways can be blocked or impaired. The idea is to decrease their burden with life-giving, nutritious foods, rather than add more stress to a body that is already maxed out.

Corn Syrup/High Fructose Corn Syrup: Simply because corn is a permitted food does not mean corn syrup/HFCS are "legal." Both of these shut down the immune system, as refined sugar does. They are chemically similar in composition. There is much controversy surrounding the use of mercury in the refining process, and how much if any, is in the final product.[12]

I wanted to update you on everything with my daughter.

We had a mishap 2 days ago. A substitute teacher gave my daughter a regular granola bar and a flavored beverage containing sucralose. You know what Kerri, when she came home from school that day she was in her own world and was ignoring me. I knew right away she had something she shouldn't have had. I was angry and saddened by what I was witnessing. Is there anything we should do since she had those 2 items that she's not supposed to have. Or just continue to move forward??

After a while on the diet it becomes obvious when an infraction happens, if you are present when it happens you can give an enzyme to help break down the food, if not, we move forward and learn how to prevent it from happening in the future.

Common Errors:

"It's no big deal if we break the diet every once in a while."

Not True!   Every time you break the diet, further inflammation is caused in the brain and gut. When gluten and casein proteins are not properly broken down, the resulting peptides reach the brain as gluteomorphin and casomorphin. It takes three days for casein to be eliminated by the body, but months for gluten to be eliminated by the body.

"My child can drink milk as long as it doesn't have casein."

Not True!   As long as the milk comes from a cow, your child cannot drink it. It doesn't matter how it's labeled. If it comes from a cow it's off limits. Cow's milk can provoke the body to produce mucous, thus providing an ideal environment for pathogens which can cause chronic inflammation.

"The allergy panel says my child isn't allergic to gluten or casein, therefore he can eat them."

Not True!   If your child has autism, or is on the spectrum, he must avoid gluten, casein, and soy. You should also observe your child carefully after adding a new food, or a food he hasn't eaten in a while. In one particular case, even though the child didn't test positive for an orange allergy he continued to produce symptoms of an allergic reaction whenever he ate one. We must remember that the body is changing constantly and that any test is only good for a couple of months, if at all.

I have seen the same story repeated over and over again with mangoes, oranges, bananas, apples, and corn, etc. Observing the conduct of your child after consuming a food you suspect he may have an allergy/intolerance to is the best way to measure whether the food is acceptable or not. As our children move towards healing, foods that at one point produced allergy-type symptoms can be tolerated without an immune system response.

"My doctor says that autism has no cure, and that the diet doesn't work."

Not True! Run from any doctor who says he will take your money even though he feels that autism is incurable. The first question you need to ask a doctor is:

> *"How many children have your recovered from autism?"*

If the answer is zero, keep looking!

The Diet is free—no one earns money if your child is on *The Diet*—so do it! You have nothing to lose, and everything to gain. However, if you choose not to do it, you may further lose the health or your child. Commit 100% to *The Protocol*, and your child may be one of the next recovery stories.

> My son had what can only be described as a miraculous reaction to the GF/CF/SF diet. Since starting 2 weeks ago, all the bumpy red areas on his face disappeared, tantrums went from about a 10 to a 2, and diarrhea is all but gone.

"We tried the diet, but Johnny didn't get any better."

The Diet is only one piece of the puzzle. However, it is the foundation of everything we are going to do. Without maintaining *The Diet*, it is difficult to know which intervention is actually helping.

Candida will be dying and a reaction to *The Diet* may be a Herxheimer. We must go beyond the diet to heal autism, but diet is the first piece of the recovery process.

When I receive an email complaining that a child isn't getting better I ask for a detailed list of exactly what the child is eating. I always find errors in parents' application of the GF/CF/SF + diet. What I typically uncover is that *The Diet* did not fail but that the application was flawed.

"I should remove gluten and casein from my child's diet gradually."

Not True!!! Remove them from the diet immediately and watch your child improve before your very eyes. Foods that cause IgG or IgE allergic reactions cause many other problems in the body including inflammation and psychotic behaviors, in response to gluteomorphin and casomorphin. The sooner you can remove these foods the faster your child will recover.

> As soon as we started working on the diet, my son received a developmental evaluation, although he was 20 months old, the results were that of a child of 15 months. 4 months after implementing the diet, the changes have been dramatic. My boy smiles again, he speaks in his own way, he points, has eye contact, interacts with others, he is very close to being recovered, although he is still missing a little bit. He is occasionally nervous and sometimes distant, but the most important thing is that the therapist reapplied the developmental test and my son is now reacting like a child of 24 months (his current age), even in some areas surpassing it! And this is only with the diet because he hasn't taken any supplements, just a probiotic that was ineffective.

"A gluten-free/casein-free/soy-free diet is good enough."

It's Not! Like I said before, I always find errors when a parent goes step-by-step with me through their child's diet. The list on page 52 is a detailed list of what our children should not eat under any circumstances. Many of these foods contain neurotoxins/excitotoxins. These foods can negatively affect developing and mature nerve tissue. Keep them out of your child's diet.

Beyond GF/CF/SF +

Sometimes, *The Diet* as explained is not enough and we need to go beyond it. If your child suffers from constipation, diarrhea, or seizures it is recommended to do a period on the Specific Carbohydrate Diet™ (SCD™). The following text was sourced from the website...

www.breakingtheviciouscycle.info

...by Elaine Gottschall. A complete list of references is also available at that website.

The Specific Carbohydrate Diet™ has helped many thousands of people with various forms of bowel disease and other ailments vastly improve their quality of life. In many cases people consider themselves cured. It is a diet intended mainly for Crohn's disease, ulcerative colitis, celiac disease, diverticulitis, cystic fibrosis and chronic diarrhea. However it is a very healthy, balanced and safe diet that has health benefits for everyone. The foods that are allowed on the Specific Carbohydrate Diet™ are based on the chemical structure of these foods. Carbohydrates are classified by their molecular structure.

The allowed carbohydrates are monosaccharides and have a single molecule structure that allow them to be easily absorbed by the intestine wall. Complex carbohydrates which are disaccharides (double molecules) and polysaccharides (chain molecules) are not allowed. Complex carbohydrates that are not easily digested feed harmful bacteria in our intestines causing them to overgrow producing by products and inflaming the intestine wall. The diet works by starving out these bacteria and restoring the balance of bacteria in our gut.

Autism & GI Problems

Altered intestinal permeability was found in 43% of autistic patients, but not found in any of the controls (Harvard University). Intestinal permeability, commonly called "leaky gut", means that there are larger than normal spaces present between the cells of the gut wall. When these large spaces exist in the small intestine, it allows undigested food and other toxins to enter the blood stream. When incompletely broken down foods enter the body, the immune system mounts an attack against the "foreigner" resulting in food allergies and sensitivities. The release of antibodies triggers inflammatory reactions when the foods are eaten again. The chronic inflammation lowers IgA levels. Sufficient levels of IgA are needed to protect the intestinal tract from clostridia and yeast. The decreasing IgA levels allow for even further microbe proliferation in the intestinal tract. Vitamin and mineral deficiencies are also found due to the leaky gut problem.

In a healthy intestinal tract the small intestine and stomach are not inhabited by bacteria. When the flora balance in the colon is lost, the microbes can migrate into the small intestine and stomach, which hampers digestion. The microbes compete for nutrients and their waste products overrun the intestinal tract. One of the toxins produced by yeast is actually an enzyme that allows the yeast to bore into the intestinal wall. The yeast also produce other toxins such as organic acids, which can also damage the intestinal wall.

Bacterial growth in the small intestine destroys enzymes on the intestinal cell surface, which prevents carbohydrate digestion and absorption.

The last stage of carbohydrate digestion takes place at the minute projections called microvilli. Complex carbohydrates that have been broken down by the enzymes embedded in the microvilli can be absorbed properly and enter the blood stream. But when the microvilli are damaged, the last stage of digestion cannot take place. At this point only monosaccharides can be absorbed because of their single molecule structure.

In the small intestine, the body should absorb the nutrients needed from what is eaten. But in the case of malabsorption, the undigested carbohydrates left in the small intestine cause the body to draw water into the intestinal tract. This pushes the undigested carbohydrates into the colon where the microbes can feast on it. This allows for even more proliferation of the unwanted microbes and continued increase in malabsorption problems.

Low intestinal carbohydrate digestive enzyme activity was found in 43% of patients with autism. (Horvath) Recent studies point out that ongoing carbohydrate malabsorption keeps the digestive system constantly weakened, leading to systemic disorders. Suspected carbohydrate malabsorption should be treated to ward off further damage to the body's digestive system. (GSDL)

Most intestinal microbes require carbohydrates for energy. The Specific Carbohydrate Diet™ limits the availability of carbohydrates. By depriving these microbes of their food source, they gradually decrease in number. As the number of microbes decreases so do the toxic by-products they create.

The Specific Carbohydrate Diet™ (SCD™) is intended to stop the vicious cycle of malabsorption and microbe overgrowth by removing the source of energy from the microbes. The SCD™ allows simple monosaccharides that do not need to be broken down in order to be absorbed.

By following the SCD™, malabsorption is replaced with proper absorption. Inflammation is decreased and the immune system can return to normal. Once the immune system is returned to adequate levels, it can begin to keep in the intestines microbes in proper balance.

The SCD™ allows simple carbohydrates, but prohibits complex carbohydrates. The diet is started by following an introductory diet, which consists of a limited selection of foods. After the introductory diet, the next stage of the diet allows many more foods, but requires that all fruits and vegetables be peeled, seeded and cooked in order to make them more easily digested. Raw fruits, vegetables, nuts and seeds are added to the diet later. To properly follow this diet, it is imperative to read Breaking the

Vicious Cycle by Elaine Gottschall. The book details the progression of allowed foods as well as providing many delicious recipes.[13, 14]

Salicylates/Phenols

Phenol is a naturally occurring chemical found in many of the foods we eat, such as fruits and vegetables, nuts, and in bioflavonoids and cartenoids (carotene, lutein, lycopene, xanthophylls, and zeaxanthin), etc. Phenols can be found in toothpaste, hair dye, and disinfectants, etc. Many foods have phenols, and they are impossible to avoid completely. Salicylates are a subgroup of phenols, related to aspirin. There are several kinds of salicylate, which plants make as a natural pesticide to protect themselves from insects, fungi, and harmful bacteria. Foods high in natural salicylates are tomatoes, apples, peanuts, oranges, cocoa (chocolate), red grapes, coffee, all berries, and peppers, to name a few.

You may also need to consider a low salicylate and/or phenol diet, as many children on the spectrum may have issues with these items. The following was sourced from *www.scdlifestyle.com*.

> Dr. Feingold is probably the most widely known individual to study this chemical, as he developed what is now referred to as the Feingold Diet. He started out in the 1960s as a pediatrician and allergist studying children's negative reactions to aspirin. Through his work, he found that many other dietary chemicals were causing physical and even behavioral reactions in his patients. He developed the Feingold Diet to eliminate all food additives, colorings, and salicylates.

> ### Why Do People React to Them?

> In a normal body that has the correct levels of sulphates and liver enzymes, phenols and salicylates are easily metabolized. The body utilizes what it needs from the chemicals and properly disposes of the rest through the bowels. In those whose levels are not normal or in the case of "leaky gut syndrome", intolerance to this chemical family can occur rather quickly.

> Many people with gut issues such as yeast/bacteria overgrowth or digestive diseases can develop salicylate intolerance as a result of "leaky gut" syndrome. Leaky gut is a result of various digestive problems and occurs when the small intestine becomes too damaged to properly filter the size and types of food particles or chemicals that enter the bloodstream. [For more on leaky gut syndrome see http://scdlifestyle. com/2010/03/the-scd-diet-and-leaky-gut-syndrome/] When these improper particles are allowed to repeatedly enter the bloodstream the

body tries to get rid of them by triggering an immune system response. Because phenols/salicylates are so common in most foods, a person with a leaky gut will have much higher than normal levels of these chemicals in their blood and can very quickly develop intolerance´s to these specific particles.

Why Can Phenols Affect Children on the Autism Spectrum More Than Others?

Research by Dr. Rosemary Waring at the University of Birmingham found that children on the autism Spectrum have low levels of the enzyme phenol-sulfotransferase-P (the enzyme that breaks down the phenol and amine families, also known as PST) and the substrate it uses: sulfates. Sulfates are a key tool that the body uses in the process of detoxification and break down phenols such as salicylates. Without normal levels of sulfates in the body, the sulfotransferase enzyme cannot do the task it was created to do: metabolize salicylates. So there are two problems with PST deficiency: low sulfate levels and low enzyme levels. PST deficiency alone can cause problems in children (remember phenols are normal) but factor in any intestinal damage resulting in leaky gut along with it and your child's body can easily be overwhelmed. The end result is a salicylate intolerance and the subsequent physical and behavioral reactions that come with it.

Reactions Caused by Phenols

Salicylates stimulate the central nervous system in people that react to them. This can often bring with it an emotionally extreme high followed by a very low, low. Other reactions to the phenol family can occur anywhere from immediately after consumption up to 48 hours after the consumption of the chemical, depending on the immune response. Physical reactions can include: dark circles under the eyes, red face/ears, diarrhea, headache, difficulty falling asleep at night, night waking, and in some cases excessively tired and lethargic. Behavioral symptoms of a reaction can be: hyperactivity, aggression, head banging or other self-injury, and even inappropriate laughter. Hyperactivity is more common in children's reactions, while adults generally experience symptoms similar to chronic fatigue.[15]

For additional information on leaky gut syndrome you may wish to look at (search for) Dr. Peter Osborne:

www.glutenfreesociety.org

If your child suffers from self-injurious behaviors limit these foods that are moderate to high in phenols:

- Almonds
- Apples
- Avocados
- Bananas
- Cacao
- Cantaloupes
- Cherries
- Cider vinegar
- Coconut oil
- Colored fruits
- Dates
- Food coloring
- Honey
- Mangos
- Mint
- Oranges
- Oregano
- Peanuts
- Pineapples
- Powdered chili pepper
- Processed meats
- Raisins
- Strawberries
- Tangerines
- Tomatoes

For more information on this you can visit:

www.scdlifestyle.com

and

www.feingold.org

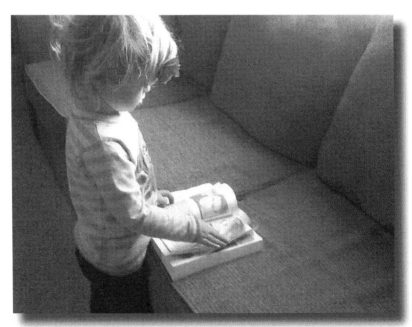

She's quite the book worm and has an impressive collection which includes classic favorites such as Brown Bear, Llama Llama Red Pajama, Barnyard Banter and Goodnight Moon... But lately, she has been drawn to her Mama's new favorite read... Perhaps she is hoping that someday her story of recovery will be told too...

Gluten Syndrome

For many parents of children on the spectrum, having their children on *The Diet* is something that is second nature to them. However, as more and more people are using the protocol in this book to heal their own health ailments we have decided to include the following section on how gluten can negatively affect many more than just the autism community. You will get a very interesting look into how the immune system works and why so many sufferers have misunderstood gluten syndrome. Thank you Olive for contributing to our understanding of the subject.

Molecular Mimicry
What It Is & How It Relates to the Gluten Syndrome
by Mrs. Olive Kaiser

Who am I?

I am a married stay at home mom, blessed with a wonderful husband and seven fantastic kids. In 2003, after decades of searching, we learned about gluten reactivity through our daughter's nursing school training and eventually confirmed that we are a gluten syndrome family. Our daughter and my husband had the most obvious symptoms, but we all had manifestations and antibodies. Additionally our oldest son reacted to his MMR vaccination and probably other shots, which added high functioning ASD/ADD to the mix, and he developed type 1 diabetes at age 19. Two other sons had various shades of ADD/ADHD. My own school age vaccinations in the 1950's may have led to repeated bouts of strep throat until I reacted to a strep antibiotic injection about age 10. I developed PANDAS from that reaction (Pediatric Autoimmune Neuropsychiatric Disorder Associated with Streptococcus). What a struggle! Decades later it has responded somewhat to diet changes and now the CD/parasite protocol. I give thanks to God for His guidance along the way.

How did I get into this community and this health project?

We tested for gluten syndrome (we called it celiac disease back then) using standard tests recommended by celiac experts and received confusing results. Then, our daughter had a troubling experience with a gluten challenge that did not match the celiac story we'd been taught. I delved into medical literature and networked extensively with the gluten syndrome community looking for help. In that desperate discovery and prayer process I found practitioners and researchers who stepped outside the "villi damaged celiac only" box. They were able to explain why we received, in the midst of obviously gluten-induced incidents, false negative results from our celiac blood tests and villi biopsy. Those tests significantly led us astray and eventually I put up a website...

www.TheGlutenSyndrome.net

...to warn others of discrepancies we stumbled upon in the diagnostic process.

What is Molecular Mimicry?

Molecular mimicry is a recognized medical theory which explains very nicely why gluten reactions may potentially inflame and damage so many different parts of the body, leading to very different symptoms in different people. It also clarifies why gluten antibodies may cross react with other foods and infections, and why it only takes a small exposure to trigger them.

When we understand molecular mimicry we are better equipped to deal with tempting social situations. Gluten syndrome has its own rules, which do NOT make sense unless this concept is understood.

The following is a brief introduction to Appendix 5, page 449, which goes into much more detail, along with references, about the following questions:

1. How does the gluten syndrome reaction actually damage our bodies?

Molecular mimicry. The molecular structure of gluten resembles the molecular structure of many of our body tissues. When the immune system attacks gluten it may also attack body tissues that "look like" gluten. Even if you do not read the other detailed answers, learn the details for this question on page 450.

2. Does gluten always damage the villi of the small intestine as the celiac story teaches? Many other tissues such as thyroid, pancreas, liver, joint, brain, nerves, heart, bone, blood vessel walls, etc., are involved in this disorder. Does all that other damage only arise from poor nutrient absorption from injured gut villi?

No, according to published research, many researchers and practitioners believe the villi are not always damaged in an autoimmune gluten reaction. Where there is no villi damage, injury to other organs CANNOT be due to nutrient deficiencies caused by villi damage. Molecular mimicry provides a mechanism for direct autoimmune gluten damage to many other tissues and organs when the villi are fine, OR other tissues/organs, *including villi*, may be directly damaged through molecular mimicry.

Dr. Vojdani's abstract in his editorial *The Immunology of Gluten Sensitivity Beyond the Intestinal Tract*, supports that the villi are not always injured. To quote his editorial abstract, "Evidence has been accumulated in literature demonstrating that gluten sensitivity or celiac disease can exist even in the absence of enteropathy [gut/villi damage], but affecting many organs."

3. I don't have damaged villi, and my tTG/gliadin tests were negative, but I feel so much better gluten-free. Why?

The tests were likely false negative. That is very common. As gluten digests, it breaks into more pieces than we have tests developed to check them, and the immune system makes a separate antibody for each piece. Standard tests only check 2-3 antibodies. You may have others (Cyrex Labs tests 28 antibodies). Your villi may be fine, but you may be injured somewhere else—for example: thyroid, nerves, heart, etc.

4. Why do many gluten syndrome patients not only react to wheat, barley, and rye but also at times to other foods, particularly oats, milk, corn, soy, egg, yeast, coffee, sesame, rice, chocolate and others?

These foods "look like" gluten closely enough in their structure that the immune system may mistake them for gluten. This situation may also cause your gluten antibodies to run high after you go gluten-free. The immune system may misrecognize other foods, such as yeast, corn or milk, and others for gluten because they resemble gluten molecularly.

5. The diet seems excessively strict? Why does it take so little gluten to start a reaction?

Our perspectives are skewed. We accept that miniscule amounts of venom injected by a bee sting, or a tiny exposure to peanuts in allergic individuals can set off immediate life threatening allergic reactions. Many medications are contained in very TINY pills, but they have powerful effects in our bodies. Immune gluten reactions are also that sensitive. "Crumbs matter."

6. Why do many people react to gluten, proven by antibody tests, but they have few or no warning symptoms for a long time and then they crash with something serious, usually autoimmune?

Gluten is famous for slowly injuring nerves by molecular mimicry, and in many cases, the nerves are silenced by that injury. The patient does not realize there is a problem until the tissue or organ that those nerves supply begins to fail.

7. Why do so many of us react to gluten today, when for centuries most people appeared to be fine with wheat, barley, rye and oats? After all, wheat and barley are mentioned positively in the Bible and other historical documents.

Today's gluten is altered, violently, by nuclear radiation and chemical mutation within the past 60 years*, plus our toxic and poorly nourished bodies do not have optimal digestive capabilities to break it down. Weak, toxic, leaky body barriers/membranes, particularly leaky gut, set the stage for gluten induced molecular mimicry.

*Nina Federoff, *Mendel in the Kitchen*

8. Why do specialists and researchers insist that the gluten-free diet must be life long? Can't we heal this problem and go back to our beloved wheat bagels, croissants, and brownies?

Our scientists still insist that gluten-free is a strict lifelong commitment. I agree. For me it is not worth playing with today's wheat. There is something strange and unpredictable about it. The memory B cells in the immune system never forget what the enemy "looks like", and fresh exposure retriggers antibodies.

9. Traditional peoples soaked and/or sprouted their wheat berries and then made sourdough bread with them. Does that process alter the gluten sufficiently for gluten syndrome patients to safely consume this bread, particularly spelt or einkorn?

No. These processes and ancient wheat grains do make the bread more digestible, but not gluten-free and still unsafe.

10. Should I substitute all the gluten foods I routinely eat with gluten-free substitutes?

No, not routinely. The gluten-free community finds that they are still mainly expensive high carb processed food (i.e., junk food).

11. What are gluten withdrawals?

Occasionally, gluten breaks into specific "pieces" in the gut that resemble opiate drugs. When a person goes gluten-free, they may experience temporary, but unpleasant, withdrawal symptoms for a few days as these pieces disappear from the blood stream.

12. What are the risks of formal gluten challenges?

Many patients avoid these challenges. Occasionally a patient tries the gluten-free diet for an extended period of time and then the patient or doctor decides to run tests to confirm gluten reactivity. The standard advice to restart the production of antibodies is to consume gluten products 4 x per day for 4-6 weeks, and then run the standard blood test, followed by a villi biopsy if the blood work is positive. This is called a gluten challenge and has created some very dramatically unhappy reactions, some of them neurological/psychological.

Please see Appendix 5 (page 449) and www.GlutenSyndrome.net for more info and references. When we understand molecular mimicry our understanding of the gluten syndrome comes into focus. It explains why gluten-free diets and beyond are important tools to reduce inflammation and promote healing. As time goes on, gluten-free diets are easier to manage in public, tests are better and social awareness has grown. The Just Eat Real Food movement and others play into healthy gluten-free dining with wonderful recipes that avoid processed foods and incorporate healthy fats and nutrient density. This is a happy, encouraging era as we watch our children heal and adults find better stability in the midst of a health crisis. Bon Appetit!!!

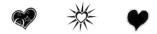

The Diet - FAQs

The following FAQ's were printed with permission from gfcfdiet.com:

Slight changes were made to match the formatting of this book; however, the content remains unaltered. Please visit gfcfdiet.com for complete list of the references contained within the following text.

1. My doctor has never heard of any of this and she is extremely skeptical. I'm embarrassed to tell her I'm considering this approach. What do you think?

Skepticism is a good thing in a medical doctor or scientist. However, since there is preliminary evidence to support this safe, non-invasive intervention, it is up to you to educate her, state your wishes, and ask for her support. For a doctor, it is better to wait until all of the data is published in peer-reviewed journals before advocating a treatment. However, for a parent, it is reasonable to want to help one's child without waiting for all of the results of the "double-blind placebo" studies. Because this approach does not include any unusual supplements, invasive drugs, or expensive treatments, your pediatrician should be supportive. Explain that you would like to try this for a few weeks, and agree that you will be objective about recording your child's progress while on the diet.

If you feel that you need to support your case legally with the scientific and medical documentation that is currently available, please see the medical links at www.gfcfdiet.com or at www.autismndi.com.

2. What is casomorphin?

Casomorphin (or caseomorphin) is a peptide derived from casein, a milk protein. Casein is one of the major proteins in the milk of all mammals including cows, goats, and humans. When casein is digested properly, it breaks down into large peptides like casomorphin, and should then be broken down further into smaller amino acids.

However, Dr. Reichelt in Norway, Dr. Cade at the University of Florida, and others found that urine samples from people with autism, PDD, celiac disease, and schizophrenia contained high amounts of the casomorphin peptide in the urine.[4] In its peptide form, casein has opiate properties similar to morphine, and may plug into the same opiate receptor sites in the brain. Researchers have found that these peptides may also be elevated in other disorders such as chronic fatigue, fibromyalgia, and depression based on anecdotal reports of symptom remission after exclusion of wheat and dairy.

3. What is gliadorphin?

Gliadorphin (also called alpha-gliadin or gluteomorphin) is a substance that resembles morphine. Ordinarily, this is a short-lived by-product from the digestion of gluten molecules (found in wheat, barley, rye, oats, and several other grains). Gliadorphin is very similar to casomorphin. Gliadorphin has been verified by mass spectrometry techniques to be present in unusual quantities in urine samples of children with autism, and are believed by many to be a central part of the system of causes and effects that cause autistic development.

The most probable reasons for the presence of these molecules are:

- One or more errors in the breakdown (digestion) process caused by enzyme deficiency and/or
- Abnormal permeability of the gut wall (that would allow these relatively large molecules to enter the bloodstream from the intestine in abnormal quantities).

4. I am confused about allergy vs. intolerance. I understand that our children may be sensitive to corn, soy, and other foods as well as gluten and casein. Does this mean that they will eventually start turning these foods into the morphine-like compounds too? If this were the case, would they show up as an allergy on a RAST test? Or were our children always allergic to these foods (a regular allergy

that may cause behavioral changes in our children), and we just didn't know because the gluten and casein were hiding the allergy?

To a traditional physician or allergist, "allergy" is used to describe a reaction of the IgE part of the immune system, resulting in hives, swelling, or breathing problems. However, the words "allergy" and "intolerance" are often used to describe any inappropriate reaction to foods or substances that should normally be harmless to the body.

There are at least three different ways that a child with autism may have a problem with foods that contain gluten or casein, and it's important to understand the distinction:

1. An IgE ALLERGY commonly results in skin problems, hives, swelling, and breathing problems, etc. This can be tested using a skin test or blood test.

2. An INTOLERANCE (usually mediated by the IgG or IgA part of the immune system, or by an enzyme insufficiency such as lactose intolerance) has more varied or vague symptoms like discomfort, stomach problems, sleep problems, joint pain, ear infections, or hyperactivity and behavior problems. Sensitivity to these substances can be tested with an ELISA blood test.

3. PEPTIDUREA (peptides in the urine) is caused by the inability of the body to properly break down certain proteins. It is hypothesized that certain peptides, notably from milk and wheat proteins, are plugging into the opiate receptor sites of the brain and disrupting brain and nervous system function. Urine testing for this is still experimental, and many parents believe that the best way to find out if this is what is causing a child's autism is a strict trial period on the GF/CF diet.

On the GF/CF diet, gluten and casein are avoided because they are strongly suspected of having a direct pharmacological effect. When these proteins are only partly broken down, some of the resulting fragments can be strikingly similar to morphine, and act in more or less the same manner. (This type of reaction can co-exist along with a classic type of allergy towards the same foods.)

Recent research indicates that protein from both corn and soy may also contain some molecular sequences that could, if the patient has an enzyme deficiency, be broken down into something closely resembling opioid peptides. Even spinach protein has been found to have some opioid activity.

Products made from soy or corn will also often contain metabolic end products made by microscopic organisms like bacteria, molds, or other fungi. Some of these are suspected of being harmful to a small number of people who are genetically predisposed to autism. The amount of danger will depend on individual conditions AND on the quality of the corn or soybeans used in the production process. Soy OIL (lecithin) may be worse than most other soy products since this product will look and taste okay, even when made from moldy raw material, and since it is commonly made from the "bottom grade" of the harvest.

Some people also think that one of the natural pigments in corn (lutein) may cause problems for reasons that are not properly understood (see: "Sara's Diet"). This must be regarded as highly speculative.

5. I don't think my child has allergies, or that allergies could cause autism. Why should I try removing foods from his diet?

Although parents have been reporting a connection between autism and diet for decades, there is now a growing body of research that shows that certain foods seem to be affecting the developing brains of some children and causing autistic behaviors. This is not because of allergies, but because many of these children are unable to properly break down certain proteins.

6. Milk and wheat are the only two foods my child will eat. His diet is completely comprised of milk, cheese, cereal, pasta, and bread. If I take these away, I'm afraid he'll starve.

There may be a good reason your child "self-limits" to these foods. Opiates, like opium, are highly addictive. If this "opiate excess" explanation applies to your child, then he is actually addicted to those foods that contain the offending proteins. Although it seems as if your child will starve, if you take those foods away, many parents report that after an initial "withdrawal" reaction, their children become much more willing to eat other foods. After a few weeks, most children surprise their parents by further broadening their diets.

7. Isn't milk necessary for children's health?

Americans have been raised to believe that this is true, largely due to the efforts of the American Dairy Association, and many parents seem to believe that it is their duty to feed their children as much milk as possible. However, lots of perfectly healthy children do very well without it. It is calcium children need, not milk. Cow's milk has been called "the world's most overrated nutrient" and "fit only for baby cows." There is even evidence that the cow hormone present in dairy actually blocks the absorption of calcium in humans.

Be careful. Removing dairy means all milk, butter, cheese, cream cheese, and sour cream, etc. It also includes product ingredients such as "casein" and "whey," or even words containing the word "casein." Read labels—items like bread and tuna fish often contain milk products. Even soy cheese usually contains caseinate.

For more information on dairy-free living, there's a very good book called *Raising Your Child Without Milk* by Jane Zukin. Another great book called *Don't Drink Your Milk* by Frank Oski (the late head of pediatrics at Johns Hopkins and author of *Essential Pediatrics*). This book cites the results of several research studies that conclude that milk is an inappropriate food for human children. It is available for $4.95 from Park City Press, PO Box 25, Glenwood Landing, NY 11547, ISBN #0671228048.

8. How do I know which foods he's allergic to?

Try an allergy elimination diet. For example, keep common allergens out of his diet for a few days and then re-introduce them, one-by-one. If you see symptoms, either physical or behavioral, try again in a few days. By being systematic you will be more certain of which foods are causing problems and correctly rule them out. Two excellent resources, probably available at your library, are Doris Rapp's book, *Is This Your Child*, and William Crook's, *Solving the Puzzle of Your Hard to Raise Child*.

9. Aren't eggs dairy?

Many years ago, most of us were taught that eggs and dairy were part of the same section of the food pyramid under "dairy." However, they are not. Eggs are free of any dairy. Dairy can be from cows, sheep, or goats. The eggs we eat are normally from chickens. Dairy and eggs happen to be side-by-side in the refrigerator section of the grocery store, which may add to the confusion.

10. What do I do when we go to a party or out to another person's house and are trying to maintain my child on a GF/CF diet? At times we find it impossible to catch him before he ingests something he shouldn't.

It is a good idea to bring some favorite GF/CF goodies with you. Keep them hidden until that moment of "competition." Show the surprise treat to your child before your child eats one of the gluten and/or casein laden foods. Bring more than one goodie to be on the safe side. Also, there are two small pamphlets that are great for handing out to friends and family members that give a simple explanation for your child's special dietary requirements. These are: "Alternative Treatments for Children Within the Autistic Spectrum: Effective, natural solutions for learning disorders, attention deficits, and autistic behaviors," by Deborah Golden Alecson, and "Leaky Gut Syndrome: What to do about a health threat that can cause arthritis, allergies, and a host of other illnesses," by Elizabeth Lipski, M.S., C.C.N. Both of these books cost $3.95 each and can be found at health food stores.

11. Do we need to worry about gluten-containing lotions, shampoos, and toothpaste being absorbed through the skin?

Nicotine patches, birth-control patches, and other transdermal applications of medications are proof that the skin does absorb many things (and pass them to the bloodstream). However, the molecules in gluten are too large to pass through the skin, according to John Zone, MD (a dermatologist quoted in the Spring 2003 issue of *Living Without* magazine).

Most often the problem occurs from hand to mouth (i.e. touching colored modeling dough and then touching one's face), which is a good reason to avoid giving our kids much access to anything that poses a threat. If your child's school has a sensory table, you can request that it be filled with rice or dried beans, instead of macaroni or gluten grains. Likewise, we suggest that you volunteer to be the "Play-Doh™ parent" and keep the classroom supplied with a safe version that you don't have to worry about.

We are not too concerned about shampoo, unless you have a child who is likely to try to drink the stuff. But toothpaste is an entirely different matter, since some of it is likely to be ingested, rather than spit out.

12. I'm already worried about my child's nutrition, and his "allergies" are causing me to further reduce his choices. If apple juice and bananas are the only fruits he will eat, and he's reacting to them, how is he supposed to get by?

Fruit contains water, sugar, fiber, and vitamins. If he will not eat other fruits then he needs to get these things from other sources.

13. I am wondering if anyone else is having problems with school and keeping them on the diet? I have sent a note saying: "Please don't give my son dairy, wheat, corn, or soy." Today I came in and they were giving him Popcorn!

My kid doesn't eat ANYTHING that isn't sent from home. He's almost ten now, and this policy has been good for him because succumbing to temptation outside of the house has simply never been an option. I don't think it would occur to him to take food from anybody without our permission.

We always made sure there are backup snacks and birthday party treats at school for emergencies. I think the school has always taken this seriously because they can see how seriously we take it.

We once got a note from a mom who said that her son had been strictly GF/CF for months without an improvement. I asked what he was eating, and she gave me a long list including expensive GF pre-packaged products. Then she ended her letter by saying, "Of course, that's just what he gets at home. I have no idea what he gets in his school lunch, or what they're using for food reinforcers in his ABA program."

Definitely try this—you might see a real difference.

14. What percentage of children will respond to dietary intervention?

DAN! doctors used to try to be conservative about this, and say at least a third of children, and then, after seeing more patients, they said two thirds. Now that they have seen hundreds or thousands of patients, most tell us that they believe that almost every ASD child will benefit from this diet. Many will need further modifications (i.e. removing grains or sugar) before the full benefits are realized.

However, age plays a big part in how quickly results will be seen. We can probably say that the response will be dramatic in more than two thirds of the children under three, and perhaps more subtle, but still helpful, in at least two thirds of older children. We think those are pretty good odds.[3]

Some Additional FAQs...

Kerri, yesterday the therapist was playing with Play-Doh™ with my daughter. She could not resist eating it. We tried very hard to stop her with no luck. In the end we had to stop her from playing with it. People say this is due to a zinc deficiency. Do you know if this is correct? Will giving her Zinc stop her from wanting to eat Play-Doh™? If yes, how much should I give?

She is not eating Play-Doh™ because of a zinc deficiency. Play-Doh™ contains wheat. She is addicted to gluteomorphin, a by-product of her eating gluten, which is contained in Play-Doh™. So, she broke her diet. She cannot touch nor eat Play-Doh™.

What exactly is Candida?

Candida albicans is an opportunistic fungus (or form of yeast) that is the cause of many undesirable symptoms ranging from fatigue and weight gain, to joint pain and gas.

The Candida yeast is a part of the gut flora, a group of microorganisms that live in your mouth and intestine. When the Candida population starts getting out of control it weakens the intestinal wall, penetrating through into the bloodstream and releasing its toxic by-products throughout the body.

What Causes Candida Overgrowth?

Candida is an opportunistic pathogen that can rapidly take over when a person is under a course of antibiotics. Antibiotics destroy beneficial gut flora but have little effect on Candida, giving this normally harmless yeast the chance to take over dominance of the gut environment very quickly.

Babies born via C-section, or to mothers who were treated with IV antibiotics during labor are especially vulnerable to the ravages of Candida overgrowth. This is because they are not exposed to a healthy balance of gut flora on the way through the birth canal prior to the moment of birth.

...disaccharides, or double sugars, are present in many carbohydrates including ALL grains—not just gluten containing ones. An inflamed, imbalanced gut overridden with Candida is unable to digest double sugar molecules completely because the lack of beneficial gut flora has compromised the function of the enterocytes.

According to Dr. Natasha Campbell-McBride MD, author of *Gut and Psychology Syndrome*, and one of the key scientists at the forefront of gut restoration research today, enterocytes are the cells that reside on the villi of the gut wall and produce the enzyme, disaccharidase, which breaks down the disaccharide molecule into easily absorbed monosaccharide molecules. When the enterocytes are not nourished and strengthened properly by adequate beneficial flora, they become weak and diseased and may even turn cancerous. Unnourished, enterocytes cannot perform their duties of digesting and absorbing food properly.[16, 17]

The critical importance of the enterocytes to health cannot be overstated!

Weak and diseased enterocytes also have trouble digesting starch molecules, which are very large molecules that consist of hundreds of monosugars, connected in long branchlike strands. People with weak digestion due to Candida overgrowth and messed up enterocytes have a terrible time digesting these complex molecules leaving large amounts of it undigested—the perfect food for pathogenic yeasts, bacteria, and fungi like Candida to thrive upon. Even the starch that manages to get digested results in molecules of maltose, which is—you guessed it—a disaccharide! This maltose also goes undigested due to a lack of the enzyme disaccharidase and becomes additional food for Candida.

We are a few days into the diet. Can someone comment on what they send to daycare with their kids for snacks? Our daycare is nut free as well. We are ok for lunches but what should we take for snacks. The gluten-free pretzels, etc. we were taking he can't have now because of yeast and soy.

Here a few suggestions: Hard boiled eggs, cut up raw veggies and fruit, air popped popcorn, apples, bananas, dried fruits (with no sugar added). Also you can join "CD/CDS MOMS WHAT IS MY KID EATING TODAY" Facebook group. You can find more ideas there.

Chapter 4

An Introduction
to Chlorine Dioxide
by Jim Humble

"Condemnation without investigation is the height of ignorance"
                                                    -Albert Einstein

Jim Humble, the man behind chlorine dioxide for healing, was kind enough to write the following introduction to our CD section...

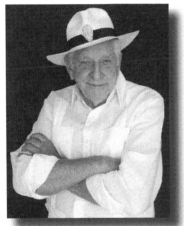

I just can't tell you how pleased and proud I am that Kerri has developed protocols using chlorine dioxide as the main ingredient to bring health and normalcy to many children who had the symptoms called autism. Their resulting healing is one of the greatest stories of this and the last century. Kerri's ability to look at something new and to evaluate the value of the new item without being totally affected by the dictates of present established medical science is truly rare. Kerri decided to do something since modern medicine has yet to come up with a reasonable priced globally available solution to the problem of autism that yielded good results. Medical science says that autism is incurable, that millions of children have to be left to suffer and live without reaching their potential. At this writing 115 children have recovered, hundreds more are near recovery and thousands have had documented improvements as a result of being treated with Kerri's protocol.

Here are some basic points:

Chlorine dioxide (the molecule) was discovered in 1814, with many giving credit to Sir Humphrey Davy for its creation, and today several patents exist for healing various ills with it (see list on page 85).

MMS (Master Mineral Supplement) – I rediscovered chlorine dioxide in 1996 and since then more than 1,020 people have traveled from more than 95 countries to the Dominican Republic, Mexico, and other countries, to be trained in its use. By our estimation, more than 10 million people worldwide have used chlorine dioxide.

The highest cost of a set of bottles of sodium chlorite + activator is less than $25 for 4 ounces of each. This means that almost any place in the world the average dose of chlorine dioxide is less than 4 cents, or less than $.40 a day or $25 for 2 months. In most places it is even less than that. So far there is no one in the world who can't afford it or who wouldn't be able to get it merely by asking if they can't afford it.

The chlorine dioxide molecule is the weakest of all oxidizers used in the human body and thus has very little effect on human cells. This molecule has the unique ability to recognize and oxidize (kill) harmful bacteria. Hans Christian Gram, a scientist of the 19th century, discovered that most harmful bacteria have a negative charge. He was able to dye positive and negative bacteria two different colors. His techniques are still used in laboratories and universities. All oxidizers, including chlorine dioxide, have a positive charge that will attract and kill negatively charged bacteria while repelling positively charged bacteria. Chlorine dioxide is thusly able to kill bad bacteria without destroying the good bacteria. This is simple high school science; like charges repel and unlike charges attract.[1]

Most chemicals and many foods in this society are tested to determine their poison index, which is designated by giving them a toxicity number known as LD_{50}. Sugar, table salt, butter, arsenic, cyanide, vinegar, wine, Clorox, window cleaner, and dozens of other household and industrial chemicals are rated as to their toxicity by force feeding 10 rats with the food or chemical in question until ½ of them die. The amount of chemical or food that it takes to kill 5 of the 10 rats determines the LD_{50} number. Every chemical has a toxic rating and is indicated as an LD_{50} number. All chemicals are toxic in large enough quantities and there are a lot of unlucky rats in our society.

There has never been a recorded death caused by ingestion of chlorine dioxide or sodium chlorite in humans. In the case of chlorine dioxide, it would take 1000 times more chlorine dioxide than is used in a daily treatment dose to reach a toxic dose for a human being. The following information is from the *Toxicological Profile for Chlorine Dioxide and Chlorite* (published by the U.S. Dept., of Health & Human Services) which contains LD_{50} toxic numbers for chlorine dioxide along with documentation that no deaths have been caused by chlorine dioxide (Emphasis in italics is the author's):

No information was located regarding death in humans following oral exposure to chlorine dioxide or chlorite. Shi and Xie (1999) indicated that an acute oral LD_{50} value (a dose expected to result in death of 50% of the dosed animals) for stable chlorine dioxide was > 10,000 mg/kg in mice.[2]

I should say something about bleach as a number of critics insist that MMS (chlorine dioxide) is a bleach and thus is a poison. Chlorine dioxide, the chemical that is MMS, has never been used domestically as a bleach for cleaning toilets. It is an industrial bleach when used 4000 times more concentrated than MMS. It is never used for bleaching purposes in the homes of people of this world.

Legally, ethically, morally, and logically, if any item does not have the characteristics of a particular item, it cannot be said to be that kind of an item. This means that a chemical that does not have the characteristics of bleach cannot be called bleach. So a chlorine dioxide solution being 4000 times weaker than that of bleach cannot be called bleach. This is a fact accepted in courts of law of the world.

I sincerely hope you will take the time to understand the basics of chlorine dioxide as explained here. Any time one has helped someone overcome the symptoms of autism he has helped save a life, as those suffering from the symptoms of regressive autism are not living their full lives. The end result of learning this data is that the time may come when you will need chlorine dioxide to save your own life or that of a loved one.

Jim Humble

Archbishop Jim Humble

A message from Kerri to Jim Humble

"With all my love, respect and gratitude. You have swum against the current for so long, and I am so fortunate that you waited for me. I will continue to recover these generations of children that are the victims of a senseless epidemic. As you have done, I will do. We can't change the past, but the future is ours. You have brought light to where there once was none."

Chapter 5

<u>Step 2 – Chlorine Dioxide (CD)</u>

"All truth passes through three stages. First, it is ridiculed. Second, it is violently opposed. Third, it is accepted as being self-evident."
*~ **Arthur Schopenhauer***

CD (chlorine dioxide) is the most amazing intervention that I have ever tried with my son. It by far packed the biggest punch in the shortest amount of time—we saw the positives in under a week with no side effects! (A Herxheimer reaction is not a side effect.) After seven days on CD, my son was looking at me in the eyes and requesting non-preferred activities using four word sentences. I have never, with any other intervention, seen a change in my son come about so quickly, especially since Patrick was your typical non-responder before CD.

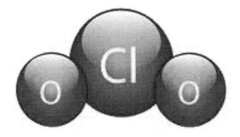

The chlorine dioxide molecule (CD).

Why CD for Autism?

We know that the symptoms known as autism are caused by:

- Viruses
- Bacteria
- Candida (yeast)
- Parasites
- Heavy Metals
- Inflammation
- Food allergies

CD catapults children into recovery because it kills these exact things. As of this writing, over three years since we started using CD in our protocol to heal autism, 115 children have lost their diagnosis. Thousands of children around the world are healing, and that means their families are healing as well, and for this I am eternally grateful.

CD has confirmed my faith and has shown me time and time again that autism IS curable. My life has changed since the day my son was able to look me in the eyes, smile, and request things. I could not keep information of this magnitude a secret. I absolutely had to share it with anyone who would listen.

CD is very affordable as you can purchase a two to three month supply from multiple worldwide suppliers on the Internet for around $25USD. The cost difference between the CD Autism Protocol and a megavitamin/supplement based biomedical protocol for a family living without insurance (or in a third world nation) could be the difference between recovering their child and not recovering their child. The results are also vastly different.

You can think of CD as a shortcut to recovery because it kills all pathogens with one shot. Hypothetically, you could use antibiotics, antifungals, and antivirals to get the same results; however, you could also cause damage due to harmful side effects from these products (liver and kidney stress, etc.). Also, antibiotics, antifungals, and antivirals can only target certain bacteria, viruses, and fungi. CD targets all types of pathogens based on their electrical charge and pH. The particular strain is irrelevant.

CD causes no side effects, leaves no toxic residues, and causes no liver damage. It causes no new stress to already stressed bodies. Everything else we use to kill pathogens leaves something behind. For example, antibiotics also kill your beneficial bacteria, and antiviral use comes with contraindications and side effects. CD is gone from the body one hour after your last dose, leaving no trace behind. We dose hourly throughout the day because CD is only active in the body for up to one hour. We must continue to dose if we want to stop the proliferation of pathogens and eliminate them from the body.

A few children with autism in Venezuela recovered using only CD, The Diet, and a probiotic. That doesn't happen every time, but it can.

False Information and the Fear it Creates

The most common reason that families have told me they are afraid of trying CD is because of false propaganda. The FDA, anti-biomed parents, and others have claimed that MMS (Jim Humbles term for a weak concentration of chlorine dioxide in aqueous solution) is a "poison," comparing it to chlorine or chlorine bleach, which it is not.

If you are interested in a deep dive into the science behind chlorine dioxide therapy (also known as MMS), please spend some time on Dr. Andreas Kalcker's websites...

www.medicasalud.com

...mostly in Spanish, though it has a few pertinent documents in English, and...

www.andreaskalcker.com

Also check Jim Humble's website:

www.jimhumble.org

There, you can also find a forum (G2Cforum.org) of people discussing the use of CD (MMS) for the healing of a multitude of ailments.

In a nutshell, chlorine (Cl) and sodium hypochlorite (NaOCl, aka chlorine bleach) are as different from chlorine dioxide (ClO_2) as "required-for-life" oxygen (O_2) and "will-damage-the-lungs" ozone (O_3) are different from each other. Chlorine (Cl) and sodium hypochlorite (NaOCl) destroy pathogens through "chlorination," while chlorine dioxide (ClO_2) destroys pathogens by "oxidation." The by-products of chlorination can bond with other molecules and form potentially carcinogenic trihalomethanes. The only byproducts of oxidation by chlorine dioxide are two neutral oxygen atoms and a chlorite ion, which can bond with sodium in the body to form table salt (NaCl).

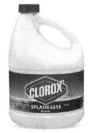

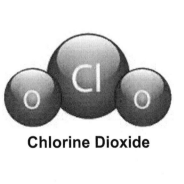

Chlorine Dioxide

IS NOT

Laundry Bleach
OR

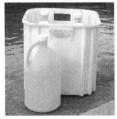

Pool Chlorine

Your doctor is most likely not a chemist, and may or may not be fluent in the language of oxidizers. If you are working with a doctor, please take the science to them when you speak with them about adding CD to your child's protocol. The best thing we can do for our sick children is to make informed decisions. Understanding the difference between chlorine and chlorine dioxide, or chlorine bleach and chlorine dioxide may mean the difference between your child recovering or not.

I have shared this with thousands of families around the globe whose children have used chlorine dioxide in very dilute aqueous solutions, and NONE have had any injuries from CD. Sure, we have had discomfort in the form of a Herxheimer reaction. This is something we have learned to minimize, and can often be prevented by going low and slow. I have learned that what may appear negative at the outset, often turns out to be a healing crisis that leads to incredible gains in the long run.

Many of the first world children who have done the CD protocol have done it in parallel with other autism protocols. They have had regular blood, urine, and stool tests and generally test healthier while using CD than before they started. CD is fortifying immune systems, improving liver function, reducing bacterial and viral loads, *Candida* markers, and inflammation.

> Just did round of blood tests on my son,
> Liver Function Test best ever after 7 months of MMS.

Critics also frequently cite the fact that sodium chlorite and chlorine dioxide can be used for industrial bleaching processes, as a way to frighten parents out of using it. Just because a substance has the power to remove color, or bleach something, doesn't mean it's "bleach." Lemon, sunlight, hydrogen peroxide, and toothpaste all remove color from textiles. We would never call toothpaste bleach, even though it's capable of removing color, nor would we call sunlight bleach, even though that's what it can do to your clothes if you leave them outside long enough. From here we can draw a very similar analogy to using chlorine dioxide for health. The dilutions we are using for internal consumption in aqueous solution (water) are very weak. Day one starts with just one drop in eight fluid ounces of water.

The 1984 study, *Controlled Clinical Evaluations of Chlorine Dioxide, Chlorite and Chlorate in Man*, found no deleterious effects when taking a concentration of up to 50ppm over several hours a day for three weeks.[1] As Jim Humble mentioned (see page 79), the concentrations used for industrial purposes are are thousands of times more concentrated than what families have been using for their children on the spectrum.

Any substance can become toxic if taken in too high a concentration—even water.[2,3] Chlorine dioxide is no exception. We always increase CD dosages, *low and slow*, and have a respect for the power that chlorine dioxide can have over pathogens, always resisting the urge to ramp up our dosing too quickly.

> We started MMS 68 Days ago and my son's ATEC has dropped from 50-23... Now that's a MIRACLE!!! He is So much more "with us" and I'm seeing improvements daily. He is just so much more fun to be with now:) He did have a plateau, but is back on track. We have only done 4 enemas to date, but they made a big difference! Baths do as well:) I can't wait to see what he is like on his 4th birthday (still 39 days away).

Chlorine Dioxide was discovered in 1814 by Sir Humphrey Davy as an effective disinfectant. Since then, numerous companies have patented its use for countless applications, including food and health.

The following is an excerpt from Jim Humble's Nov 21, 2012 newsletter:

Dr. Andreas Kalcker spoke of patents obtained by different multinational pharmaceutical companies, to cash in on this product or to prevent it from being marketed.

Some of those patents include:

- Nontoxic Antiseptic (Pat 4035483/1977)
- For combatting human amoebas (Pat.4296102/1981)
- Against dementia caused by AIDS (Pat.5877222/1999)
- For curing all types of illness of the skin (Pat 4737307/1988)
- For disinfecting live blood (Pat. 5019402/1991)
- For curing injuries more rapidly (Pat. 5855922/1999)
- For all types of oral care (Procter & Gamble) (Pat. 6251372B1/2001)
- Against infections caused by bacteria (Pat. 5252343/1993)
- For treatment of severe burns (Pat.4317814/1982)
- For the regeneration of bone marrow (Pat. 4851222/1989)
- Treatment of Alzheimers, dementia etc. (Pat. 8029826B2/2011)
- To stimulate the immune system in animals (Pat. 6099855/2000)
- To stimulate the immunological system (Bioxy. Inc.) (Pat. 5830511/1998)

...The danger that may occur is if one mistakenly used a highly concentrated form. Highly concentrated forms of virtually every substance can cause death. In his conference, Dr. Andreas Kalcker points out that 70g of even plain table salt can cause death.

There have been thousands of reports worldwide of excessive doses of MMS being ingested, however, with the hundreds of millions of tons of this substance used each year worldwide for water purification, preservation of vegetables, sterilization of slaughtered meat, and hundreds of other uses, there has never been a report of a death caused by ingestion of chlorine dioxide.

This proves chlorine dioxide to be one of the safest products known.

There are many products that contain chlorine dioxide (ClO_2) that are currently approved by the Food and Drug Administration (FDA) in US. They are manufactured by *Frontier Farmaceutical, Alcide, Bioxy,* and others for skin and oral care. A number of these product names are listed below: [4]

- DioxiRinse™ Mouthwash
- DioxiBrite™ Toothpaste
- DioxiWhite™ Pro Teeth Whitener
- WhiteLasting™ Maintenance Gel
- BioClenz™ Dental Unit Waterline Cleaner
- Penetrator™ Periodontal Gel
- Simply Clear™ Acne Treatment
- DioxiWhite™ Home Teeth Whitener
- Cankers Away™ Canker Sore Cure
- DX7™ Skin Protectant Gel
- Periodontitis Treatment
- DioxiSmooth™ Facial Exfoliant
- Gingivitis Treatment Surface Disinfection
- Fire Fighter™ Burn Pain Reliever
- DioxiGuard™ Spray Disinfectant
- Nail-It™ Nail Protector

Chlorine Dioxide is an Oxidant...
But aren't <u>Anti</u>oxidants Good for Us?

In 1954, Denham Harman published an article called the "Free Radical Theory of Aging," [5] claiming antioxidants would slow the aging process. However, he later found that mitochondria determined life span, and that antioxidants do not enter the mitochondria, and subsequently published the

"Mitochondrial Theory of Aging,"[6] in 1972. The "Free Radical Theory of Aging" is still responsible for billions of dollars in antioxidant supplement sales a year. While writing this book, a fascinating article was published in the journal *Open Biology* by Dr. James Watson (of Watson and Crick) called "Oxidants, antioxidants and the current incurability of metastatic cancers."[7]

Watson sets forth a hypothesis that links the presence of antioxidants in the body with late-stage (metastatic) cancer. He points out that some successful cancer treatments use "free radical" molecules to treat cancer—the very same molecules that antioxidants attack and kill. Watson urges his readers of the new paper to consider the following: "Unless we can find ways of reducing antioxidant levels, late-stage cancer 10 years from now will be as incurable as it is today."[8]

The following was excerpted from the same article in *Open Biology*.[8] Please see the original document for references contained within the text.

> Free-radical-destroying antioxidative nutritional supplements may have caused more cancers than they have prevented.
>
> For as long as I have been focused on the understanding and curing of cancer (I taught a course on Cancer at Harvard in the autumn of 1959), well-intentioned individuals have been consuming antioxidative nutritional supplements as cancer preventatives if not actual therapies. The past, most prominent scientific proponent of their value was the great Caltech chemist, Linus Pauling, who near the end of his illustrious career wrote a book with Ewan Cameron in 1979, *Cancer and Vitamin C,* about vitamin C's great potential as an anti-cancer agent [52]. At the time of his death from prostate cancer in 1994, at the age of 93, Linus was taking 12 g of vitamin C every day. In light of the recent data strongly hinting that much of late-stage cancer's untreatability may arise from its possession of too many antioxidants, the time has come to seriously ask whether antioxidant use much more likely causes than prevents cancer.
>
> All in all, the by now vast number of nutritional intervention trials using the antioxidants β-carotene, vitamin A, vitamin C, vitamin E and selenium have shown no obvious effectiveness in preventing gastrointestinal cancer nor in lengthening mortality [53]. In fact, they seem to slightly shorten the lives of those who take them. Future data may, in fact, show that antioxidant use, particularly that of vitamin E, leads to a small number of cancers that would not have come into existence but for antioxidant supplementation. Blueberries best be eaten because they taste good, not because their consumption will lead to less cancer.

Don't Oxidants Cause Oxidative Stress?

Not necessarily. Dr. Andreas Kalcker presented us with another theory explaining why oxidative stress is caused by pathogens and parasites rather than oxidants. If you take an oxidant such as CD, it is likely to upset the parasites living in the intestinal tract, causing them to defecate. Waste from worms can contain many toxic substances including MDA (malondialdehyde), formaldehyde, and ammonia. These toxins are known to cause oxidative stress.[9,10,11,12] When parasites are present in the body they are releasing these toxins, even if we don't kill them. Parasitic presence in the body is responsible for many of the symptoms known as autism.

Oxidants themselves are not directly responsible for oxidative stress in the body. However, they can exacerbate oxidative stress, which can cause parasites in the body to release toxins. The solution is to get rid of the parasites. Please see Chapter 8 for an effective Parasite Protocol.

Chlorine Dioxide & Antioxidants

Although antioxidants have their place in personal health and are common in many foods and supplements, they cannot be taken at the same time with chlorine dioxide—they negate each other. This is why vitamin C, juices, and other antioxidant containing foods are prohibited in *The Diet*.

Just a testimonial to MMS: For those of you new to the group and still unsure of the MMS protocol I wanted to tell you about us. I was afraid at first, but we decided to try MMS. Within 3 weeks my son went from an ATEC of 36 to 18! That was amazing. Then we were afraid of the enemas. We said no way, we would just do oral MMS. Of course, after seeing others progress here we decided to do them. He would calm down! Then for months we agonized over the PP. We were afraid of it. We were scared of the meds, everything. Finally we decided to try it too. We are in the middle of our first PP and our son, who used to hit, kick, bite and scream at me over the smallest things all the time, has now been a perfect joy. When he gets mad it is over quickly and does not escalate into world war 3. Also these bumps he had on his face have cleared up along with his attitude! So if you are unsure of MMS like I was, here is one more testimonial of just how good the protocol really is. Thanks Kerri, and all the other moms that came before me!

Herxheimer Reaction (Die-Off Reaction)

There are many stories on the Internet about the "side effects" of CD. The definition of a side effect is:

The unintended or secondary effects of a substance.

When people describe what they believe to be side effects of CD, they are actually talking about a Herxheimer reaction. Jim Humble's original chlorine dioxide (MMS) protocols called for higher doses per hour ramped up much faster than we titrate up for autism. In some cases that resulted in nausea, vomiting, and/or diarrhea. Critics of CD claim that a Herxheimer reaction, which is the result from ramping up too quickly, is the body's reaction to being 'poisoned' by chlorine dioxide.

This is absolutely not the case, as the aforementioned study by Judith R. Lubbers and colleagues found that when healthy individuals were given minimal doses of chlorine dioxide in increasingly higher concentrations, no deleterious effects were noted.[2]

A Herxheimer reaction indicates that the patient is suffering from an overload of pathogens/toxins. If the person taking CD has a fair amount of pathogens, the rapid killing of these invaders produces excess toxins in the bloodstream. It is these substances that the body wants to rid itself of in short order. People with autism often have impaired methylation cycles that reduce their ability to eliminate toxins, making it even more difficult to handle an influx of toxins. So LOW AND SLOW is the way to go.

Children with autism typically don't (or can't) tell you they have nausea. However, discomfort may be visible from seeing that they're eating less, their eating habits have changed, or they're more listless than usual. That's usually a sign of detox, and in which case, we won't give the child any more CD that day. Detox is great, it's what we want, but without stressing the body further. We need to stay just beneath a Herxheimer reaction.

A Herxheimer reaction can present itself in many forms including:

• Blisters	• Fatigue	• Hiccups
• Bloating	• Flatulence	• Nausea
• Burping	• Flushing	• Runny nose
• Chills	• Headache	• Sleep changes
• Diarrhea	• Heart Burn	• Vomiting

If any of these symptoms appear, suspend the remaining doses of CD for the rest of the day. The following day, return to the number of doses given when the child was stable, which is usually the dose that was given the day prior to the Herxheimer reaction.

To mitigate a Herxheimer reaction from chlorine dioxide, you can give vitamin C or orange juice, as either one of these will cut the effects of CD immediately. To help bind the excess toxins you may want to try activated charcoal, bentonite clay, (be aware that these both can cause constipation), or burbur (a liquid detox extract).

Using Chlorine Dioxide for Autism

As I developed this protocol, it became clear to me that we needed to focus on excesses causing the symptoms of autism, rather than deficiencies caused by them. In the autism biomed world, we are accustomed to supplementing deficiencies (low iron, low B_{12}, low calcium, etc.), without questioning why the deficiency exists in the first place (i.e., presence of pathogens/parasites).

As soon as a family completes one week on *The Diet*, we get right into CD. Everyone starts with the "baby bottle" method, one drop of CD in eight fluid ounces of water, which makes the first day's dose 1/8 of a drop at a time. We have greatly minimized Herxheimer reactions by using this method, but it remains very important to monitor your child while they are using chlorine dioxide. It's very important to go low and slow. Every drop we give is helping to heal our children.

What is Chlorine Dioxide (CD)?

Refer to the diagram on the right for a visual overview.

You can't actually buy CD. You have to make it. Fortunately, it's not a big deal. If you can make coffee... you can make CD, which stands for *chlorine dioxide*.

Chlorine dioxide (ClO_2), is a gas produced through a chemical reaction when two liquids, sodium chlorite ($NaClO_2$) and an acid (such as hydrochloric acid (HCl) or citric acid ($C_6H_8O_7$)), are mixed. The acid brings the combined pH level below five, causing the sodium chlorite to become unstable and release chlorine dioxide (ClO_2).

If any of this sounds complex, it isn't. Go through the following explanation and don't get bogged down by the chemical symbols.

Conceptual Overview of Chlorine Dioxide (CD)

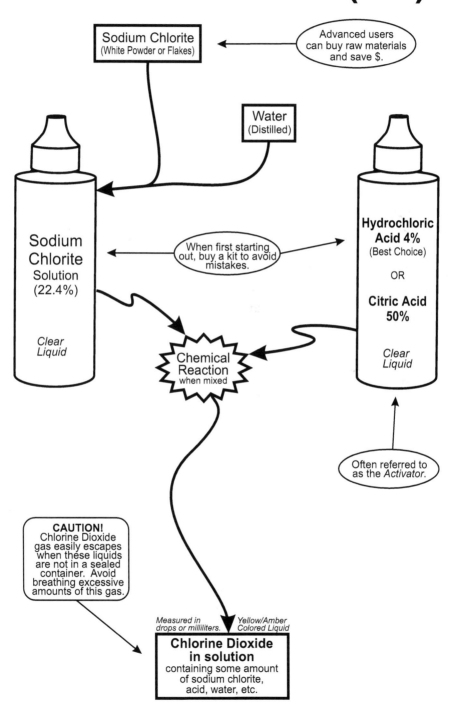

Sodium Chlorite
(White Powder or Flakes)

Advanced users can buy raw materials and save $.

Water
(Distilled)

Sodium Chlorite Solution (22.4%)

Clear Liquid

When first starting out, buy a kit to avoid mistakes.

Hydrochloric Acid 4%
(Best Choice)

OR

Citric Acid 50%

Clear Liquid

Chemical Reaction when mixed

Often referred to as the *Activator*.

CAUTION!
Chlorine Dioxide gas easily escapes when these liquids are not in a sealed container. Avoid breathing excessive amounts of this gas.

Measured in drops or milliliters.   *Yellow/Amber Colored Liquid*

Chlorine Dioxide in solution
containing some amount of sodium chlorite, acid, water, etc.

Sodium Chlorite (NaClO₂)

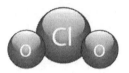

This is the first chemical you must have to make CD.

You can get it in one of two forms:

- **Sodium chlorite liquid in water:**
  - If you are beginning, get a starter kit of this.
  - Expect to pay about $20-$30 for a 4 fl. oz. bottle set (usually includes acid activator).
  - 22.4% sodium chlorite solution (from 28% technical grade sodium chlorite salts).
  - Recommended: Buy quart or liter sized quantities of liquid once you understand the principles.

- **Sodium chlorite powder or flakes:**
  - FOR ADVANCED USERS ONLY!
  - Cheaper in the long run.
  - Recommend buying 5 lbs. of flakes/powder for a cost of about $100-$200.
  - Look online or check with your supplier for mixing instructions.
  - Avoid buying 90% sodium chlorite flakes. You want 80%. Most suppliers that sell liquid also sell flakes.
  - NEVER mix any acid directly with powder/flakes!

What's the 28%? 22.4%?

This is not a critical thing for you to worry about unless you are mixing your own. But here is the jist: sodium chlorite powder is not 100% sodium chlorite. It's usually 80% sodium chlorite and 20% salt and other inert ingredients. When diluted in water, you end up with 28% solution of powder, but only 22.4% is sodium chlorite. Labels usually show one or both of these numbers.

Sodium Chlorite Flakes vs. Powder

Sodium chlorite flakes and sodium chlorite powder are the same thing. The resulting physical consistency may vary by different manufacturers. We've even seen clumps of powder. It's still the same chemical. The important part is that it is technical grade, and 80% of the powder/flakes should be sodium chlorite (NaClO₂). Mixing info is at: *www.youtube.com/watch?v=t0C8XVm9QVE.*

Acid - The Activator

To produce CD, you must add the second chemical, which is a food acid, to the liquefied sodium chlorite (22.4% solution in water). Chlorine dioxide gas is produced when the pH of the sodium chlorite goes below five. We call the acid used to lower the pH of sodium chlorite an "activator" because it activates the sodium chlorite to produce the chlorine dioxide.

There are several activators to choose from. These are food acids in that they are commonly found in food preparations, or are actually food:

- **Hydrochloric Acid (HCl)**
  - The same acid found in your stomach, and therefore, the most biocompatible option.
  - Working concentration is between 4% and 10%.
  - Available on the market in liquid concentrations of 4%, 5%, 10%, 32%, 35%, and 37%.
  - Any concentration over 10% must be reduced to a working concentration of between 4% and 10%. See Appendix 7, page 471. (Note: We use 4% for CD and CDH; & 10% for CDS.)
  - Only available in liquid form.

- **Citric Acid**
  - Commonly available around the world.
  - Often found in soft drinks to give them a tangy flavor.
  - Some people have problems tolerating this acid.
  - Usually used in 50/50 concentration by weight mixed in water.
  - Available in liquid and powder form.
  - Inexpensive; can be purchased online.

- **Lemon or Lime Juice**
  - Consider this an emergency alternative to be used if the first two choices are not available.
  - Can be found in most stores carrying produce.
  - Should be from pure, organic and freshly squeezed lemons (or limes).
  - Relatively weak acidity requiring five drops of lemon juice to every one drop of sodium chlorite solution.
  - Substantially longer activation time.
  - Lower ClO_2 output.

The amount of acid used, and the length of time you wait to dilute the mixture, will depend on the acid activator and its strength. The following chart gives you an idea.

Activator	Strength	Ratio	Time
Hydrochloric Acid	10%	1:1	40 secs
Hydrochloric Acid	4%	1:1	60 secs
Citric Acid	50%	1:1	60 secs
Citric Acid	33% or 35%	1:1	60 secs
Lemon Juice	Pure	1:5	120+ secs

You are unlikely to be using lemon juice, but we've included it here for completeness.

Families should use whichever activator is available to them depending on where they live and what they have access to. All kids are different, so if yours doesn't respond well to 4% HCl, by all means, try citric acid, or vice versa.

If the HCl you purchased is anything other than 4% or 5%, then see Appendix 7 for instructions on reducing concentration.

If you are using one of the two most commonly available activators, then you are likely to be using a 1:1 mixing ratio (1 drop sodium chlorite + 1 drop activator).

In the case of 10% citric acid or pure lemon juice, you would be using five drops of activator to one drop of sodium chlorite, and waiting about three times as long as if you were using one of the newer, more concentrated activators.

Purchasing Product

When you first start out, you should buy a starter kit and get familiar with the chemistry. A starter kit usually comes in two bottles of four fluid ounces each.

1. Sodium chlorite, (4 fl. oz.)
2. Activator (hydrochloric acid or citric acid), (4 fl. oz.)

The bottles look something like those shown in the diagram on page 91. Getting the hydrochloric acid activator is slightly preferable.

You will also need an 8 fl. oz. baby bottle. This is a handy tool for storing a day's worth of CD doses with the added benefit of having marks that show how much it contains. Glass bottles are much better than any kind of plastic bottle. Lifefactory.com (shown on the right) produces a bottle we especially like. It is made of silicon-covered glass and has a reliable top. This particular bottle is marked as having a capacity of nine fl. oz., but we use it up to only eight fl. oz. Plastic should only be used for lids; avoid bottles with metal tops. Over time, CD will oxidize metals so they can't be used.

Another item that most people have at home is a shot glass or wine glass that tapers down in the middle like a "U" shape. This will be used to mix the chemicals and the tapered shape insures that even as few as two drops will find each other. You can also use a cup with a flat bottom, but must tilt it so both solutions pool together.

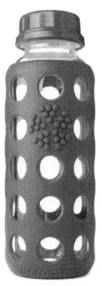

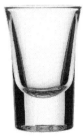

A standard shot glass with a "U" shaped bottom is the preferred mixing container for CD & activator. A glass baby bottle, such as the one made by Lifefactory®, is the ideal dosing bottle.

Terminology of Available Products

There can be a bit of confusion for some as to what to look for and buy. The following chart shows the actual chemical, and some of the common names found on the label. There may be other names we are not aware of. In most cases, the chemical and its strength are identified on the bottles.

Common Activators & Their Various Names on the Market

Chemical	Common Names
Sodium Chlorite	Chlorine Dioxide – Part 1 (Purifier) Master Mineral Solution Miracle Mineral Solution Miracle Mineral Supplement MMS MMS Drops MMS Solution MMS Water Purification Drops MMS1 NaClO2 Natriumchlorit (German) Pathogen Biocide Sodium Chlorite 28% Water Purification Drops Water Purificator
Hydrochloric Acid	Activator Chlorine Dioxide – Part 2 (Activator) MMS Activator
Citric Acid	Activator Citric Acid – 20% Citric Acid – 50% MMS Activator

Checklist for Preparing a CD Dose

Assuming you have received the starter kit, it's time to make your first dose. Here's the check list of what you now should have on hand before you begin:

- ❑ Bottle of sodium chlorite solution (28% sodium chlorite salts / 22.4% sodium chlorite)
- ❑ Bottle of acidic activator (hydrochloric acid or citric acid)
- ❑ A clean and dry shot-glass with a "U" shaped bottom.
- ❑ 8 fl. oz. glass baby bottle.
- ❑ Distilled or reverse osmosis water (filtered water will do, but no alkaline water!).

A Few Points Worth Noting!

Looking at the short checklist above, it should be apparent that this is not going to be rocket science. Nevertheless, a few pointers are in order:

- In the past, people who used CD for various things would mix a fresh batch each time they took CD. This involved a lot of extra work that could be avoided by producing one batch big enough to last the entire day. For this exercise, we are assuming you are starting out and going to do things low and slow. We are going to produce 8 fl. oz. of water solution containing one drop of CD, with the intention of your child consuming one fl. oz., of water (containing 1/8 drop of CD) eight times throughout the day.

- When you mix sodium chlorite solution and the acidic activator, you are mixing equal drops of each substance (unless you are using one of the less concentrated activators mentioned earlier).

- CD doses are measured in drops of sodium chlorite. So one drop of sodium chlorite + one drop of activator = one drop of CD.

- On your first day, start with one drop of sodium chlorite and one drop of activator (in other words—ONE drop of CD).

- If you put in too many drops of one solution or the other, start over with a clean and dry shot glass.

- A batch of CD is good for 24 hours. <u>However, you must keep the cap on tight!</u>

- Keep the bottle with the daily CD batch out of direct sunlight. A brief exposure won't ruin it, but it will become weaker. Why? The chlorine dioxide gas will come out of the water and sometimes form a cloud in the air pocket of the bottle. No need to worry if you see the cloud—it's a common occurrence.

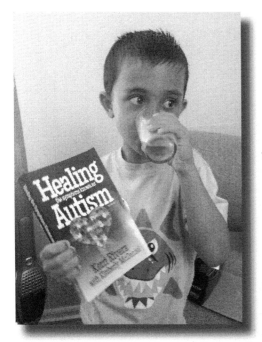

Vincent taking his hourly dose.

Preparing Your First One drop CD Batch for the Day

1.	Start by filling the baby bottle with 8 fl. oz. (237ml) of water (distilled or reverse osmosis). NO alkaline water!	
2.	Place 1 drop of sodium chlorite solution into the CLEAN and DRY shot glass.	
3.	Add 1 drop of acidic activator (hydrochloric acid or citric acid) to the shot glass containing the drop of sodium chlorite. The number of drops may be higher if you are using a weaker activator. See chart on page 94.	
4.	Now wait the appropriate time for the mixture to react (see chart on page 94). You should see the color change from clear to slightly yellow. If there were more drops in the shot glass, the color change is more noticeable. You are also likely to notice the chlorine-like smell coming from the shot glass. Remember, this is NOT chlorine, but rather chlorine dioxide.	
5.	After the activation time has passed, pour a little water from the baby bottle into the shot glass and let it mix. This mostly stops the chemical reaction and insures you get most of the mixture out in the next step.	
6.	Lastly, pour all of the watered down mixture in the shot glass back into the baby bottle, and seal it tightly with the cap—don't leave it sitting open for any length of time. Think partially used soda pop and how you would want to keep that closed.	

Voilà! You have just produced your first batch of CD!

This is now a ONE drop batch, that makes EIGHT hourly doses—each 1/8 of a drop in strength. If your batch is larger; your hourly dose is stronger:

- 2 drop batch = 8 hourly doses of 1/4 drop
- 4 drop batch = 8 hourly doses of 1/2 drop
- 8 drop batch = 8 hourly doses of 1 drop

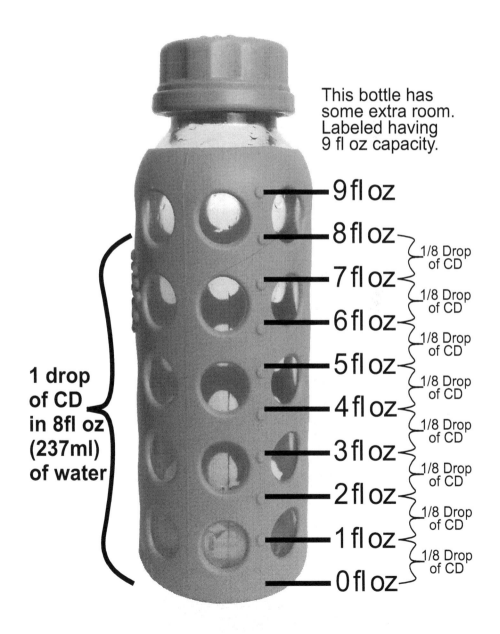

This bottle has some extra room. Labeled having 9 fl oz capacity.

9 fl oz

8 fl oz
1/8 Drop of CD

7 fl oz
1/8 Drop of CD

6 fl oz
1/8 Drop of CD

5 fl oz
1/8 Drop of CD

4 fl oz
1/8 Drop of CD

3 fl oz
1/8 Drop of CD

2 fl oz
1/8 Drop of CD

1 fl oz
1/8 Drop of CD

0 fl oz

1 drop of CD in 8fl oz (237ml) of water

Oral Protocol for CD in
Autism Spectrum Disorders (ASDs)

In the previous exercise, you learned how to prepare the dose for Day One. Children and adults all start by taking only one drop of CD divided into eight hourly doses. On Day Two, you make a batch of two drops sodium chlorite plus two drops activator and mix that into eight fluid ounces of water. Increase this dosage by one drop per day, unless you see a Herxheimer reaction (see page 89 for more information).

The chart on the right allows you to determine the estimated full oral CD dose based on the weight of the individual. This gives you an idea of the maximum goal number of drops per day for your child. Once the child has been at the full suggested dose for several months, we may need to increase again, by a few drops, to prevent a plateau.

Important Note: Some children can't go up by one drop each day and need to go slower. A child may have a relatively higher toxic load, or he may be extremely sensitive. Whatever the case, resist the urge to try to get to full oral dose as quickly as possible. This is not a race! Some children need to spend a few extra days at the same dose to avoid a Herxheimer reaction. Even if you must remain at one level for a few days or more does not mean you are making no progress. Whatever the level of dosage, you are detoxing the body.

When you get within two to three drops of your child's maximum dose by weight, go ahead and spend three days at each dose, while carefully observing your child, moving up only when your child is stable. For example, if the full dose is 16 drops in the 8 fl. oz. (237ml) baby bottle, stay at 14 drops for a few days to see how that dose level is tolerated, and then increase every third day till reaching the full dose. If the person is better at a drop or two below the calculated full dose, go back to that lower dose that they tolerated best.

> Just had a fascinating appointment with my son's functional neurologist. My son had this third Qeeg today, which clearly showed that previously under-stimulated parts of his brain are 'waking up'. I told our doctor about CD very early on and he believes that it is THIS that is having such a huge impact on his brain. He got quite emotional and said 'every time you get a worm, you are saving your son. Keep doing what you're doing, cause he clearly isn't autistic. He's poisoned'. Goosebumps!!

Estimated Full Oral CD Doses by Weight

Use these numbers as a guide only. You may need to go up by as much as 50% or more over the indicated drops. Read chart as: **POUNDS / KILOGRAMS → DROPS OF CD (per 8 fl. oz. water)**

25/11→8	62/28→17	99/45→24	136/62→29	173/78→33	210/95→37
26/12→8	63/29→17	100/45→24	137/62→29	174/79→33	211/96→37
27/12→9	64/29→17	101/46→24	138/63→29	175/79→34	212/96→37
28/13→9	65/29→18	102/46→24	139/63→30	176/80→34	213/97→37
29/13→9	66/30→18	103/47→24	140/64→30	177/80→34	214/97→37
30/14→9	67/30→18	104/47→25	141/64→30	178/81→34	215/98→37
31/14→10	68/31→18	105/48→25	142/64→30	179/81→34	216/98→37
32/15→10	69/31→18	106/48→25	143/65→30	180/82→34	217/98→37
33/15→10	70/32→19	107/49→25	144/65→30	181/82→34	218/99→38
34/15→10	71/32→19	108/49→25	145/66→30	182/83→34	219/99→38
35/16→11	72/33→19	109/49→25	146/66→30	183/83→34	220/100→38
36/16→11	73/33→19	110/50→26	147/67→31	184/83→35	221/100→38
37/17→11	74/34→19	111/50→26	148/67→31	185/84→35	222/101→38
38/17→11	75/34→20	112/51→26	149/68→31	186/84→35	223/101→38
39/18→12	76/34→20	113/51→26	150/68→31	187/85→35	224/102→38
40/18→12	77/35→20	114/52→26	151/68→31	188/85→35	225/102→38
41/19→12	78/35→20	115/52→26	152/69→31	189/86→35	226/103→38
42/19→12	79/36→20	116/53→26	153/69→31	190/86→35	227/103→38
43/20→13	80/36→21	117/53→27	154/70→31	191/87→35	228/103→38
44/20→13	81/37→21	118/54→27	155/70→31	192/87→35	229/104→38
45/20→13	82/37→21	119/54→27	156/71→32	193/88→35	230/104→39
46/21→13	83/38→21	120/54→27	157/71→32	194/88→35	231/105→39
47/21→14	84/38→21	121/55→27	158/72→32	195/88→36	232/105→39
48/22→14	85/39→21	122/55→27	159/72→32	196/89→36	233/106→39
49/22→14	86/39→22	123/56→27	160/73→32	197/89→36	234/106→39
50/23→14	87/39→22	124/56→28	161/73→32	198/90→36	235/107→39
51/23→15	88/40→22	125/57→28	162/73→32	199/90→36	236/107→39
52/24→15	89/40→22	126/57→28	163/74→32	200/91→36	237/108→39
53/24→15	90/41→22	127/58→28	164/74→32	201/91→36	238/108→39
54/24→15	91/41→23	128/58→28	165/75→33	202/92→36	239/108→39
55/25→16	92/42→23	129/59→28	166/75→33	203/92→36	240/109→39
56/25→16	93/42→23	130/59→28	167/76→33	204/93→36	241/109→39
57/26→16	94/43→23	131/59→28	168/76→33	205/93→36	242/110→39
58/26→16	95/43→23	132/60→29	169/77→33	206/93→37	243/110→39
59/27→16	96/44→23	133/60→29	170/77→33	207/94→37	244/111→40
60/27→17	97/44→24	134/61→29	171/78→33	208/94→37	245/111→40
61/28→17	98/44→24	135/61→29	172/78→33	209/95→37	246/112→40

Serving Cup Dilution

Don't have your child drink out of the baby bottle. Pour the hourly dose into a separate cup and add extra water if needed. Make sure to add water to each dose to ensure that there is a **minimum** of one fluid ounce of water per activated drop of CD. However, there is no maximum amount of water for dilution. To be absolutely clear about this, note the following chart which assumes eight fl. oz., daily batches containing eight hourly doses.

Drops of CD in Batch	Hourly Dose	Min. Water Dilution
1	1/8 drop	1 fluid ounce
2	2/8 drop	1 fluid ounce
3	3/8 drop	1 fluid ounce
4	4/8 drop	1 fluid ounce
5	5/8 drop	1 fluid ounce
6	6/8 drop	1 fluid ounce
7	7/8 drop	1 fluid ounce
8	1 drop	1 fluid ounce
9	1 1/8 drops	2 fluid ounces
10	1 2/8 drops	2 fluid ounces
11	1 3/8 drops	2 fluid ounces
12	1 4/8 drops	2 fluid ounces
13	1 5/8 drops	2 fluid ounces
14	1 6/8 drops	2 fluid ounces
15	1 7/8 drops	2 fluid ounces
16	2 drops	2 fluid ounces
17	2 1/8 drops	3 fluid ounces
18	2 2/8 drops	3 fluid ounces
19	2 3/8 drops	3 fluid ounces
20	2 4/8 drops	3 fluid ounces
21	2 5/8 drops	3 fluid ounces
22	2 6/8 drops	3 fluid ounces
23	2 7/8 drops	3 fluid ounces
24	3 drops	3 fluid ounces
25	3 1/8 drops	4 fluid ounces
26	3 2/8 drops	4 fluid ounces
27	3 3/8 drops	4 fluid ounces
28	3 4/8 drops	4 fluid ounces
29	3 5/8 drops	4 fluid ounces
30	3 6/8 drops	4 fluid ounces
31	3 7/8 drops	4 fluid ounces
32	4 drops	4 fluid ounces

CD is active in the body for about one hour and, as result, hourly doses give us the best progress. This is difficult on school days, but we recommend that you dose two to three times before school and the rest after to distribute the pathogen-fighting more evenly. Eight doses a day is the minimum requirement, but the more you can fit in the better. Try to dose every hour as much as possible.

Special Cases: "The Double Dose"

As a child goes through the detox process, they may exhibit conduct which can include hyperactivity, anxiety, OCD, aggressiveness, and night wakings. In these cases, a double dose is 2 fl. oz. (60ml) of the baby bottle given at once. For example, if your child receives one drop per fluid ounce of the baby bottle method, they will be receiving 2 drops. Let's say for example your child wakes up at 1am, give them a double dose. If your child is still awake at 2am, give another dose. The most common scenario is that after 1 or 2 double doses, the child will fall back asleep. This helps oxidize the toxins from the die-off. During the day if your child has a tantrum or other issues with conduct, we can double dose every hour as well.

CD has two functions with pathogens; one is that is oxidizes the pathogen itself, and the second is that it oxidizes the toxins released by the pathogens while they are living, dead, or dying.

Advanced Protocol – The Enema!

In early 2011, we added enemas to the protocol to kill the pathogens causing dysbiosis in the large intestine (we didn't know about parasites yet). We wanted to get the chlorine dioxide into the blood stream so it could kill the biofilm that exists in the blood. In this way, the blood can carry the CD past the blood-brain barrier to kill pathogens in the brain

When we are detoxing, it is absolutely critical to keep the colon moving and avoid the reabsorption of toxins through the intestinal walls. Enemas allow us to do just this. Some toxins can exit the intestine through the intestinal wall (more so if leaky-gut syndrome is present), and cross the blood-brain barrier, therefore affecting cognition and behavior. When we cleanse the colon, we get those out before they can cross into the brain, and we detoxify the lymphatic system, liver, and gallbladder.

The Enema Stigma

When I say the word enema to a family new to the protocol, I often hear things like "*I could never do that!*," or "*My son would never let me do an enema.*" I assure you it's not traumatic as it has been hyped up to be. Modern society has gotten away from it, but for millennia, cleansing the colon was considered part of daily hygiene. Enemas were mentioned in the Vedas, the Bible, and by the Mayans. The reason for doing CD enemas is NOT for relief of constipation. Of course, when constipation is present, CD enemas can relieve the cause of constipation.

> *Great news! First enema today...*
>
> *My son was so happy that we did and the first thing he said while sitting on the toilet was: "Mommy! IT WORKED!!!" hahaha He is so used to sitting on the toilet and having such a hard time. Poor thing, he was so happy that IT WORKED!*
>
> *And he even said he wants to do it again tomorrow. He felt so much better and ate so much more for dinner with an empty stomach. I think he got rid of stuff that was there for ages! His tummy is now soft and not hard as usual. Quite amazing and it didn't bother him at all.*
>
> *Today his molar hasn't bothered him so a perfect day to start the enemas! His appetite has gone up quite a bit. He has seldom asked for food before and now he asks a few times a day for something to eat. The diet is going wonderfully and he is now used to the change of foods. He asks about cheese and milk but I try to talk about something else to distract him so he eventually stops asking. hahaha He hasn't gotten upset about food he wants (that he can't have) not even once. YAY!*

I would like to clear up one thing here before we get in the mechanics of the enemas. More than one person has asked in the blogosphere, "*If Kerri Rivera loves enemas so much, why doesn't she do them on herself???*" As a matter of fact I do! I have done my own enemas for years, so has my husband, my sister, and plenty of the parents using this protocol for their children. We understand the benefits of a fit colon, and have no problem applying our own enemas or going for a colonic from time to time.

Actually, I would strongly advise you to practice on yourself. That way you know from first-hand experience that this is really no big deal. You will also discover how much better you feel after cleaning out your colon, and you will understand when your child feels better as well.

When to Start Giving Enemas

Enemas should be started when the child reaches full oral dose.

However, if your child suffers from constipation you can add enemas and baths on day one (see page 113), before you get to the full oral dose. However, alternate them on opposite days or opposite ends of the day.

Frequency of Enemas

I recommend enemas no less than once every other day. You may need to do them more often, particularly if you see parasites coming out. Doing as many as four in a day is not uncalled for if each one results in parasites being released. Some of the older children seem to pass a lot of parasites in one day, typically in or around a full or new moon.

Timing of Enemas

If your child is going to school, avoid giving an enema in the morning since they may need to visit the toilet a few times after. If the child is homeschooled or too young or sick to attend, the timing is up to you. Ideally, do the enema after the child has a bowel movement.

Enemas — What You Need

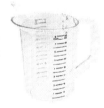

The first thing you are going to need is some kind of a large plastic, liquid measuring container. Glass is not recommended since it can get knocked over and break in the confines of a bathroom.

You will also need all the same things you used for making CD batches:

- Water. Use reverse osmosis, filtered, or distilled. DO NOT use tap water or alkaline water!
- Sodium chlorite solution
- Acidic activator
- Shot glass
- Natural lubricant (coconut oil or any other simple food oil). NO perfumed baby oil or chemical lotions such as Petroleum Jelly or K-Y® Jelly.
- Enema kit (see your options on the following page)

Enema Options (Most to Least Preferred)

Gravity Bag or Bucket with hose

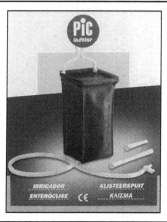 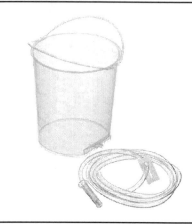

Pros:
- Holds plenty of liquid
- Can be refilled without taking it down
- Flow is easy to control
- Can be hung on a door
- Can be used for both enema and douching
- PIC Indolor: Folds for easy travel
- PIC Indolor: Has valve
- PIC Indolor: Two sizes of cathetors

Cons:
- Bucket doesn't fold for easy travel

Enema / Douche Bag / Hot Water Bottle

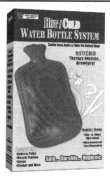 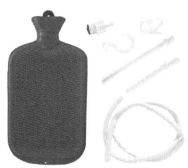

Pros:
- Holds plenty of liquid
- Flow is easy to control
- Can be hung on a door
- Can be used for both enema and douching
- Easy travel
- Has two sizes of cathetors

Cons:
- Can't be refilled without taking down
- Usually made of rubber, which tends to dry out quickly, especially from CD.

Syringe & Catheter

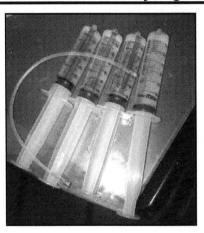

Pros:
- Flow is easy to control
- Can be used for both enema and douching
- Good for small children

Cons:
- Holds only 60ml-140ml
- Need more than one.
- Have to swap them out to go beyond the capacity of one syringe.
- The graduations rub off easily (suggest putting clear shipping tape over them to protect the markings if they are important to you).

Enema Bulb

Pros:
- Portable
- Can be used for both enema and douching
- Good for "implants" of mebendazole

Cons:
- Volume too small for an effective treatment.
- Hard to clean inside
- Can't tell if dirt is on the inside.
- Holds only about 200ml.

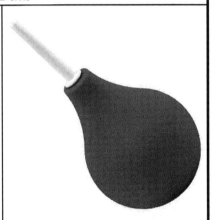

Fleet Enema (Last Resort)

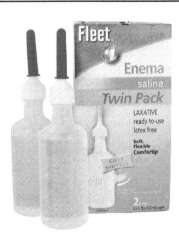

Pros:
- Cheap
- Can find it in most pharmacies
- Portable
- Can be used for both Enema and Douching

Cons:
- Volume too small for an effective treatment.

Enema Kits

As shown in the previous two pages, here are your enema kit options listed from best to less than good. Prices are estimates in US Dollars and are likely to be higher outside the US:

★★★★★ PIC Indolor Gravity Bag (~$15-$30)

★★★★☆ Enema Bucket (~$5-$10)

★★★½☆ Multipurpose Enema/Douche Bag/Hot Water Bottle (~$15-$30)

★★★☆☆ 100ml+ Syringes plus Catheter (~$5-$10)

★★☆☆☆ Enema Bulb (~$5-$15)

★☆☆☆☆ Fleet Enema (emptied out) (~$5-$15)

You must have a separate enema kit for each person doing enemas. This insures that you are not cross-contaminating parasites.

In my own home we have recently started using the PIC Indolor enema/douche bag. This has made the process faster, and we can tolerate more water before feeling full and desiring to release the enema. This is probably the most practical kit, especially because of the built-in shut-off valve. The enema bucket is a close second, but the sliding clamp that comes with it doesn't last long and breaks easily. You can always just kink the hose and control the flow that way.

The multipurpose enema/douche/hot water bottle type is a good option, but it is usually made of rubber. This material often goes bad over time and CD just speeds up that process. Rinse it out several times before and after use to insure that no breakdown or CD residue is left. Don't use if you notice the rubber becoming brittle.

Even two-year-olds still use about 400 to 500ml in an enema. The intestine is long. Parents with small children sometimes like the 100ml syringe/catheter method. The enema bulb or fleet enema are not really practical for our purposes due to the small volumes they hold. However, if you want to get started right away, they are usually available in most major pharmacies.

You can find syringes, catheters, gravity bags, multipurpose enema/douche bags on various online sites, pharmacies and medical supply stores around the world.

Preparing and Administering the Enema

Make all your supplies easily accessible in your work area before bringing your child in the bathroom. If this is your first time and you are working out the process, you may wish to ask your spouse or someone else for assistance. It's a good idea to do a dress rehearsal without the child, to insure that it goes smoothly when the child is present. Once you and your child have the process down, it will be easy. Being prepared is the key to success.

Please note: The eight fluid ounce baby bottle is NOT involved in any way with enemas!

1. Ideally, time the enema just after a bowel movement.

2. Start by washing your hands to insure you are not introducing any new bacteria into the colon. Everything you are working with should be clean. Wearing gloves and a face/surgical mask is HIGHLY recommended.

3. Assuming you are using one of the suggested gravity bags, find a good and stable location to hang it up. The best location really depends on your particular bathroom's layout and where you are going to place the child during the procedure. I hang mine from a towel hook in the bathroom, or you can use the shower curtain rod. The idea is to have the bag/bucket about three feet (~one meter) over where the enema will be administered. Most parents put a towel on the floor of the bathroom and lay their child on the towel (smaller children can lay across your lap).

4. Refer to the chart below and measure out the appropriate amount of water for the individual receiving the enema. The ratio is two drops of CD per 100ml of filtered warm water.

Age/Size	Water Volume	Drops of CD
Child	1/2 Liter (500ml)	10
Adolescent	1 Liter (1000ml)	20
Teen/Adult	up to 2 Liters (2000ml)	40

5. <u>Don't add any CD yet.</u> The next step is to heat the water to body temperature (98°F / 37°C). The water should feel warm to the touch—NEVER hot! Similar to the temperature of milk in a baby bottle... test it on your wrist. If you are concerned about getting the temperature right use a quality thermometer. Be aware... many cheap thermometers are notoriously inaccurate!

6. After the heating step, pour the water back into the big measuring cup.

7. Referring again to the chart on the previous page, prepare a CD mixture in the clean dry shot glass that's appropriate for the volume of water needed. For example, if you have an adolescent and are preparing one liter, then you will need to mix 20 drops of sodium chlorite and 20 drops of acidic activator to end up with 20 drops of CD! Note: The most important part of the enema is the **water**. Resist the urge to add more than two drops per 100ml of water.

8. After the appropriate activation time, pour the concentrated CD from your shot glass into the large measuring cup. You may want to rinse out the shot glass with some water from the large mixing cup so you get all the concentrated CD solution into the water.

9. The bag/bucket should now be in its working location with the hose firmly attached, Place the end of the hose so it is over the top of the bag/bucket. A clothes pin can come in handy to hold it up over the bag/bucket. Now, fill the bag/bucket about 3/4 full with the CD water mixture you just prepared.

10. Make sure the hose is filled with water. You may want to let a bit run out into the sink or some other container and then clamp it. The bucket type enema has a plastic clamp for this purpose. The bag type has a valve where the catheter attaches. What you don't want is for there to be a bunch of air in the hose that then is transferred into the colon.

11. If all of the above is ready, it is time to bring your child into the bathroom.

12. Explain what you are going to do. Some parents say that they are going to put the catheter in his bottom, and that it has "special water" in it to help him feel better. One little boy called it "butt medicine" while another called it "butt wash." We recommend you say that you are the only person who is allowed to give this to him. Just say whatever you need to say to explain what is happening.

13. If the child is on the floor (on a rug or towel), they should lie on their stomach. If the child is small then laying them on your lap is best. You can also have them in a doggy position on the floor.

14. Place one or two drops of coconut oil (or similar) on their anus so the area is well lubricated.

15. Now take the hose and gently insert the tip, (one to two inches is plenty—more is not necessary) as the sphincter muscle will hold the tip of the catheter in place. If you are having any problems getting the catheter in, then you may need to add a bit more oil and/or adjust the angle.

16. Release the clamp or open the valve to allow the liquid to flow. The goal is *fill & release.*—NOT *fill & hold.* We are imitating the colonic process that is made up of gallons of water, yet in the home environment.

17. Your child will most likely hold the contents on their own—they will squeeze hard so as not to "go." This kind of happens naturally.

We do a fill and release method. The first part of the enema is usually stool. After that, we usually see parasites and or biofilm.

It's a learning experience and as time goes on, you will get the hang of it.

Quote from a teenager using the Protocol: "I like the enemas. Before them I am mad. But then when I get one, I feel better. My mad leaves in my poop.

Syringe/Catheter Method

Before I started to use the gravity bag, the syringe/catheter method was my favorite. We have a YouTube video on our channel that shows how to fill the syringes and switch them out while using the catheter. If you don't have access to that video here is an explanation on how to do it:

1. Fill a bowl with body temperature filtered water and fill your syringes. If your child uses 500ml for an enema, fill all five syringes and dump out whatever water is still left in the bowl.

2. Squirt all the water from the syringes back into the bowl. You now have exactly 500ml of purified water.

3. Activate your drops of CD in a clean dry shot glass. If you are using ten drops, activate them and then use the water from your bowl to stop the activation process.

4. Pour the contents of the shot glass back into the bowl.

5. Refill your syringes with the activated CD solution.

6. Lubricate the tip of your catheter with coconut oil, and attach the first syringe.

Note: If you wish to preserve the graduation marks on the syringes, cover them with some clear plastic shipping tape. The printed on marks are often easily rubbed off and the tape will prevent that.

Fleet Enema Method

The third option for enemas is to use a Fleet enema, which can be purchased at any drug store. This method is acceptable if you don't have access to the other items but want to start immediately, as, generally speaking they are easy to find. An enema bulb is a fancy fleet enema without being prefilled with saline solution. Skip step one if that's what you are using:

1. Dump out the contents of the enema (basically saline water). Since a Fleet enema only holds 137ml, two drops of CD are the maximum number you can add. To use more water, empty additional Fleet enemas.

2. Activate your two drops of CD and dilute them with filtered water (not tap water).

3. Funnel the activated CD solution back into the Fleet bottle. Insert the applicator and squeeze the bottle until all or most all of the contents are empty.

Comments & Suggestions from Parents

Most people are surprised at how well this goes. Some parents have asked if they can do the Protocol without the enemas, and I say yes, but why? The results are just that much better with them. Enemas have, in fact, been around for thousands of years, and colon hydrotherapy is becoming a growing trend in autism recovery.

I was really intimidated at first by the enemas. The syringe/catheter system, however, is brilliant. I lube the tip up with coconut oil, attach a filled syringe, and ask my son to put it in. He's 7 and very low verbal. He started inserting the tip by himself maybe on our 3rd or 4th enema with this system and I would depress the syringe. A few months later of every other day (ish) enemas, and he's doing the syringe depressing part himself. All I do is fill and swap syringes out. We are now to 11 100ml syringes, with 3-5 releases per enema (4 months into enemas). He requests enemas frequently on days I don't plan to give him one by getting the box of supplies and handing it to me.

Here are one mom's enema guidelines:

> *Be low-key about it, your attitude sets the tone. Have all your enema gear ready to go and in the bathroom for when the moment strikes. Put a nice, fluffy, washable blanket on the floor; bring in iPad, iPhone, whatever occupies your child for a few minutes. I've been doing my son's enemas after an afternoon poop if I get one because I figure it is easier as he is already in the bathroom, the bowel should be emptier, leaving more room for CD. Also the one time I did an enema close to bedtime, I swear he was up for an extra hour, however, another child might have the opposite reaction. I kneel on the floor, lay a beach towel over my lap, lay my son across me so he's on the ipad, pull his knees up a bit and then in it goes. You can put coconut oil on the anus or on the tip of enema. I ask my son to count to try to hold it in. (On the 4th enema, we only got to 40 seconds.) Then plop them on the toilet, and there you go.*
>
> *If possible, start the enema while lying on the left side, then rolling to the right. In this way, more water is able to reach the colon. (However, this may not be possible for all children.)*

CD Baths

Taking a bath with CD is another good way of detoxing your child. The CD gets into the pores and helps with skin rashes common with autism detoxification. This additional process can be added when you start with the enemas after reaching full oral dose, but avoid giving the child a CD bath right after an enema.

CD baths are done on non-enema days, unless you are doing daily enemas, in which case they are done on opposite ends of the day.

Enemas Every Other Day						
Sun	**Mon**	**Tue**	**Wed**	**Thur**	**Fri**	**Sat**
Enema	Bath	Enema	Bath	Enema	Bath	Enema

Enemas Every Day (Enemas can also be in the morning and baths at night.)						
Sun	**Mon**	**Tue**	**Wed**	**Thur**	**Fri**	**Sat**
Morning Bath	Morning Bath	Morning Bath	Morning Bath	Morning Bath	Morning Bath	Morning Bath
Evening Enema	Evening Enema	Evening Enema	Evening Enema	Evening Enema	Evening Enema	Evening Enema

The CD baths can go from as low as 10 drops to as high as 80 to 100 drops; it just depends on the person, and the size of your tub. With younger/smaller children we start with ten drops. Since we're doing baths every other day, start with ten drops on Monday, 11 drops on Wednesday, and 12 drops on Friday. Just keep going up until you get to 20 drops. The bigger and older the person is, the more drops they can tolerate.

Fill the tub to a level that maximizes skin contact.

If they start getting nauseous/listless or have loose stool, you should back down and find out what their signature dose is on the baths. Some people who have suffered from chronic constipation have done CD baths with up to 100 drops and had a BM during the bath or immediately after, without the use of drugs, laxatives, or suppositories.

CD Steam Bath

Inhalation of CD for children is generally impossible, because you just can't tell a child, especially a child with autism, "just inhale a little bit." That's not going to work. So we do the following:

In a bathtub, with the bathroom door and windows closed, plug the drain, put 20 activated drops on the floor of the tub, and turn on a hot (to tolerance) shower water. The steam will bring the CD into the air, making a really nice steamy bathroom.

When the tub is full, turn it off and place the child to soak in the water for 20 minutes. This way, the child is absorbing it through their skin as well as inhaling it through the air. This technique creates a very dispersed, low concentration dosage. I've seen a lot of children that were going back and forth to the hospital, getting steroid injections and lots of antibiotics due to bronchitis, coughs, asthma, etc., and it was rounds and rounds. This is how this particular method of steam baths came to be a very gentle way of inhaling the CD. It works beautifully; particularly if the child has a really bad cold and is congested, do the oral, enemas, and steam baths. Steam baths are great for asthma, flu, first signs of a cold, runny nose, coughing, etc., putting an end to running to the hospital or pharmacy.

CD Foot Baths

Sometimes it is impossible to give a CD bath, and in some places not all homes have bathtubs. To remedy this you can use a CD foot bath. Fill a small plastic container with hot (to tolerance) water and add your activated drops of CD.

If you have a smaller child, start with ten activated drops, and work up from there. If you have a larger child or an adult, start with 20 drops and go up. Soak feet for 20 minutes every other day, alternating with enemas, or opposite ends of the day if using daily enemas.

72/2 Protocol (Weekend Protocol)

When we give a child eight oral doses of CD throughout the day we are killing more and more pathogens. But at night when we sleep, the pathogens don't. So in order to get ahead of them, we can dose throughout the night. Imagine the progress we can make if we don't give them the chance to gain strength overnight!

Hence, the 72/2 Protocol, which involves giving one dose of CD every two hours for 72 hours straight—including the middle of the night. Here are some additional thoughts and guidelines:

- Start protocol when you pick up your child from school on Friday.
- Give them the last 72/2 dose when you drop them off at school on Monday.
- Avoid giving CD enemas or CD baths during this protocol, UNLESS they are dumping parasites, in which case you might need to reduce the amount of CD on both the oral and enema dose to insure the child doesn't have a Herxheimer reaction.
- Why not give hourly doses during the day at the usual dose? It's simply too much if you are doing it all night as well.
- Watch for improvements on Tuesday or Wednesday each week.
- Ideally, get your spouse or significant other to help with every other nightly dose.

The key is to observe your child and their reactions to the various treatments while keeping the pressure on eliminating the pathogens. You can do this every weekend or not at all. Some families are so happy with the results that they dose throughout the night for months on end.

Ocean Water

This protocol concentrates on excesses and not deficiencies. While we are using CD to reduce pathogen populations and heavy metal toxicity in the body, we need to remineralize the body. Remineralization is extremely important as vital nutrients may be lost along with toxins while detoxing. Children with autism are often mineral deficient to begin with due to these same pathogens and parasites, as well as gut dysbiosis which can prevent adequate nutrient absorption. We need to fortify our cells and tissues so that they can overcome the deficiencies and eventually return to a state of vitality.

Ocean water has helped us achieve mineralization and has led to increased brain connectivity; not to mention the parasites hate it. The importance of ocean water to this protocol cannot be understated. On page 388 of the Testimonials appendix you will see before and after lab tests proving that this protocol, when used correctly, can correct imbalances. More than one family has reported healthy nails, hair and skin as well as appropriate growth and weight gain.

We've all been taught that drinking salt water from the ocean is dangerous. Let me make it clear: We are not advocating drinking glasses full of straight ocean water nor water mixed with table salt. That would most likely make anyone sick, since it would be too much salt for the body. Rather, we are talking about diluted ocean water. Also, there is no comparison between real ocean water and just taking plain salt and mixing it into a glass of water!

The ocean is a complete source of minerals that are bioavailable to the human body. I prefer ocean water to any synthetic minerals, since the body easily recognizes and assimilates it.

Ocean water contains trace amounts of over 74 bioavailable elements including:

- sodium
- iron
- selenium
- sulfur
- calcium
- molybdenum
- cobalt
- boron
- silver
- fluorine
- potassium
- chromium
- zinc
- silicon
- chlorine
- vanadium
- nickel
- lithium
- iodine
- magnesium
- manganese
- copper
- phosphorus
- bromine
- gold
- etc.

We can use water directly from the ocean (diluted to 25%) and drink this to remineralize ourselves. However, the water must be from clean locations where schools of small fish swim and/or near ocean vortices. These locations provide safe and clean ocean water from which we can harvest. Most of us do not have access to oceans. Fortunately, clean ocean water is available commercially from multiple vendors online.

For further information about how and why ocean water is specifically beneficial to all of us, please research Rene Quinton's work on how he healed the sick using ocean water.

Using Ocean Water with CD

You can add ocean water in before starting CD, or after reaching full CD dose. We use a one part ocean water plus three parts drinking water mixed together (1:3). If we take too much ocean water, we can get loose stool. Start low and slow, 5ml ocean water mixed with 15ml drinking water and go up to tolerance.

Use the following chart as a rough guide:

Ocean Water Dosing				
Size	When	Pure Ocean Water	Purified Water	Total Volume
Child	Start at	5ml	15ml	20ml
	Go to	30ml	90ml	120ml
Adolescent	Start at	10ml	30ml	40ml
	Go to	50ml	200ml	250ml
Teen / Adult	Start at	15ml	45ml	60ml
	Go to	75ml	225ml	300ml

Ocean water should be given three times a day, with the first dose being given in the morning, after the first dose of CD. You want to separate the dose of ocean water from doses of CD by at least five minutes. Larger children can take anywhere from between 70 and 120ml, depending on the child. Some adults take up to a cup (plus dilution water) per day. It is important to watch for loose stool/diarrhea when you are increasing the dose of ocean water, as that will be an indicator that the person is at their upper limit. The ratio of ocean water to drinking water is 1:3 (one part ocean water to three parts drinking water). It is important to stay under diarrhea. So we need to add slowly, and to tolerance. If someone suffers constipation, with the right amount of ocean water that will quickly change. So low and slow as we increase the ocean water.

Some parents have reported that their children will not drink ocean water, even when diluted, due to its salty taste. You can try adding a little flavored SweetLeaf® Stevia, or if necessary adding it into a beverage or soup. As some ocean water purists say, heating it kills some qualities of the ocean water. Nevertheless, your child will still be receiving all of the minerals.

Biofilm

One of the pioneers in autism recovery, Dr. Anju Usman gave the autism community one of the critical pieces of the puzzle—biofilm. The following information is used with permission from her presentation, *Gut Biology and Treatment*.

What is Biofilm?

A biofilm is a collection of microbial communities enclosed by a matrix of extracellular polymeric substance (EPS) and separated by a network of open-water channels. Their architecture is an optimal environment for cell-cell interactions, including the intercellular exchange of genetic material, communication signals, and metabolites, which enables diffusion of necessary nutrients to the biofilm community.

The matrix is composed of a negatively charged polysaccharide substance, held together with positively charged metal ions (calcium, magnesium, and iron). The matrix, in which microbes in a biofilm are embedded, protects them from UV exposure, metal toxicity, acid exposure, dehydration, salinity, phagocytosis, antibiotics, antimicrobial agents, and the immune system.

Ok, so in layman's terms, these are microbial (bacteria, Candida, virus, etc.) communities that have a protective layer around them, which makes them 100 to 1000x harder to kill than if they did not live in these protected communities.[13]

Why are they so hard to get rid of?

- Microbes impart genetic material to one another to maintain resistance.
- Colonies communicate with one another through the use of quorum sensing molecules.
- Colonies fail to express OMP (outer membrane proteins).[14]

These colonies are fairly amazing in their development. They communicate with each other, share genetic material to prolong their own survival, and don't express outer membrane protections. This last statement is very important to understand. This is the main reason that the immune system doesn't attack these colonies, they don't express themselves as a threat, and therefore the immune system, which in many children with autism is already compromised, is not able to detect or eliminate them.

In addition to this we must be careful with what supplements we choose to give to our children. Some supplements and nutrients may inadvertently feed the biofilm. "When trying to kill bugs, if you take calcium, you may not be making headway," Usman said. "Calcium, iron, and magnesium block our efforts to dismantle the biofilm."

Step 2 – Chlorine Dioxide (CD)
Why CD Works on Biofilm

The microorganism communities attach to surfaces (in many cases the gut), and are held together by polysaccharides (sugars/carbohydrates) and by iron, calcium, and magnesium. EDTA is a known chelator, and can therefore break the bonds (iron, calcium and magnesium) that hold the matrix together. Neither an antibiotic alone nor a chelator alone was effective against a staph (bacterial) biofilm. However, when combined, EDTA broke the bonds exposing the bacteria to the antibacterial agent, allowing the body to expel the biomass.

Chlorine dioxide oxidizes inorganic compounds by effectively removing their charges. Here is how it works: Fe_2+, Ca_2+, and Mg_2+ are positively charged ions that hold the negatively charged matrix together. When these substances are oxidized by CD, the bacteria are then exposed to the CD which can oxidize (kill) the bacteria, allowing the body to finally expel the biofilm mass.

Many parents using chlorine dioxide orally, and with enemas, have found biofilms in their children's stool. Biofilm can look thick, mucousy, cloudy, whitish, greyish, sometimes like pantyhose, etc.

There is some more interesting information available through the AutismPedia about Dr. Usman's work with biofilm.[14]

> We had our appointment yesterday and to all our surprise when he tested her for Lyme it was negative. Just 3 months ago and before starting MMS she was testing very positive for it. He was pleased with the outcome. Thank you so much for your guidance and we owe this to the miracle of MMS and your dedication to helping me with my questions. I really, really appreciate your help in bringing us one step closer to the cure.

Also, this article "Lyme-Induced Autism Conference Focuses on Biofilm and Toxicity"[15] by Mary Budinger discusses the effects of pathogens present in the biofilm for Lyme disease and autism. The following is a notable quote from the aforementioned article by Dr. Stephen Fry of Fry Labs, which explores the possible pathogenic causes of chronic disease.

> I could be barking up the wrong tree, but maybe not. Remember that we used to think stomach ulcers were caused by too much acid production. Then Barry Marshall and Dr. Robin Warren turned medical dogma on its head by proving that a bacterium was the cause. The pair identified

the bacterium H. pylori and proved how it causes inflammation, then ulcers. Maybe in 10 years we will be smart enough to know that the 'auto' in 'autoimmune' actually means pathogen and the whole concept of autoimmunity will change. Chronic inflammation is chronic infection. In autoimmune disease, my model is that there is a chronic infection that cannot be eliminated, thus the immune system is always switched on. The self antibodies are due to apoptosis and death of host cells with host immune response.

I couldn't agree more, and am so grateful that we have CD to combat pathogens, and restore the body to a state of health.

Mitochondrial Dysfunction

Children on the spectrum are also more likely to have mitochondrial dysfunction than neurotypical children of the same age group. The following is an excerpt from *Science Daily*.[16]

> Children with autism are far more likely to have deficits in their ability to produce cellular energy than are typically developing children, a new study by researchers at UC Davis has found. The study, published in the Journal of the American Medical Association (JAMA), found that cumulative damage and oxidative stress in mitochondria, the cell's energy producer, could influence both the onset and severity of autism, suggesting a strong link between autism and mitochondrial defects.
>
> "Children with mitochondrial diseases may present exercise intolerance, seizures and cognitive decline, among other conditions. Some will manifest disease symptoms and some will appear as sporadic cases," said Cecilia Giulivi, the study's lead author and professor in the Department of Molecular Biosciences in the School of Veterinary Medicine at UC Davis. "Many of these characteristics are shared by children with autism."
>
> Dysfunction in mitochondria already is associated with a number of other neurological conditions, including Parkinson's disease, Alzheimer's disease, schizophrenia and bipolar disorder.
>
> Mitochondria often respond to oxidative stress by making extra copies of their own DNA. The strategy helps ensure that some normal genes are present even if others have been damaged by oxidation. The researchers found higher mtDNA copy numbers in the lymphocytes of half of the children with autism. These children carried equally high numbers of mtDNA sets in their granulocytes, another type of immune

cell, demonstrating that these effects were not limited to a specific cell type. Two of the five children also had deletions in their mtDNA genes, whereas none of the control children showed deletions.[10]

In our MMSAutism webinar, Dr. Andreas Kalcker mentions that CD changes the mitochondrial membrane electrical potential.[17] This leads to increased power in every cell in the body, including immune system cells. The mitochondria are the electric generator or "powerhouse" of each cell. When we turn off this electrical generator, cancer can develop. If the cell cannot produce electrical energy through oxidation it will use fermentation.

In practice, what I have seen is that children who suffered from lack of energy, listlessness, and other symptoms that can be related to mitochondrial dysfunction have perked up with the use of CD. They are able to do exercise again, walk without having to be carried, and can cognitively sustain activities without tiring. You will see a few testimonials mentioning "mito issues" at the end of the book. It is wonderful to think that this is another means by which CD can help people on the spectrum heal.

ATEC Statistics

Through some of our Facebook groups we have been collecting ATEC data for the past year. Just to give you an idea of what others are experiencing in terms of test results, here are some statistics:

- 246 parents have given us 2 ATEC scores. Of those, the average drop between ATEC1 and ATEC2 is 15 points. We take ATEC data quarterly, so in general that drop is in three months or less. The more impacted a child is the bigger their initial drop – kids starting with an ATEC over 100 averaged a 26 point drop between ATEC1 and ATEC2.

- Of those 246 ATEC reports, we had 32 children (13%) gain in points in the first quarter. The average gain among those 32 was 7 points. All 32 reported ATEC scores three months later, and 29 of them dropped points between their ATEC2 and ATEC3 scores. Further, 13 of those 29 dropped enough points to put them at or below their ATEC1 starting number. Which means at the 6 month mark, only 19 out of 246 (or 7%) had gained points. 93% of children who do this protocol have improved their ATEC score at the six month mark.

- We have now had 163 parents provide four consecutive ATEC scores (encompassing one year on the protocol). Of those 163, the average ATEC drop between ATEC1 and ATEC4 was 24 points.

- Of those 163, a total of 9 or 6% reported an increase in ATEC score between ATEC1 and ATEC4. The average increases was 6 points. 94% of children who do this protocol have improved their ATEC score at the one year mark.

- In a Facebook group collecting ATEC data, we have 25 recoveries as defined by the ATEC dropping to 10 or under in a year. So we have a rate of 15% recovery as defined as ATEC score under 10 in the parents who have taken this protocol through one year.

Thus showing that the longer they are on the protocol the more points they lose.

Although we all would like to see "high level" statistical research done, this is no doubt a major step in the right direction, and demonstrates that the protocol does work. But, research takes money.

DOs & DON'Ts of CD for Autism Recovery

DO review all current supplementation that your child is taking and remove all supplements which contain any antioxidants including vitamin C, vitamin E, vitamin A, vitamin K, ALA, Coenzyme Q_{10}, and colloidal silver as these will neutralize the CD, rendering it ineffective.

DO consider removing supplements that include iron and vitamin B_{12}. These are principal foods for the parasites, which explains why many children are low in them. If you are seeing a chronic iron or vitamin B_{12} deficiency, revisit the parasite chapter. These levels should normalize when parasites are no longer consuming nutrients.

DO use the Baby Bottle Method in an eight-ounce glass bottle with a completely sealing lid and start at one drop, regardless of weight. Increase by one drop/day, until you reach the optimal dosage.

DO dose frequently throughout the day. The less time we leave the pathogens to proliferate the better. Do a minimum of eight doses a day, but try to get in more doses if possible. Go for 16 in cases of PANS/PANDAS and acute situations like colds and flu.

DO activate CD for the proper amount of time for the acid you use. HCl and citric acid both activate sodium chlorite in 60 seconds.

DO supplement minerals using ocean water.

DO completely avoid the following: citrus fruits, corn syrup, fruit juices, green tea, pineapple, vitamins C, E, A, and K. Only give coconut milk and coconut water a minimum of one hour after the last CD dose at night so they will have no chance of affecting the CD. Coconut milk and coconut water are very alkaline.

DON'T give fruit juice of any form—not fresh, organic, homemade or store bought.

DON'T give highly antioxidant foods including chocolate (cacao/cocoa), coffee, green tea, kombucha, citrus fruits, pineapple, mango, or kiwi. Berries (if you have to give them at all) can only be given at night, one hour after the last CD dose.

DON'T mix anything but water with your CD drops.

DON'T give CD with food.

DON'T use a vitamin C shower water filter—yes, there is such a thing to neutralize chlorine in tap water. Unfortunately, it also neutralizes chlorine dioxide.

CD Troubleshooting Checklist

Before you decide that CD isn't working for your child please take a look at following list of common errors. If it looks like you are doing everything right, but you aren't seeing gains, please, before giving up, use one of the support options shown in Appendix 17, page 521. You are NOT alone! We have a network of parents who are ready and willing to help you.

❑ Are you preparing your CD in a clean, dry shot glass, or other type glass container that insures both chemicals are mixing?

❑ Is the CD mixture turning yellowish brown? There should be a chlorine-like smell. If there isn't, something is not right. Perhaps you have bad or incorrect chemistry? Maybe the supplier did something wrong in preparing the solutions.

❑ Are you using the correct ratio of sodium chlorite to acidic activator drops? See chart on page 94 for the correct mixture ratio depending on the type and concentration you are using.

❑ Are you allowing the correct activation time before dilution with water after mixing the sodium chlorite and acidic activator? See chart on page 94 for the minimum activation time you must wait for the chemical reaction to occur.

❑ If you question the potency of your CD, then you may wish to test its strength. See Appendix 6, page 467 for testing information.

❑ Is your CD or activator cloudy or not changing color after they are mixed? If so, there is something wrong with one or both chemicals. Check with your supplier.

❑ Did you leave your baby bottle solution in direct sunlight? A brief exposure to light is no big deal, but if you left it in a hot car for an hour, it may have lost potency.

❑ Are you keeping the same baby bottle solution for too many hours? It should be used on the day it was prepared.

❑ Are you giving antioxidant supplements or a multivitamin containing antioxidants? Vitamin C, vitamin E, etc., should not be given. Cod liver oil and fish oil supplements in general have lots of antioxidants to keep them from spoiling. Make sure those are out as well. Mixing any of these will cancel out the effect of the CD—and the vitamin. You CAN give them a few hours apart.

❑ Have you checked all your labels of supplements and foods to make sure they don't contain antioxidants?

❑ Have you removed all juices and all citrus fruits from the diet (including oranges, pineapple, mango, kiwi)? Berries (if you have to give them at all) can only be given at night, no less than one hour after the last CD dose.

❑ Are you dosing CD 30 minutes apart from food, as a minimum (one hour is optimal, but not always possible)? Grazers do 15 minutes and we dose CD 16 times a day.

❑ Are you mixing anything with your CD, such as baking soda, juice, etc.? The only thing you can add into your dose of CD is more water!

❑ Are you using alkaline water to prepare your CD? Alkaline water kills CD. Some expensive water filtration systems are designed to produce alkaline water, which we must totally avoid!

❑ Are you breaking The Diet? Could there be dietary infractions at school or with relatives while you're not there?

❑ Are you dosing so high that you are detoxing your child too fast and getting a Herxheimer reaction? Some people need to increase every three days—NOT every day.

❑ Are your doses too low to accomplish anything?

❑ Are you giving too few doses of CD? We need a minimum of eight doses per day or more.

❑ Have you started the Kalcker Parasite Protocol? If you have done three Parasite Protocols (PP) it is time to start looking into supplements, chelation, HBOT, GcMAF, etc.

Frequently Asked Questions (FAQs)

Can I use less than one ounce (30ml) of water to administer a dose of CD?

One ounce of water, or more, is best. You can always add more water, but at least an ounce is the minimum per drop.

We have been on the Protocol and are at five activated drops of CD in the baby bottle. My son's "usual" autistic symptoms got exacerbated to the maximum. He has horrible constipation, stimming, scripting, and he seems to be in a bad shape. Our target dose is 15 drops. What should I do?

The general protocol is to wait with CD enemas and CD baths until one is at their full target oral dose. His negative symptoms are probably from reabsorption of toxins from his unpassed stool. You need to resolve his constipation to stop this vicious cycle. You can administer CD enemas and CD baths on consecutive days. This should help the constipation, and flush the toxins out of his system. Then, once he is stable you can resume slowly titrating up to full dose.

What should I do if my child can handle "double doses" (two ounces of the baby bottle) all day with no herxing?

If your child is taking "double doses" all day, then it is NOT a double dose—it's his actual dose! Depending on his gains and what else you are folding into your protocol you can consider going up from there.

Is 72/2 only if you have done the parasite protocol? We are full oral dose but won't do PP until next full moon.

You can do 72/2 protocol before the Parasite Protocol, but you must have reached full dose of CD.

We are really struggling to get in enough doses of CD with school. We do well to get in 8; we really need more (way, way more). Night dosing is not an option (he won't go back to sleep; our mornings start early enough around here as it is), nor is coming to school during the day to dose him (we both work). Advice?

Some parents are dosing every 45 minutes to get in their doses when they are with their children. However, we need to be killing pathogens around the clock. It is not possible to be effective at killing pathogens when we are giving them 16 hours without a dose of CD. You need to get 1 to 2 doses in before school starts. Then get the other 6 (ideally more) in after school is over and in the evening.

My child hates the flavor of CD. Can I give Stevia with CD to improve the taste?

We recently discovered that some brands of Stevia are compatible with CD, CDS and CDH (i.e., SweetLeaf® & KAL® brand)—it doesn't reduce the potency. However, past tests were not so positive. Some added ingredients may be why this was so in our initial tests. Try to use only pure Stevia or check with the Facebook groups on what others are using successfully.

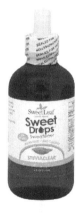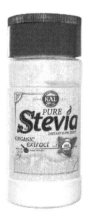

Preliminary tests show that some brands of Stevia can be used with CD to improve taste without losing potency. The two brands we have tested in-house are SweetLeaf® and KAL®. Some of our moms report having successfully used flavored versions of SweetLeaf®.

When you say do two back-to-back baby bottles of 11 drops... you mean do a total of 22 drops in 16 hours? Correct? I'm going slowly up on oral CD because of behaviors. If I go from 11 to 22 drops overnight, won't he have strong detox and behaviors?

> This is spread out over 16 hours or more, such that every 60 minutes it is the same amount. It is different than putting 22 drops in 8 fl. oz. Behaviors associated with bacteria (PANDAS/PANS) are often reduced with the tolerated dose spread over longer periods of time. Remember that CD is only active in the body for about one hour.

My child seems very uncomfortable. What should I do?

> If you see a detox like this, stop dosing for the day. The next day, return to the last dose when the child was stable. Pathogens are dying and toxins are being released into the bloodstream on their way out of the body. This causes discomfort in some people.

How do you know if I should go past full oral dose of CD?

> A Herxheimer reaction will be your biggest indicator if you have gone too far. If you have reached full oral dose and it seems like your child has plateaued, please schedule a consult with Kerri to discuss your options. Note: The full oral dose chart (page 101) is only a general guide and not a one size fits all.

Is an hour enough time to separate CD neutralizers from the CD dose?

> CD is only active in the body for about one hour, however, supplements like vitamins A, C, E, K and ALA, CoQ10, and GSH (glutathione) need to be avoided. Also, orange juice, pineapple juice, and other high antioxidant fruits are a problem even after one hour. So, the best thing to do is eliminate everything that kills the CD. If not, it is pretty much like not using CD. I have seen it too many times and it's not worth it. Antioxidants destroy CD. There is no period of time that is safe to use antioxidants with CD.

I know you have to start the parasite protocol on a certain day of the month, but how about the first dose of CD?

> You can start giving CD any day of the month. That said, it might be easier to start on a weekend, or a day when you will be with your child all day to make sure to get in all of their doses, and keep an eye on them to make sure they tolerate it well, i.e. no Herxheimer reaction.

What is 72/2?

72/2 is when you give a dose every two hours around the clock for 72 hours. We use a baby bottle and a half to get through the night hours. This can be added in once you are comfortable at your full oral dose and have added in enemas and baths. See page 115 for more information.

Do you recommend 72/2 for everyone?

Once a child is at 100% of their target oral CD, enema, and baths then they can do a 72/2 weekend. They are exhausting for the parents, but some kids do wonderfully. A lot of families get a nice boost. But, if you do a couple of weekends and you don't see anything afterwards, then forget it. The benefits are usually seen two to three days after the 72/2 is over.

My son suffers from constipation. Can I start the enemas before I get to his full oral dose?

Anyone who suffers constipation needs enemas right away. These can be combined with oral doses. Still start low and slow, but it is important to get the bowels moving with any detox protocol. When constipation is present, we do not wait to start enemas.

What is the maximum amount of water to use with enemas? How many times do you hold and release?

First of all, we don't encourage holding. Rather we do a fill and release, which is kind of a home colonic. If your child can hold for a few seconds without fuss, then great. The number of cycles depends on the results of each. If all you are getting out is water, you may be finished, unless the person is seriously constipated. The amount of water really depends on the individual's size and the number of cycles administered. My basic philosophy is: *Any enema is a good enema*. So, even if not much comes out, you are still getting some water and CD in.

Is it possible that my son has been getting rid of mucous after his CD enemas? What is up with the mucous? Why is it there in the first place? And, is it a good or a bad thing that it is coming out?

Mucous is always a sign of inflammation and can contain pathogens and parasites. Mucous gives a home to pathogens. The inflammation and mucous can be caused from the allergies and pathogens. It is common to see mucous come out in the beginning of the enemas since our children have so much intestinal dysbiosis.

What is a good enema method for a 17 year old boy? I am having trouble understanding the enema part of the book. The video in the file really helps, but I am having a hard time imagining doing it on my son. How do other people with older children do it? Can it be self-administered eventually? Kerri mentioned a gravity bag, so you don't have to keep changing syringes. Has anyone tried that? Where do you get the bag?

Here is some advice one mom gave to another mom on one of our boards:

My son is 14 and tends toward constipation. I had done suppositories in the past to help him have a bowel movement. So, I told him that the enema was "fanny medicine" to help him have a BM and make him better. I started with just showing it to him after a BM after I wiped him. Then, I just put it next to his anus the next day. Then closer every day. He was still constipated so just inserting the tip would help him poop and then later I was able to push the liquid with him standing next to the sink and it would run all down his leg. After several weeks of this, it was a full moon and he could not poop at all and was lying on his bed in pain. I said let's try it here because it will really help you. I got out a hundred towels and did it right there and he pooped. It was a slow process over two months but now we do them AM and PM always right after the shower. I counted over 20 feet (of parasites) coming out this last PP. And that is just what I could see. I don't dig, just pull out obvious ones that are a foot long. Main advice is keep calm with soothing voice and have tons of patience and keep telling your son how much you appreciate his patience too. I also tell him this will get rid of his autism. He is non-verbal but said with RPM that he is mad he has autism. Also, the soft tip is key. I use syringes because they go fast.

My son is not having daily bowel movements. What should I do?

Do CD enemas every day until the stools normalize to daily. If you absolutely cannot do enemas, use CD baths in high doses (50+ drops depending on the size of the tub). Ocean water in high doses will move the bowels as well. Castor oil also helps.

I am scared of the CD enemas. Will CD harm the intestinal lining?

CD stays active only for about one hour and can gently, but effectively remove biofilm and kill pathogens in the intestine. Our society has shied away from this healing method in the last few decades. However, CD enemas have been proven to be positive turning points in the treatment, time and time again. Lots of kids will actually ask for enemas, as they provide them relief and comfort. If you are nervous, apply an enema to yourself first. You will see it is no big deal, and feel more at ease applying one to your child. Some parents have shown their higher functioning children how to apply their own enemas, so no one has to be there, and to make them feel more comfortable.

What is the difference between colonics and enemas?

Colonics cleanse the entire length of the colon while enemas cleanse the lower part of the colon. Colonics involves multiple infusions of water into the colon, while enemas involve a single infusion of water into the colon (which can be repeated). With colonics, fecal material leaves the body via a tube. Colonics normally involves going to an office and receiving assistance by a trained colonics hydrotherapist, while enemas are free and done in the privacy of your own home.

I have never done an enema before. How do you administer it?

There are several positions that work well, but there will be one that works best for the individual. The enema instructions are on page 109. Some examples would be on all fours or lying on your left side on a towel, or a small child could lay across your lap.

Enema clean up question: What are we boiling? What are we spraying with *Everclear*? What are we throwing away?

After you are finished looking for worms you can throw away any plastic plates/forks you may have used. Pour boiling water on your specimen collector, enema nozzle and catheter. Then spray with *Everclear* grain alcohol. If you are using syringes, you may pour boiling water over them as well.

How far do I need to insert the catheter for an enema?

Not very far at all; one to two inches is plenty. The anal sphincter is about one inch past the anus. As soon as the catheter passes this muscle, it will hold it in place and there is no need to go further.

What is intestinal biofilm supposed to look like?

Biofilm is fluffy, cloudy, and mucousy in appearance. There are no rules on the color. It can look like pantyhose. But, it is usually mucousy and a cloudy whitish/grey color.

How far away should we be doing enema from food? If we miss the morning enema, can I give it right after lunch?

They can go together; there is no need to separate enemas from food. Any enema is a good enema.

I'm having trouble with my syringes (for enemas). One plunges really smoothly, but the other two are almost impossible to move. Do I need to grease them up somehow before each use? How do you clean them?

I use *Everclear* grain alcohol to clean them, but note, it will dry out rubber parts. You can use coconut oil to lube the plunger gasket.

Is it normal to see black specks coming out after using enemas? We saw white specks for a couple of days too.

Black specks can be heavy metals. Oxalates are known to bond to metals and would come out with metals. White dots are generally parasite eggs.

Does ocean water need to be refrigerated after opening?

No it does not, it is fine at room temperature.

If I harvest my own ocean water do I have to sterilize it?

No. Sterilizing is not necessary or desirable in our experienc—we don't want to denature it. Pouring it through a coffee filter to remove any potential particulate matter is fine. Do NOT use charcoal filters (such as a Brita® water filter), because they will alter the characteristics of the natural ocean water. Just make sure to collect the water far from any harbours or large river outlets.

I bought pure sea water in Australia. It sounds like a great mineral drink. Would this be beneficial for killing parasites or just putting goodness back into the body?

Actually, it does both.

How do I avoid feeding the pathogens?

CD kills pathogens. I would use CD to rid the body of pathogens rather than try not to feed them.

Is it possible to use CD, CDS, or CDH during pregnancy? If it is ok, how much can be used?

CD/CDS/CDH are not advisable during pregnancy or nursing.

Can I add CD to breast milk to the bottle to help the baby detox?

CD must be given in water. Mixing breast milk and CD will reduce or potentially cancel out the potency of the CD.

How many drops go in a CD bath?

It depends on the weight of the child (20-100 drops). If he is a little guy I might start at 10 or 15 activated drops and work up over the course of the following couple of weeks. The size of your tub also plays a part. The bigger the tub, the more CD you are going to need. See page 113 for more information.

I've heard that some people mix CD directly in capsules and then swallow them. Can we use that on our children?

NO! Not a good idea! Since many children with autism can't speak, they won't be able to tell you when the capsule gets stuck. CD needs to be diluted in water before taking as instructed in this chapter.

Can I use warm water instead of cold water to store CD and how long will it remain potent mixed in the baby bottle?

CD is a gas dissolved in water and therefore has to be preserved in a sealed container. If not, it will lose its potency, similar to how soda goes flat if the cap to the bottle isn't screwed on tight. Colder is better because the CD will gas out quicker at higher temperatures. If you have doubts about CD potency, get the Lamotte ClO_2 test strips to be sure. See Appendix 6, page 467 for more information.

Are purified, distilled and filtered water all the same thing?

They are different. However, we can use purified, distilled or filtered water. But, alkaline water should never be used!

Must the activated CD water mix be stored in a glass bottle, or is a no-BPA plastic bottle with an airtight cap ok?

I prefer glass to any plastic. Over time, chlorine dioxide can degrade plastic, and that means you or your child will be consuming it. Yes, the bottle needs to remain sealed. Plastic is acceptable for lids only! Metal lids should never be used because they quickly rust, even if covered with a plastic coating.

Is it a problem to transfer one ounce of CD to a steel bottle briefly before drinking it?

That is fine for a transfer, but I wouldn´t store CD in a steel bottle.

Is the GF/CF/SF "clean" diet essential to the CD protocol? My son doesn't have bad reactions and I just do not see how we could implement it.

A healthy, clean diet is very important to the healing process. Unfortunately, our "standard diet" is filled with preservatives, colorings, and other potentially harmful chemicals. When the goal is to heal, the diet is necessary. Dairy especially can cause inflammation and mucous production. Mucous provides protection to parasites.

What is a good CD-friendly multivitamin?

All multivitamins have antioxidants. What we need to supplement during detoxification are the minerals. Ocean water has 90 bio-available minerals, and it is what I prefer for this protocol.

Are there other specific foods, veggies or fruits that need to be avoided in addition to juices?

> When you are following the CD Protocol, all antioxidants need to be avoided. Chocolate is a strong antioxidant. As far as vitamins are concerned; A, E, K, and ALA are off limits. High antioxidant supplements such as curcumin have also been a problem for many people. In the case of vitamin D, it is not an antioxidant, but it has caused aggression in previously calm children. Therefore, as a supplement, it must be used with care, if at all.
>
> Vegetables and legumes which are high in antioxidants have not shown to be very detrimental to the effects of CD. However, citrus fruits, pineapple, mangoes must be avoided. Berries are best given at night, one hour after the last dose of CD, if you must give berries. Juice, any sort of fruit juice, is completely prohibited. Not only can the antioxidants involved kill CD, but the high sugar content (albeit natural) shuts down the immune system, which is already impaired in children with autism.

Can our kids drink anything other than water for the duration of the CD protocol or just not drink juices down with the CD?

> Some people are not used to drinking water and find it difficult. Some people drink nut milks or rice milk. On occasion, some folks put a piece of fruit in the blender with an apple and blend it, strain it, water it down and have that sometimes. Juicing is taking 5 apples to make a glass of juice and that is a lot of sugar (albeit natural) as well as a lot of antioxidants. Antioxidants kill CD and sugar slows the immune system. You want to totally avoid alkaline water.

Can I use rice milk to give the CD instead of water?

> Water is what we need to use to give the CD. If you are giving CD mixed with another beverage you are reducing its potential. By combining CD with liquids other than water we will not get the desired results. Rice milk might be okay, but you would need to test how it affects the potency of the CD. You can get the *LaMotte High Range Chlorine Dioxide Test Strips* (#3002) at www.amazon.com. This way you can see for yourself how mixing CD with any beverage affects its potential. However, I do not recommend putting CD in anything but distilled/purified water.

Can I give my child fresh pressed green juices (celery, kale, cucumber, apple)?

> Anything that is very nutritious to the human body is nutritious for the pathogens/parasites. So, a healthy green drink is very healthy for the pathogens. If you are giving "green" juices make sure they are not loaded with sugar from apples, carrots, etc. In my opinion, it is preferable to avoid these for the first few months of the Parasite Protocol (PP), at least.

Can I use coconut and almond milk with CD?

You can drink coconut and almond milk 60 minutes after your last dose of CD, but I would not combine anything other than purified water with the dose of CD.

Can my child drink coconut water if he is taking CD?

If you want to give your child coconut water, give it one hour after your child's last dose of CD, at night, before bed.

Does lemon interfere with CD, even after it is cooked?

Yes, in some cases. A family of a child who suffered from SIB noticed a direct correlation with lemon use in their meals with the return of his SIB. I would avoid it at all costs.

My son barely drinks anything, especially all at once. This is why we have been unsuccessful with detox programs. Is CD different?

You should make sure that your child is well hydrated, but for the CD alone one ounce (30ml) of water is sufficient. I find that it is easier to drink CD cold rather than at room temperature. Also, if the smell is a problem, put the dose in a plastic syringe and squirt it right into your child's mouth. This prevents them from having to smell it before they swallow it. Enemas are a great tool for hydration.

My child's appetite has changed since starting CD. Is this normal?

Yes. On average larger kids tend to slim down, while thinner kids tend to gain some weight.

Can I give green tea or kombucha while taking CD?

That is out of the question in my humble opinion. Green tea is high in antioxidants and caffeine. Kombucha is similar. I don`t know exactly how long the antioxidants in either one are active in the body, so with autism, if we are looking for healing, avoid them both.

Can I use original Nutriiveda™ with CD?

Nutriiveda™ is derived from whey, a dairy product. In humans, all dairy causes inflammation and mucous, which provides a protective refuge for pathogens. That makes this product contraindicated for this protocol, plus it contains antioxidants.

Can I use Chia seeds with CD?

Yes. But do not mix them directly into the CD.

How do I dose my child when he/she is at school from 8:30 am to 3 pm? I work full time so "dropping in to dose" is not an option.

Give a dose upon waking, one at the door of the school at 8:30 and the third dose of the day at 3pm at the door of the school. The last dose of the day is at bedtime, there should be at least four hours between school pickup and bedtime to get in the other four doses. Once you get the hang of it, it is not that hard, it just takes a little getting used to and some prior planning.

What should I do if my son goes away for 5 days with school? Do you think it is possible to prepare a bottle of CDS for 5 days and he takes only one portion each evening?

It's not ideal, but better than nothing.

My son is refusing the CD. What do I do?

Have you tried adding more water with the dose, using cold water, using a syringe or a straw? Here is some advice from a Mom whose daughter refused oral CD:

We just went through a REALLY rough patch with my daughter when she absolutely refused to take oral CD, and I know it gets super stressful for both you and your child if you try to force it… I had to respect her as clearly she was telling me in her own way, "Mom, this does not make me feel good!" for whatever reason and after maybe a week we were back on track. During that time I was able to give her a few doses (dropped from 14 drops of CD to 5) here and there, during really good moments. For example, in the bath or swing that she loves and I think that helped her associate CD with feeling better again. You WILL be back on track in no time!!!!! Good luck! Keep calm and dose on!

I am on 30 activated drops/day with my teenage boy. The taste is simply horrible. He refuses to drink his doses. What should I do?

You can dilute your baby bottle as far as a liter bottle if necessary; it will not impact its effectiveness. Obviously, one dose will be more like a half a cup or a full cup in this case. However, be mindful of your conversion rate so that you get your dosage right. Cold water helps with the taste. You can add approved Stevia brands to cover the taste of CD. See page 126.

If the country I live in doesn't have glass baby bottles, can I use a plastic bottle?

No, do not use plastic for storing CD. If the cap is plastic, we can live with that. In almost any country you can find a glass water bottle (with a plastic cap). You can use a shot glass to measure out eight ounces, and even mark them on the outside of the bottle with permanent marker. Many

parents in Venezuela do this, as neither glass baby bottles nor LifeFactory®
bottles are available in their country. NEVER use a Stainless steel (or
other metal) bottle or container!

**Do you think this Protocol could work for a child who already has a
low ATEC score (18)?**

Yes. I started with a 12-year-old, who last February 2012 had an ATEC of
18. He did not budge from there after years of biomedical interventions.
He could not stop with fears, phobias, anxiety (all parasitic in nature) and
we started him on CD in February 2012 and the Parasite Protocol in June
2012. His ATEC is now a one!

**My son's ATEC is not going down as I had hoped it would by now. It
has hovered around 65 the past few ATEC's. I think it is probably due
to the fact that if I am not home my husband often forgets to give
him his doses or his PP meds. Does anyone have any suggestions on
how to stress the importance of this protocol to him?**

The following responses are from moms on our public Facebook group:

*You will never know what following the protocol will do for your son until you
follow the protocol. When I first started the protocol a little over a year ago, I
remember I had been using a special juice that so many people were raving
about and I was paying $140 monthly for this miracle juice and I really wanted
to keep in in my son's protocol. I asked my husband to give it to my son at 4
am when he got up, and that was 4 hours before he would get any CD doses...
how could that effect our results? The juice was given 4 hours before starting
CD for the day, we were following the protocol exactly otherwise, and even doing
the enemas. Well, nothing happened, nothing, until about 3 weeks later when I
said, well let's stop the juice and see... BAM! Immediately my son's ATEC results
dropped and he blossomed. I mean not only did his constant pacing stop, but
his eyes lit up, he not only started talking more, more, more but even his laugh
changed to a typical sounding teenager's laugh. It was incredible. His ATEC
dropped instantly and kept dropping, 68, 25, 13, 7, 5, 3. It's a 6 today but this a
super bad new moon for him. You will never know until you follow the protocol.*

*We have also seen our son stop pacing, stop suffering minute to minute, in the
beginning we made our mistakes, missed a dose, didn't get this or that done, we
now stick to it, the cumulative effect of staying on protocol means the difference
in drops in ATEC scores and staying the same or going up, it did for us anyway.
I could feel the slipping, we are still working on getting this right, it is an evolving
protocol that requires the entire family's buy in. I have kept my son home from
school to make sure he is dosed properly but that's just us. In November he
is supposed to begin going to school full days, if they do not dose him correctly,
I will hire a homeschool teacher, that's how important this is. You will not get
your child well, Kerri told us 16 doses a day, he got better, she told us to start*

enema's early, that made a big difference, we started our first PP before he was at full dose, it's all made a huge difference, email her, keep watching your child to see what's working, this protocol works, it may take time, but what is the alternative????

My husband is not good about giving meds either. When I'm gone my older girls give it. I text them reminders. Sometimes setting a timer can help. I also set all of the meds that go along in a morning and night dose daily case. Often when I organize it all for them it's much easier for the meds to be given properly and in time.

My child has horrible nasal congestion. Can CD help?

Yes, you can use CD and make nose, eye, and eardrops. Put one activated drop of CD into one ounce of water. Use one drop of the mixture in the nose (eyes or ears) every 15 minutes till symptoms disappear. NOTE: DO NOT USE PURE ACTIVATED CD WITHOUT DILUTING IT!

You can also do a steam bath, which is done by closing off the bathroom (windows and door shut), and putting 20 activated drops on the floor of the tub. Run hot shower water on top of the drops until the tub fills; the air will be full of CD smell. Now, turn off the shower, put the child in the water to soak for 20 minutes, where he will breathe the light CD air.

Is there a seasonal-allergy protocol for using CD? I suffer from extreme itching in my eyes, redness, puffiness, sneezing, sinus congestion etc. Will CD provide relief quickly or does it need to be used over a long period of time?

Being on full CD, ocean water and the parasite protocol the allergies should begin to fade away.

Can I try the CD ear protocol if my child has not started oral doses?

Yes!! Please start the eardrops, if there is an infection, every hour until the symptoms disappear. If you catch an infection at the onset of its symptoms, give one drop of the mix every 15 minutes. We have seen earaches clear up in a couple hours. In any case, work towards a full oral dose, at least one drop eight times a day to combat the infection on all fronts. The eye, ear, and nose protocols are all the same: one activated drop of CD in one ounce of water in a sealed dropper bottle. Apply one drop of this mix every hour until symptoms diminish.

Can CD help arthritis?

Absolutely! CD is amazing for arthritis. Include CD baths in your routine. Use CD in conjunction with DMSO.

Our son has a runny nose and sneezes a lot, but has no fever. He hasn't been sick in well over a year! I'm wondering if it is from doing CD.

> This sounds like a very typical die-off reaction. Monitor his progress, make sure he is hydrated, and continue with the Protocol. If his reactions remain manageable, you don't need to back down or change much. This could also be parasites, depending on whether the symptoms are chronic, etc.

Has anyone seen kids who had never been sick start getting sick as they heal?

> Yes, it means immune system is waking up and fighting back against the crud they've been carrying around for a long time. It's called a healing crisis and is not uncommon and is actually a good thing.

Does CD, CDS or CDH work on HIV? Also, are there any contraindications of CD and HIV drugs?

> We do not focus on HIV or its treatment and therefore we cannot give you a definitive answer. Anecdotally, there are many testimonials that indicate CD having a positive impact on the disease. In addition, we have spoken to doctors in various parts of the world who use CD to treat their HIV/AIDS patients and have positive results from what we understand.

Can I use CD in a Netti pot when doing an ear, eye or nose wash?

> No. Do not use a Netti pot with CD. Instead, use the steam bath method. See page 114 for more information.

I´m wondering if CD can be used in a nebulizer? With our daughter's chronic mycobacterium issues, we can never get rid of the cough. I thought maybe it would be helpful to get it into her lungs or is this not safe?

> Try a steam bath. Inhaling CD directly has to be done very delicately. This is why the steam bath is recommended, as the particles have time to disperse into a very large area rather than being inhaled directly. Some people are using humidifiers with 35 drops of CD per gallon. See page 114 for more information.

What supplements do I need to avoid while using CD?

> Antioxidants (vitamins C, E, A, K, ALA, and CoQ10) need to be avoided because they kill CD. We avoid iron and vitamin B12 because parasites feed on these. So if you do not have something in place to kill pathogens/parasites, like CD, then the majority of your supplementation goes to strengthening the parasites instead of your child.

I really don't understand something basic... Vitamin C in food. I know not to give citrus or mangoes. Also, kiwis are rather high in vitamin C. If my child eats a kiwi or other high vitamin C containing food, how long does this impact CD? When will it wear off?

Kiwis and other fruits high in vitamin C are a tough call. We do our best to avoid the biggest offenders. Unfortunately, I have seen families lose months because they continued to give fruit juice or supplements high in antioxidants. As soon as these were pulled, their children began to improve. A few years ago, a popular omega high in antioxidants became popular for autism. Families that I was helping all over the world noted regression in their children. As soon as we figured out what the common thread was, and pulled that supplement, the improvements began again, but it was a nightmare. To answer the second part of your question, I don't know exactly how long vitamin C from a natural fruit source lasts in the body. A few different websites estimate up to 24 hours.

We have been using gluthatione every day and modified citrus pectin as a binder. Are those compatible with CD?

Gluthatione is a very powerful antioxidant and cannot be used as a supplement with CD. Modified citrus pectin is fine.

I have heard that CD helps with oxalate problems. Is that true?

Rompepiedras (RP) is very effective against oxalate-crystal formation. There are connections between parasites and oxalate problems, which this protocol seems to be helping. Ridding the body of parasites helps with high oxalates.

I know that CD neutralizes heavy metals. What does that actually mean? What is the difference between chelating and neutralizing?

The mechanism of how CD neutralizes and removes heavy metals such as mercury is not clearly known (or understood). However, a number of recovered children have had heavy metal burden tests performed before and after the use of CD, and their heavy metal burden dropped. We also know of an adult in our circles who was extremely toxic with mercury and was able to normalize his levels after all other medical interventions had failed him.

So is CD enough and we don't need to chelate?

For many it is not necessary to chelate while on CD. There are some children though who do IV chelation and CD at the same time. This method seems to have good results; there are big metal dumps, when administering chelation challenge testing. As time goes by, we add interventions until we reach recovery.

Are all chelators compatible with CD?

In many cases there is no need to do both. To answer your question, EDTA is fine as well as DMSA and DMPS with CD.

You may want to consider Bio-Chelat™, bentonite clay or zeolite clay. These are great light chelators.

We have tried every biomed option available, but nothing has helped. What makes CD different?

Biomedical treatments in general provide large amounts of antioxidants. CD is an oxidizer and kills all pathogens in the body. The premise is that once your body does not have to feed and house pathogens, it will work much better and will heal. This protocol focuses on excesses and not deficiencies, which in itself makes it different from many other biomedical interventions. With CD and the Parasite Protocol we are eliminating the pathogens and parasites that cause the symptoms known as autism.

Most biomedical interventions seem to be only applicable to small kids. Does CD work on "older" kids, teenagers or young adults?

Of course! Families with older teens and adults have had success. The body wants to heal at any age be it 7 or 70! This year, two 17-year-olds lost their diagnosis through the use of CD as part of their biomedical protocols. A 32-year-old male is doing excellent on the Protocol as well. Time will tell, and parent/caregiver dedication is the key to success.

How long should I do the protocol to see if it is working for us?

Within 30 days you will know. If you do the Protocol 100%, and in the order laid out here you should see improvements. Some see improvements with their first dose!

Has anyone had an increase in PANDAS/PANS stuff while on CD? Our ATEC didn't budge this time around and it is mainly due to the OCD and other PANDAS stuff that has increased. I get in 16 doses on weekends, but not on weekdays—maybe I get in 12 on a good day during the school week. Has anyone done anything to treat this PANDAS stuff?

Parasites typically coexist with bacteria, so it is very important to treat bacteria and parasites at the same time. It is extremely important to get in 16 doses a day, whether you get in doses earlier in the morning, or send doses to school. Also, many children with PANDAS/PANS need to be treated month long for parasites. If you are giving a probiotic, you can try doing a period without it and see if you child does not improve. We must keep in mind that if you are seeing parasites coming out with the enemas, we may not be seeing gains until we have eliminated a good number of the parasites living in the body. The toxins that they excrete—living and dead—can also cause some of the behaviors we relate with PANDAS/PANS.

Has anyone seen elevated liver enzymes while on CD?

Liver enzymes will not be high from CD. I have watched people do the liver enzyme tests for two years and the kids are in the normal range. However, when they are dumping worms or doing parasite meds is when we may see the enzyme levels go up. Within a couple of weeks they go back to normal, in the handful of times that I have seen them go up. Mebendazole and Combantrin® are non-systemic, and therefore are not absorbed; they basically travel through the intestinal system and are eliminated in the stool and urine.

My son still has a lot of mercury (DMSA provocation). Is it possible that the level can go down from using this protocol? How long should I wait before testing him again?

It is very common for the heavy metal load to go down. If you want to do labs, you can do them in three to four months.

How young is too young for CD?

There is no age that is too young. If a baby is showing signs of cold/flu, etc., you can start with the baby bottle method, one drop in 8 fl. oz. of water, so they are getting 1/8 of 1 drop per dose. The protocols are based on weight.

Ok we have had my son on this protocol for 11 months now. We started at an ATEC of 82 and had a dramatic decrease right away. Our second score was 26! Now we have had 3 consecutive ATECs of 33, most points being in the speech category. Where should I go from here? More diet changes and or supplements? We have been GFCFSF for years, considering going grain free next. We already use omegas and ocean water, and have done nine parasite protocols.

It may be time to look into hyperbarics or GcMAF, as you have *The Diet*, CD and parasite protocol firmly in place. If these 2 options are not financially possible, you need to look at the speech supplement list. Go in order, and see if your child doesn't see gains from some of those. You can also look at chelators. Also, please check that your omega does not have any antioxidants in it, as that will be killing your CD.

Is it normal to see diarrhea in the beginning of the CD protocol?

I consider there to be two types of diarrhea. One is the water faucet, which we want to avoid. If you see water faucet diarrhea, stop for the day, and give a lower dose of CD the next day, when you start up again. The other type of diarrhea is loose, unformed stool, which is normal during detox. As the body is attempting to eliminate the excess toxins quickly, the digestive process will speed up, and not all of the excess water will have a chance to be absorbed through the intestinal tract, causing loose stool.

How do you move CD through inspections at the airport?

Don't carry concentrated sodium chlorite and activator bottles into the cabin. They must go into your checked luggage. Make sure each bottle is tightly sealed. Double bag each bottle SEPARATELY and place at opposite ends of your luggage but not right up against the sides. You may wish to stick each bottle into a pair of socks as extra protection. Surround each bottle with plenty of clothes to insure they will be protected if the bag is roughly handled. According to TSA regulations, you can bring aboard up to 3.4 fl. oz., (100ml) of a liquid in your carry-on luggage, which can hold 3 doses from your baby bottle batch.

Can I use CD as a toothpaste? Should I use regular toothpaste in addition?

I use CD spray (ten drops of activated CD per ounce) on the toothbrush first. Then, brush the teeth, and follow with fluoride-free toothpaste. CD is great for healthy teeth, tongue, and gums.

Is it okay to go swimming when on CD? I worry about the chlorine.

They do have a molecule in common; however one has nothing to do with the other. Some doctors don't let ASD kids swim in chlorinated pools. But, as far as taking CD goes, the chlorine in the pool will not deactivate the CD in your body, nor react with it. A child on CD can swim in a chlorinated pool, just as a child not on CD can swim in a chlorinated pool.

Can I give colloidal silver with CD?

No. Colloidal silver is active for up to 24 hours in the body, and will lower the potency of CD. Therefore the two are not compatible.

Where is the autism clinic in Venezuela?

Puerto Ordaz, Fundacion Venciendo el Autismo. Carolina Moreno is the president and one of my best friends. Her email is venciendoelautismo@hotmail.com. We have over 36 recovered children there. It is wonderful.

My son has been sick and has really bad diarrhea. Can we skip the enemas for a few days or still do them?

We don't use enemas just for constipation, but for overall colon irrigation and health. CD kills pathogens in the colon, and thereby helps heal autism. As the sickness causing the diarrhea is most likely pathogen induced, CD enemas will continue to kill these pathogens and help your son get over this acute situation faster.

My daughter just drank undiluted CDS. What do I do?

First, get her to drink plain water right away. Next, give orange juice or vitamin C to neutralize the CDS. Give burbur or activated charcoal to mop up the toxins that were released. Considering the strong taste, it is unlikely she would have consumed very much.

Can CD be harmful?

In the past 3 years that families have been using CD for autism, we have not seen any children or adults harmed by using this protocol correctly. Liver enzyme tests, nutritional tests, metal porphyrins tests, etc., have consistently shown improvement in the health of the children. Since Jim Humble started using chlorine dioxide for health, no one has died from ingesting CD (or MMS). The story that is often shared around the internet from Vanatu, concerning a woman who unfortunately passed away, was not attributed by the coroner to be the result of ingesting chlorine dioxide. There was another case of a 25-year-old male who attempted suicide with 10g (nearly the contents of a four ounce bottle of sodium chlorite at 22.4% solution) of sodium chlorite (inactivated CD). He developed methemoglobinemia, which he received treatment for, but survived his suicide attempt. That said, as we have mentioned before... anything used incorrectly or recklessly can harm you. Water, table salt, etc. The reason we outlined the protocol in such detail is to prevent mistakes and help families use it responsibly to recover their children with autism.

Does clay or bentonite clay interfere with CD? How far apart should it be taken from CD?

One hour apart from CD is fine. I use diatomaceous earth about ten minutes apart from a CD dose.

Is ibuprofen ok to take while doing CD protocol?

We have never seen a drug that was contraindicated with CD. Always consult your physician for prescription contraindications.

Is it ok to add Epsom salts to a CD bath?

We do not use epsom salts baths in this protocol. We use CD baths. See page 113.

Is it ok to take SAMe (S-adenosylmethionine) with CD? I took out all antioxidants, but not sure about SAMe.

No, it contains magnesium and vitamin C. For a mineral supplement, we take Ocean Water. Vitamin C kills the CD. Magnesium feeds biofilm, and therefore is counterproductive to our goals of healing.

Can I use DMSO in a CD enema to help drive the CD into the parasites?

> **Warning:** <u>Never use DMSO in an enema!</u> Never introduce it into the body rectally. If it is applied rectally, it will carry toxic fecal matter into the bloodstream through the intestinal wall.

How do I use DMSO?

> Every chance you can, apply DMSO to a clean body for 20 to 25 minutes and let it soak in. Apply it to affected parts first then remove rings/jewelry to cover all parts of the hands. Allow it to dry while applying to another body area (i.e. right arm, left arm, right leg, left leg). Apply to clean skin with clean hands. Use natural fiber clothing if it is going to come in contact with the DMSO, which can dissolve synthetics. Dr. Stanley Jacob has proven that DMSO brings about healing of rheumatoid arthritis, and it is great for migraine headaches, etc. You can research his work at...

www.dmso.org

> ...or find a DMSO retailer at...

www.protocolsuppliers.com

> The 99% pure stuff is best, but never use that strength on the skin directly. It must be diluted to 70% or less for topical use.

Does DMSO neutralize CD?

> No, it does not. However, DMSO has not proven itself to be a tool for autism recovery. In general, we use it for self-injurious behavior (SIB). The "S" in DMSO (dimethyl sulfoxide) is "sulf" as in sulfur. Many children with autism have a spirochete (amongst other pathogens), which feeds on sulfur. We saw many setbacks when adding DMSO. It is used on a case-by-case basis.

Chapter 6

CDS
Another Way of
Delivering Chlorine Dioxide

There is more than one way to skin a cat.

~ Seba Smith

In October 2011, I received an email from Jim Humble. After a visit with Dr. Andreas Kalcker, he had some fantastic new information for healing autism. Jim wanted me to fly to the Dominican Republic to see him yet again that year so he could share this new information.

The big news surrounded the creation of *Chlorine Dioxide Solution* (CDS)—a new method of producing and using chlorine dioxide; substantially different from the CD mixing process we were using (described in Chapter 5). Jim was excited about all of the great things that Andreas was developing.

Andreas was contacted by a cattle farmer who was frustrated by the health problems of newborn calves he was receiving. These calves were suffering from infections, diarrhea, ear problems, cysts, coccidiosis, bovine respiratory syndrome, etc. His yearly veterinary drug bill was around €28,000, not including the cost of feed. The farmer had heard about the wonders of MMS in humans and wondered if it might help his animals as well.

Andreas thought, "Sure! Why not?" However, he quickly learned that cattle were very different from humans when it came to their digestive system. Cattle digest through fermentation, which CD disrupts, so he had to find a way to bypass their digestive system and go directly to their blood stream. But, that idea had another big problem. The pH of standard CD was too acidic and therefore not compatible with the calves' blood stream. Injecting even dilute CD caused great pain and could result in damage to the veins. There had to be another way!

After much thought and research, Andreas came up with a distillation process to extract the chlorine dioxide—the key ingredient—from the CD mixture so it would not contain any sodium chlorite or acidic activator. He named the resulting liquid *Chlorine Dioxide Solution* (usually abbreviated CDS). Note: CDS can still contain <u>trace amounts</u> of sodium chlorite and whatever acidic activator used to produce it, but usually not enough to be an issue.

This new CDS solution was injected into the 800 cattle with very positive results. The animals health improved and the vet bill dropped like a rock.

In one case, the farmer called Andreas about a particularly sick cow. He advised him on a dosage, but apparently the farmer misunderstood the instructions and gave the cow 10 times the recommended amount. The result? The cow was a bit "high" with ears and tail standing up, but subsequently became healthy with no ill effects from the accidental overdose.

On the human side, CDS also solves the problem some people have with sensitivity to citric acid as well as the taste of CD. Not having the original chemicals (sodium chlorite/citric or hydrochloric acid) in CDS makes a big difference for some. Another advantage of CDS was a drastic reduction in Herxheimer reactions.

After a long weekend in the Dominican Republic, we went home with new information to try out with Patrick.

I began by swapping out drops of CD for milliliters of CDS. Initially, I didn't notice improvements or regression, but I did notice that Patrick was waking earlier and having a less profound sleep. After about 30 days of trying the new miracle I began to think that, "If it ain't broke, don't fix it." So we went back to the original CD that had given us all of the recoveries and improvements. Patrick went back to sleeping very well and I never looked back. I was a confirmed CD user and CDS, for me, had no obvious advantages.

A little over a year later, Jim was at our home, and on December 26th, 2012, his new assistant showed up from the Middle East to help him. She could be called the "CDS poster child." We differed on this topic right away. But, she was very insistent. She asked me why I didn't like CDS and I told her. So, she told me that I had been using "unstabilized" CDS and now they "stabilize" the CDS.

When the CDS is "stabilized" (with some sodium chlorite added back into the CDS liquid), it gives an extra kick, such that when the chlorine dioxide molecule oxidizes a pathogen, there is sodium chlorite on hand to react with the acid that is created by the death of the pathogen. The result is more chlorine dioxide released on the spot.

I decided to try stabilized CDS with Patrick. We arrived at his full dose based on tolerance. His sleep has been perfect. He sleeps as any pre-teen should—like a rock. And, he has great energy all day long. I can say that there was no noticeable difference over the four months that he was taking CDS, from the days when he took CD. However, he is a little bit "lighter," as if he has no cares in the world. It seems as if something that might have made him uncomfortable no longer bothers him. Little by little, a few families switched to CDS to see if their children did better, worse, or as well as they did with CD.

After a couple of trial months with about 20 families, I think that it is safe to say that CDS has its place in the buffet of different methods of chlorine dioxide administration. We still have the original CD, made with citric acid or HCl. Now, we have CDS and CDH (Chapter 7). Today, we no longer use stabilized CDS, as I feel that CDS is only for hypersensitive individuals and to be used only until they can switch over to CD or CDH. Whatever formula we choose, it will help to heal the body of unwanted pathogens, and helps with parasites as well as heavy metals. Each person is different, and it is up to us as parents to observe and decide which method of chlorine dioxide administration is best.

You are in no way encouraged to switch to CDS if what you're doing with CD is working for you. For some people it may be better, but as of now, only one of our recoveries has come from CDS—all the rest are from CD. Some children may try CDS and come to realize that CD is still better for them.

When to Use CDS

CDS is used when someone just can't get past 1 drop divided in 8 fl. oz., over a day without experiencing a Herxheimer reaction. This allows us to get past the road block and still detoxify the body. Eventually, we want to go back to the standard CD Protocol which I believe to be more effective.

This is not a common situation, but it does occur.

Making vs. Buying CDS

Most people are a bit concerned about making CDS since it involves a distillation process where you produce chlorine dioxide gas and then cause it to go into water. When Andreas first came up with making CDS, it involved two containers, a hose, heat and lots of ventilation. There are still lots of videos on YouTube explaining that original process. However, there is now a much better, easier and safer way to produce CDS at home. So, if you see a CDS making video or read instructions that talk about using a hose—forget it! The new process is much easier and safer and doesn't involve any heat nor hoses.

There are some online sellers of CDS, but the cost of it is high and making your own is simple. It just takes a little effort in learning the process and having the right equipment. In addition, by making your own, you will have a better understanding of the behavior of chlorine dioxide.

Some Important CDS Points

When it comes to CDS, it is all in the concentration of chlorine dioxide in water; measured in *parts per million*—abbreviated **ppm**.

When buying or making your own, the goal is to end up with a bottle of CDS having a concentration strength of 3,000ppm. This bottle should ideally be made out of glass and kept in the refrigerator. You never use this concentrated solution directly. It must be diluted.

When we say, for example, use 10ml of CDS, we mean mix 10ml of 3,000ppm CDS with whatever indicated amount of water, and use that diluted mixture for the indicated purpose.

Make sure you read and understand Appendix 6, page 467 which explains more about concentration and measuring ppm.

There are several names attributed to this new, better and simpler method of making CDS, such as:

- The Shot Glass Method
- The Overnight Method
- The New Method

There are some demonstrations on YouTube showing this new method along with write-ups on various forums. These methods use a plethora of different containers having different shapes and sizes. The specific tools used to produce CDS can have a significant impact on the concentration.

It should also be noted that the concentration strength is reduced every time you open the CDS source bottle as chlorine dioxide gas escapes the liquid and evaporates into the air space above the liquid. When you open the source container, some of the chlorine dioxide gas escapes. So, the strength of a half full CDS bottle can be substantially less than what you started off with when the bottle was full. This is similar in concept to a pop bottle that loses its fizz if not used up quickly.

To substantially reduce the evaporation of the chlorine dioxide gas, the CDS source bottle should be stored in the refrigerator, which stabilizes and significantly reduces the amount of CD gas escaping the CDS solution. But, no matter what the temperature, some gas will always escape and reduce the concentration each time the bottle is opened. A narrow neck bottle helps maintain the integrity of the CDS for longer periods.

It is better to store the concentrated source CDS in smaller 300ml bottles than keep it in a larger one liter bottle. That way you use up what is in one bottle faster with less concentration loss. A good storage bottle is shown and described on page 160.

The New CDS Making Method — The Basic Concept

First, let's go over the basic principles of the CDS making process and then we will go into details.

We start with two containers (both ideally made of glass). One container is larger and has some kind of a lid that can be tightly closed. The other is a smaller container having NO lid. The relative size of each container is such that the smaller container fits comfortably inside the larger container while allowing the lid to properly close on the larger container when the smaller one is inside. See page 151 for an example of a well-made glass kit distributed by wps4sale.com.

The large container is then partially filled with filtered/distilled water. The level of water must be low enough so as to not overflow into the smaller container if it is placed into the partially filled larger container. The photos on page 151 show the concept of the two bottles visually.

Now that you have the basic idea, let's make some CDS...

Using the Overnight CDS Generating Kit

The following directions assume you have the glass *Overnight CDS Generating Kit (1000 ml)* from wps4sale.com (as shown on page 151). You are of course not required to use their kit. However, based on our own experience of looking high and low for a good one, theirs has the key features:

- Made of glass
- Smaller glass fits inside of larger container AND 1000ml of water inside the big container will not flood into the smaller container once placed inside.
- Lid fits tight and no gas escapes during the chemical reaction time.
- Lid is plastic—NEVER USE METAL LIDS!

Note: There are plastic CDS kits that work. You may be able to find a combination of containers made of plastic but not glass where you live. In fact, I made a YouTube video where I show how to make CDS using a plastic container. Just understand that chlorine dioxide will deteriorate plastic containers over time, so it should be avoided. Even if you have to use a plastic jar to make the CDS, store the final product in glass. The less time the CDS is in plastic, the better! As for lids, we have no choice. Only use plastic lids. Metal lids will oxidize VERY rapidly! Even metal lids with a plastic coating on the inside will deteriorate.

Steps to Making CDS:

1. Start by pouring one liter of distilled or reverse osmosis water into the large glass container. The water should be around room temperature.

2. Place the empty dessert cup inside the large container making sure no water spills into the cup.

3. Measure 75ml of sodium chlorite solution (22.4% $NaClO_2$ in water) and pour into the dessert cup, while being careful not to spill any sodium chlorite into the water surrounding the cup.

4. Measure 75ml of 10% HCl or 50% citric acid solution and pour into dessert cup.

5. IMMEDIATELY screw on the lid to the large container while being careful to not jiggle the container which could potentially cause the CD solution

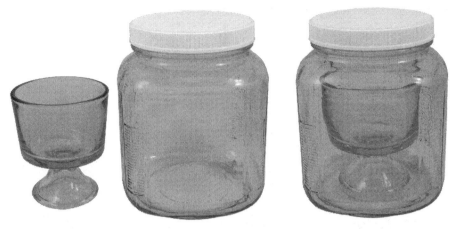

wps4sale.com sells this <u>Overnight CDS Generating Kit</u> that produces 1 liter of CDS at 3,000ppm from 75ml of sodium chlorite plus 75ml of activator. The only part not made of glass is the plastic lid. The glass dessert cup is sized just right to fit inside the larger glass jar with enough room left over for 1 L of water that won't overflow into the dessert cup.

---

to mix with the surrounding water. Make sure the cover is tightly screwed down so as to not have any leaks. If you smell chlorine dioxide (beyond the little that escapes while you are putting on the lid) then something is wrong with the lid and/or container.

6. If you did everything correctly you should see the CD solution turn a dark amber/brown within about a minute (see below) and notice that the water starts to turn a light yellow several minutes later. It is also normal to see bubbles form in the dessert cup. It is normal for the pressure to change during the chemical reaction. We find that citric acid produces a vacuum and HCl can produce a pressure at first and then a vacuum.

7. Cover the kit with a towel to reduce its exposure to light. It doesn't have to be in a pitch black location, but it definitely should not be in direct sun light. Feel free to check it from time to time and see how the colors change. Of course keep this kit out of the reach of children or anything that could disturb it. I keep mine in the cabinet overnight with a towel on it.

8. When the color in the dessert glass matches that of the surrounding water, the chemical reaction is complete. There is no harm in waiting a bit longer—nothing more will happen. This usually takes from 12-24 hours depending on room temperature and the strength of the acid used.

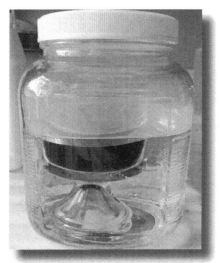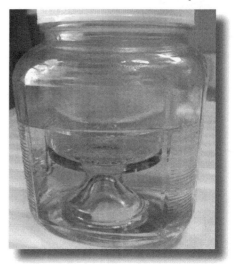

*After the sodium chlorite and activator mix, the color will
quickly turn a dark amber, almost black color (left). After about
12 hours, the color of the solution in the dessert cup and that
of the water surrounding it should be identical (right), which
indicates the chemical reaction has completed and the CDS is
ready to be poured into a storage container.*

9. Have your glass storage bottle(s) clean and ready to receive the CDS
    solution.

10. Before opening the kit make sure your work area is well ventilated.
    Perform the steps that follow outside or have the door and/or window
    open nearby. Having a fan lightly blowing any gas that escapes away from
    you is a good idea.

11. Slowly open the container being careful to not jostle it which could cause
    the CD solution to mix with the freshly made CDS. If the chemicals mix,
    you will have to start over again, so be careful! You will most likely smell
    the chlorine dioxide gas that was sitting in the air space when you first
    open it. This is normal, hence the need for good ventilation.

12. Slowly remove the dessert cup while being careful to not spill its contents
    into the CDS. Immediately dispose of the contents in the toilet and rinse
    off the dessert cup.

13. Now pour the CDS into the storage bottles while being aware that some
    chlorine dioxide gas will come out of the water into your working area.

14. Tightly seal the storage bottle(s) and place in the refrigerator.

Note: 10% HCl is the recommended activator when making CDS. However, you can also use 4% of HCl, but the reaction time will be slowed down. It may take as much as a full day before the color of the CD solution and the water match.

Dosing CDS

As mentioned earlier, CDS is particularly well-suited for unusually sensitive individuals who cannot tolerate even low doses of CD.

Start with a baby bottle filled with 8 fl. oz., of water and add 1ml of CDS. This will provide eight doses of 1/8ml. If all is well on the first day, increase to 2ml on the second day. Each day you increase by one milliliter. Increase the amount based on tolerance. If the person is having a problem with a certain level of CDS, then go down to where they were fine and stay there a few days before increasing again.

Tolerance is the key here. Once you can no longer increase you have reached that person's full oral dose of CDS.

Slowly Switching Back to CD

Once you have found the full oral dose where they are stable and cannot go higher, it is time to fold CD back in.

The goal of using CDS is not to replace CD, but rather do some fundamental detoxing so you can bring CD back and reach full oral dose of CD.

This is accomplished by taking out one milliliter of CDS and replacing it with 1 drop of CD. For example, if the individual can tolerate 20 milliliters of CDS, then an ideal transition would be represented in the chart on page 154.

Of course this chart represents an unlikely scenario where everything goes exactly as desired. However, it does demonstrate what we are striving for— switching out CDS for CD and continuing to increase the dose of CD as described in Chapter 5 (page 81).

To accomplish this process effectively requires careful observation of your child and making decisions as to when you can go up; when to hold; and when to back down.

Hypothetical CDS to CD Transition			
Transition Day	CDS in milliliters	CD in drops	Comments
1	20	0	Last CDS only day.
2	19	1	Transition starts
3	18	2	
4	17	3	
5	16	4	
6	15	5	
7	14	6	
8	13	7	
9	12	8	
10	11	9	
11	10	10	Transition continues
12	9	11	
13	8	12	
14	7	13	
15	6	14	
16	5	15	
17	4	16	
18	3	17	
19	2	18	
20	1	19	
21	0	20	Transition completes
22	0	21	
23	0	22	CD increases each day
24	0	23	
25	0	24	

CDS Enemas

CDS enemas can be useful for sensitive individuals when starting the protocol. Follow the same enema instructions in Chapter 5, page 103, keeping in mind that 1ml of CDS has a relative strength of approximately 60% of 1 drop of CD. With that in mind you can work up to 40ml of CDS per liter of enema water.

Chapter 7

<u>CDH - Going Beyond CD & CDS</u>

"The progressive development of man is vitally dependent on invention. It is the most important product of his creative brain."
~ Nikola Tesla

This protocol is constantly evolving, and until every person with autism recovers, we will continue to search for things to add or tweak to the protocol so we reach that goal. A few months before the release of this second edition, I was made aware of a new method of CD preparation, known as *Chlorine Dioxide Holding (solution)* or simply CDH.

CDH can almost be described as a hybrid between classic CD and CDS. Where CDS has no raw material left in the final product, but only chlorine dioxide gas dissolved in water, CDH contains some raw material (similar to classic CD) along with the chlorine dioxide in the final product. This new process allows the sodium chlorite to react with the acid for a significantly longer period of time, thereby reducing much of the remaining amount of unactivated sodium chlorite and activator. Some people cannot tolerate citric acid so CDH is usually made with 4% HCl. Initial reports indicate that CDH is better tolerated than CD.

Another interesting benefit of CDH is that it appears to mix well with the permitted natural sweetener stevia (SweetLeaf® brand) without reducing the potency of CDH. This can help children who have an aversion to the taste of CD. Many families have also reported that they were able to increase their child's dose without producing a Herxheimer reaction, in contrast to classic CD. Older children and severely affected children have benefitted as well from the CDH preparation; you can read more about that on page 221.

Currently, this new method is being used by a relatively small group of families (around 70 as of November, 2013). Many of them are reporting that CDH continues to produce results for their children on the spectrum, and they are seeing even better things than before.

As with all new things, it is important to test with a diverse group of families over a long enough time period to make sure that gains are sustained. So we ask that you please keep in mind that CDH is literally the bleeding edge of this protocol. While we are excited to share a new option with you, the decision to use CDH must not be taken lightly. If you are doing well with classic CD you may never need to use CDH. Consider the old saying, "If it ain't broke, don't fix it." Of the 115 children who have lost their autism diagnosis, 114 have done so with CD and 1 with CDS. So far, 0 with CDH (4 months in use for ASD). I expect this number to change soon as we are seeing good things from CDH. Time will tell. Stay tuned.

Scott McRae, his wife Brenda, and Charlotte Lackney have been pioneers in developing the CDH method. The following section is written by Scott where he discusses how CDH evolved along with detailed instructions on how to prepare and use it.

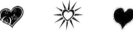

My wife, Brenda, and I first learned about CD early in 2009, through Bhante Vimalaramsi, an American born Buddhist monk. He's now a very close friend of ours, and even as I'm writing this, I'm at a meditation retreat which is based upon his understanding of the open-minded, experiential teaching of the Buddha.

After receiving our first set of CD bottles from an online seller, we started by trying to get to 15 drops of CD activated with lemon juice for 3 minutes, twice a day, which was the protocol at the time. Though we gave it a good effort, we couldn't get past 6 drops before vomiting and having diarrhea, and this caused us to initially stop taking CD. Then, after moving to Jakarta, Indonesia (Brenda's home town), I experienced almost monthly illnesses, which I believe was due to being in a new and tropical part of the world (I'm from San Diego, CA), riding in public transportation twice a day and teaching in a school of over 300 students. After a year and a half of constantly being sick, I remembered our bottles of CD which we had fortunately brought with us from the US, and I started on Protocol 1000. By that time, *Protocol 1000* had been developed to be what it is now—3 drops of CD (activated for 20 seconds with 50% citric acid) per hour, 8 times a day—and so I decided to do the 3 week cleanse. By doing the cleanse, I experienced a huge improvement in my health. Not only did I immediately stop getting sick, but I also felt that my energy level had increased by about 25%! Obviously, I was excited by these great results and so was my wife because she had started taking CD again as well. However,

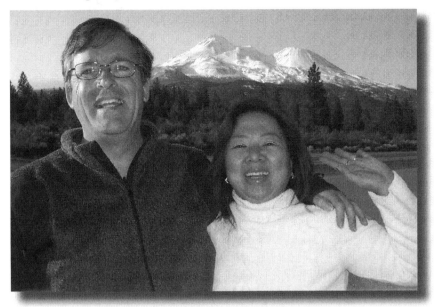

Scott & Brenda McRae from Jakarta, Indonesia

even though our results were great and our experience was far better than before with the old, "try to get to 15 drops twice a day protocol," we still were having some nausea and bouts with diarrhea when we took CD. This was especially true at the times when we felt the symptoms of a cold or flu and tried to take more than the 3 drops doses in order to overcome it. Still the results we were getting with CD on Protocol 1000 outweighed the nausea and diarrhea that we experienced and so we continued using it, especially when we felt some sickness coming on.

After taking CD for about a year in this way, CDS hit the CD world. Being the experimental type, I decided to give it a try. After searching all over Jakarta for the plastic tubing for a couple of days and finally finding it, I made our first batch of CDS. We both tried CDS for about six months but found it to be less effective than CD, so we stopped with CDS and went back to CD and Protocol 1000.

Nevertheless, there were 2 things I really liked about CDS: (1) it NEVER caused us any nausea or diarrhea, and (2) it was so easy to use since it was pre-made (no mixing of chemicals before each use). The main thing for me was not having any more nausea because I really disliked feeling sick. So, I started thinking about CDS and my experience with making it and I came to the conclusion that possibly, the reason why CDS wasn't nauseating was because there wasn't any unactivated sodium chlorite in the solution—it was just chlorine dioxide dissolved in water. I remembered that when I made CDS myself, even after the activation process had gone on for an hour in a heated condition, if I stirred or swirled the activation chamber bottle, more ClO_2 would still come out of it. This got me to thinking... if the chemical reaction between the sodium chlorite and the 50% citric acid solution used to make the CDS was still able to produce more chlorine dioxide after an hour in a heated condition, then surely the 24 drops that I was using to make my daily CD dosing bottle weren't being fully activated after just 20 seconds.

Therefore, I decided to increase the activation time and tried it out on myself first and then my wife (aren't I considerate?). We both found there was no longer a nausea problem, even when taking more drops per hour than we had ever taken before.

Since I was in an experimental mode, I decided to see if I could make larger quantities of concentrated CD all at once to make it more convenient. I mixed equal amounts of sodium chlorite and 50% citric acid in a bottle, let it activate for about a minute, and then added a specific amount of hot water to further encourage the activation process. In the end, I had a total of 140 ml of this concentrated CD solution. Later, I found that hot water wasn't necessary and that room temperature water worked even better because there was less CLO_2 gas lost in the process.

The finished chemistry was indeed very strong and still didn't cause any nausea, so I was compelled to post my discovery on the Genesis II Forum. I named it *7 Day Fridge MMS (CD)* because it provided a 7 day supply of Protocol 1000. The ingredients added up to 140 ml, so each 20 ml was 1/7th of the total, or a one day supply of "pre-activated" CD similar to Protocol 1000. This made taking CD every day really easy. Just pour out 20ml of the new concentrated solution into a water dosing bottle, and then pour out 1/8th of the bottle every hour into some water in a glass, and drink it.

The *7 Day Fridge MMS (CD)* method worked great for my wife and me. Others on the Forum also tried it and liked it. In addition, I gave it to some people at the school where I work to overcome their colds (usually overnight) as well as other diseases within a short time.

About 18 months later, Charlotte, my Forum friend, began testing the *7 Day Fridge MMS (CD)* process to determine the actual ClO_2 content using her *Sensafe*™ Chlorine Dioxide Photometer. Over several months, we worked together to further refine the 7 Day Fridge method. The result of all of our testing and refinements is this new and exciting CDH product.

The final formula to produce CDH using the 1 Bottle Method came out to be:

22 parts water	91.6%
1 part sodium chlorite	4.2%
1 part HCl (4%) or Citric Acid (35%)	4.2%
Total Solution	**100%**

I believe this new way of making CD will be of great benefit to humanity because it will allow people to gradually double or even triple the amount of CD they can take with little or no stomach upset. By increasing their doses to higher levels, people will be able to overcome CD treatable diseases more quickly than ever before.

As with any new technology, more changes and developments are likely. For example, we now know that CDH tastes much better if activated with hydrochloric acid instead of citric acid.

Producing CDH Using the One Bottle Method

Making CDH is really quite simple. You can use any size of bottle, and produce any quantity you wish, as long as you follow the basic instructions and keep the proportions the same. However, before diverting into different quantities, it is recommended you follow these directions exactly to insure you have the process down correctly.

Note the following volume equivalents:

Fluid Ounce (U.S.) Approximate Equivalents

30ml	=	1 fl. oz. US (2 Tablespoons)
660ml	=	22 fl. oz. US
720ml	=	24 US fl. oz. US
750ml	=	25 US fl. oz. US

Equipment Needed

- One 750ml (25 fl. oz. US) glass bottle with an airtight cap. DO NOT use a metal cap (even if it is lined with plastic). The best caps are plastic or even a synthetic cork in good condition. A common 750ml wine bottle is ideal for this as you can get them colored to reduce possible UV exposure (the darker the better). But, a colored bottle is not absolutely necessary and using a clear one will allow you to actually see the chemical reaction as it turns from clear to yellow.

- Three 240ml (8 fl. oz. US) bottles ideally made of colored glass to protect the CDH from UV light (the darker the better), but colored bottles are not absolutely necessary. You can also use smaller bottles if you like—these are just used to divide up the resulting 720ml of CDH into smaller bottles to help retain the ClO_2 concentration while opening and closing the bottles during dosing. *Schweppes*™ sells 6-packs of Ginger Ale, Club Soda and Tonic Water in 10 fl. oz. glass bottles with plastic lids that are great for this purpose, and hold 300ml easily. Only the Ginger Ale is in a colored bottle (green), the others are clear.

- One measuring cup or graduated cylinder to accurately measure liquid in either milliliters or fluid ounces.

Ingredients Needed

Ingredients should be at room temperature—not cold. If CD and/or activator are right out of the refrigerator make your water warmer to offset, or allow ingredients to warm up before using.

- 660ml of distilled or purified water at about 70°-90°F (21°-32°C).

- 30ml of sodium chlorite (22.4% solution) near room temperature or slightly above.

- 30ml of 4% Hydrochloric Acid (HCl) or 35% Citric Acid ($C_6H_8O_7$) near room temperature or slightly above.

Note: The amounts indicated above add up to 720ml, while the wine bottle easily has room for an additional 30ml and more. Refer to the chart on right if you wish to produce a different batch amount.

The CDH Formulation Table
and Different Acid Concentrations

What if you have 10% Hydrochloric acid or 50% Citric Acid (very common)? Or, you wish to use a different size of bottle? Not a problem. These acids can still be used. However, the formula changes accordingly.

The table below is a great tool for determining the formula for a given bottle size. To use the table, start by circling the size of the bottle you wish to fill in the left most column. Next look at the acid you have and its labeled concentration. Match that with one of the 4 options across the top. Below the matching acid/concentration you will find the 3 formulation numbers for water, sodium chlorite (labeled "SC"), and whatever acid you are using. Just go down the appropriate 3 columns to where the bottle size line intersects and you will have the numbers you need. Substitute these numbers in the following preparation instructions if your situation calls for it.

CDH Formulation Table
(Applies to the One Bottle Method of making CDH ONLY!)
SC=Sodium Chlorite / HCl=Hydrochloric Acid / CA=Citric Acid

Water Bottle (ml)	Hydrochloric Acid 4%			Hydrochloric Acid 10%			Citric Acid 35%			Citric Acid 50%		
	Water (ml)	SC (ml)	HCl (ml)	Water (ml)	SC	HCl (ml)	Water (ml)	SC (ml)	CA (ml)	Water (ml)	SC (ml)	CA (ml)
10	9.2	0.4	0.4	9.4	0.4	0.2	9.2	0.4	0.4	9.3	0.4	0.3
20	18.3	0.8	0.8	18.8	0.8	0.3	18.3	0.8	0.8	18.6	0.8	0.6
30	27.5	1.3	1.3	28.3	1.3	0.5	27.5	1.3	1.3	27.9	1.3	0.9
40	36.7	1.7	1.7	37.7	1.7	0.7	36.7	1.7	1.7	37.2	1.7	1.2
50	45.8	2.1	2.1	47.1	2.1	0.8	45.8	2.1	2.1	46.5	2.1	1.5
60	55.0	2.5	2.5	56.5	2.5	1.0	55.0	2.5	2.5	55.8	2.5	1.7
70	64.2	2.9	2.9	65.9	2.9	1.2	64.2	2.9	2.9	65.0	2.9	2.0
80	73.3	3.3	3.3	75.3	3.3	1.3	73.3	3.3	3.3	74.3	3.3	2.3
90	82.5	3.8	3.8	84.8	3.8	1.5	82.5	3.8	3.8	83.6	3.8	2.6
100	91.7	4.2	4.2	94.2	4.2	1.7	91.7	4.2	4.2	92.9	4.2	2.9
150	137.5	6.3	6.3	141.3	6.3	2.5	137.5	6.3	6.3	139.4	6.3	4.4
200	183.3	8.3	8.3	188.3	8.3	3.3	183.3	8.3	8.3	185.8	8.3	5.8
250	229.2	10.4	10.4	235.4	10.4	4.2	229.2	10.4	10.4	232.3	10.4	7.3
300	275.0	12.5	12.5	282.5	12.5	5.0	275.0	12.5	12.5	278.8	12.5	8.7
350	320.8	14.6	14.6	329.6	14.6	5.8	320.8	14.6	14.6	325.2	14.6	10.2
400	366.7	16.7	16.7	376.7	16.7	6.7	366.7	16.7	16.7	371.7	16.7	11.7
450	412.5	18.8	18.8	423.8	18.8	7.5	412.5	18.8	18.8	418.1	18.8	13.1
500	458.3	20.8	20.8	470.8	20.8	8.3	458.3	20.8	20.8	464.6	20.8	14.6
550	504.2	22.9	22.9	517.9	22.9	9.2	504.2	22.9	22.9	511.0	22.9	16.0
600	550.0	25.0	25.0	565.0	25.0	10.0	550.0	25.0	25.0	557.5	25.0	17.5
650	595.8	27.1	27.1	612.1	27.1	10.8	595.8	27.1	27.1	604.0	27.1	19.0
700	641.7	29.2	29.2	659.2	29.2	11.7	641.7	29.2	29.2	650.4	29.2	20.4
720	660.0	30.0	30.0	678.0	30.0	12.0	660.0	30.0	30.0	669.0	30.0	21.0
750	687.5	31.3	31.3	706.3	31.3	12.5	687.5	31.3	31.3	696.9	31.3	21.9
800	733.3	33.3	33.3	753.3	33.3	13.3	733.3	33.3	33.3	743.3	33.3	23.3
850	779.2	35.4	35.4	800.4	35.4	14.2	779.2	35.4	35.4	789.8	35.4	24.8
900	825.0	37.5	37.5	847.5	37.5	15.0	825.0	37.5	37.5	836.3	37.5	26.2
950	870.8	39.6	39.6	894.6	39.6	15.8	870.8	39.6	39.6	882.7	39.6	27.7
1000	916.7	41.7	41.7	941.7	41.7	16.7	916.7	41.7	41.7	929.2	41.7	29.2

Preparation Instructions

Follow the steps of mixing ingredients in this order (assuming you are using the 750ml glass bottle):

1. Pour 660ml of purified water into the 750ml glass bottle.
2. Add 30ml of sodium chlorite to the 750ml glass bottle.
3. Add 30ml of 4% HCl or 30ml of 35% citric acid to the 750ml glass bottle.
4. Immediately cap/cork the bottle tightly so that no ClO_2 gas can escape and give it a good shake to thoroughly mix the ingredients (and a few more times later on if possible).
5. Store the bottle in a dark place with a temperature of 70°F to 90°F (21°C to 32°C) for 12 to 24 hours or more (24 hours or longer if you're in a cold environment—below 70°F (21°C)).
6. After the storage time has passed, place the bottle of CDH into the refrigerator (not the freezer) and allow it to cool down for 3+ hours before opening it for the first time. The temperature of the solution should be no more than 51°F (10.5° C). Note: If you are using a significantly smaller bottle, cool down time can be reduced because the smaller volume of solution will cool faster.
7. Finally, pour the CDH from the 750ml bottle into the smaller bottles, cap tightly and keep refrigerated until ready to use. The smaller bottle are easier to dose from and they also help reduce the number of times gas can escape and reduce the potency of the solution.

Using CDH

The CDH is now ready for use. Each milliliter of CDH solution contains 1 pre-activated drop of CD. It can be used for ANYTHING that CD is used for; viruses, bacteria, yeast, parasites, heavy metals, enemas, tub baths, gums & teeth, skin care, infections, etc.

When used orally, each 1ml of CDH should be added to at least 30ml of water. You can add even more water if you notice slight throat irritation with higher doses. If taste is an issue, a little bit of stevia may be added to each dose to improve taste by sweetening it. Some of the moms are adding SweetLeaf® Natural Stevia Sweetener to their daily bottle and report no negative impact on ppm level.

Although CDH is strong, it has shown to be gentler on folks who have issues with nausea when using traditional CD. You should be able to start at whatever drop dose you were on with CD and switch to an equivalent milliliter dose of CDH and gradually increase to tolerance. Typically, people are able to take 2 to 3 times as much of CDH as traditional CD, without experiencing nausea.

The CDH bottle should be kept refrigerated and only taken out to extract doses. Since 720ml is a fairly large quantity that may take many days to finish, it's a good idea to take the 720 ml and divide it up into 3 smaller 240ml bottles (720ml ÷ 3 = 240ml) so you won't lose much of the ClO_2 each time you open the bottle. By doing this, you will conserve as much of the ClO_2 as possible. It's also easier to extract doses from a smaller bottle using a syringe or pipette.

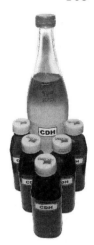

Also, keep the CDH bottle out of direct or indirect sunlight to prevent loss of ClO_2. If you make a dosing bottle <u>for the day</u>, it's best to keep it cold, but it is not absolutely necessary.

A little note about taste: Most people who complain about the bad taste of CD, CDS or CDH (which does not have any taste at low doses) are actually reacting to the smell of the ClO_2 which can lead to developing a long-term aversion to any of the treatment solutions. So, if you can minimize the gas floating around your nose, you will have an easier time with drinking the CD, CDS or CDH dose. To accomplish this, Charlotte suggested avoiding the use of a cup or wide mouth drinking bottle. Instead, use a bottle with a small opening such as a common water bottle (preferably made of glass). Of course, if the smell doesn't bother you, this is a moot point, but at least you have this little trick if it does.

Well, that's all you need to know to get started on this great new way to make and use CD. May this new CDH formulation bring you and your family much health and happiness.

Scott McRae
Jakarta, Indonesia
November, 2013

We appreciate Scott, Brenda and Charlotte's contribution to the variety of ways to produce and use chlorine dioxide. Be sure to check the Facebook groups and forums for the latest developments on CDH.

Some of you may feel overwhelmed by what you just read. So, let me give you my "Easy-Peasy" single paragraph method of making CDH: I take a 600ml Lifefactory™ bottle, put in 550ml of water; add 25ml of sodium chlorite; followed by 25ml of 4% HCl (or 50% citric acid). Leave it 12 hours in a cabinet, after which it goes in the fridge for 2 or more hours. Done! ☺

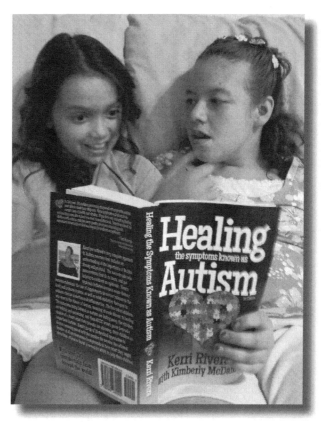

Healing & beating autism.

Chapter 8

Step 3
The Kalcker Parasite Protocol

All of our fathers had a treatment for parasites as a part of their cultural practice. We have gotten away from this because of our reliance on modern practice. We would do quite well to relearn the ways of our ancestors in this area and keep ourselves in relatively good health always.
~ ***Chief Two Trees***

The word "parasite" comes from the Greek word meaning, "one who eats off the table of another." Parasites, to Ancient Greeks, were those who sat at another's table, and paid for their meal with flattery.

As I mentioned earlier in the book, a very interesting thing started happening with the CD enemas. What we had previously believed to be mucous or biofilm coming out with the enemas, turned out in many cases to be worms (helminths) (aka parasites)—in rare cases they were still alive and wiggling in the toilet! We believed the most common were *Ascaris lumbricoides* (roundworm). However, what we are now seeing more and more appear to be rope parasites, a potential new species of helminth discovered by Dr. Gubarev, Dr. Alex Volinsky, and coworkers (submitted January 14, 2013). DNA testing is the only way to definitively say, but at $25,000 USD for each analysis, with a minimum of 100 test cases, it is rather cost prohibitive at the moment.[1]

In addition to Ascaris and rope parasites, parents have also seen hookworms, pinworms, tapeworms, and flukes, among others. This is an extremely important piece of the puzzle for so many of our children. We have been led to believe that in first world nations, parasites are not a problem. This is absolutely not the case.

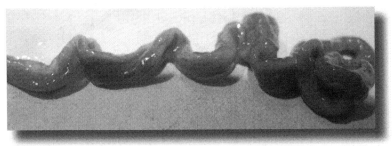

A well washed parasite. You can almost feel the texture.

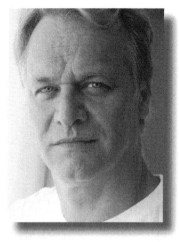

Andreas Kalcker,
co–author of the
Kalcker Parasite Protocol

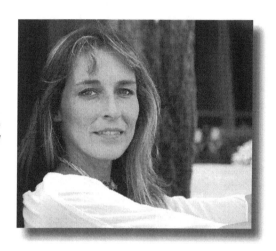

Miriam Carrasco Maceda,
co–author of the
Kalcker Parasite Protocol

I was honored to have Dr. Andreas Kalcker and Miriam Carrasco Maceda share a chapter from their upcoming book, *Parasites: The Silent Enemy.* Andreas explains the importance of lifelong deworming, and shares with us a protocol that has helped many children and adults become healthier; and for some children on the spectrum was the last piece added that led them to recovery. The version included here has been tailored specifically for children and adults with ASDs. The original protocol can be found at:

www.andreaskalcker.com/
index.php/en/health/parasite

Very few details have been changed, but it is important to note that the Parasite Protocol here is what has been proven to help many of our children on the spectrum, including many of the recovered children.

Thank you Andreas and Miriam for your valuable contributions to this movement, selflessly sharing your findings, and for always taking the time to help.

HOW TO DETECT AND
TREAT A PARASITIC INFECTION

Parasitic infections are more common than most people think, and may or may not result in serious health problems. We may be infected with multiple types of parasites, which vary in size and location, on or in the body.

Parasites can be classified as either microparasites, such as malaria that are only visible under the microscope, or large macroparasites such as round or flat intestinal worms (roundworms, tapeworms, etc.). These can be seen by the naked eye, and can reach great sizes. Internal parasites are found, not only in the intestines, as is generally thought, but anywhere in the body, including the lung, liver, muscle, stomach, gallbladder, brain, blood, skin, joints, and even in the eyes.

In recent history, the great migratory movements of the human population via rapid transportation and widespread trading have shortened the distances that previously had separated people and diseases. Formerly localized diseases have thus become universal ailments. Parasites previously confined to very specific geographical areas now appear in other locations, far away from their initial homelands. Unfortunately, conditions typical of the lower socioeconomic strata, (under which a large percentage of the global population lives) tend to favor the transmission of diseases and parasites.

A high percentage of the world population suffers from infections by parasites, which the WHO (World Health Organization) estimates are responsible for 15 million child deaths annually. In addition to the great cost represented by deaths, chronic and persistent infections have increased as parasites have developed multiple mechanisms of evasion and resistance to specific immunity. This allows them to circumvent and cancel the host immune response.

Persistent parasitic infection in human hosts leads to chronic immune reactions, which can result in tissue damage and altered immune regulation. Ninety percent of the world population is infected with one or more parasites, and up to five different types may coexist in the same host.

This situation becomes dangerous when the internal balance within the host is upset, the number of parasites skyrockets, and the host begins showing signs of serious illness that may even result in death. However, in some cases, parasitic worm infections do not result in disease, in fact, a number of carriers are found to be healthy.

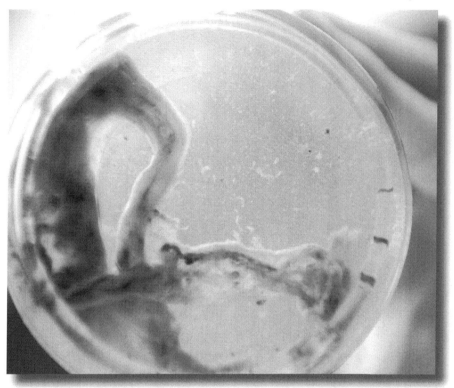

A really good look into a parasite. You can see the actual intestines of the parasite. Also known as a helminth.

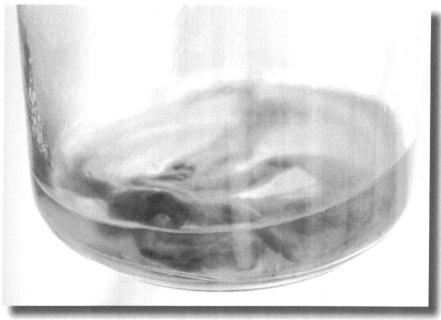

The same parasite (as above) from a different angle.

Considering that most people are not even aware of their infections, parasites have become silent killers, claiming the lives of many unsuspecting victims going about their lives oblivious to the danger. Some doctors in Western Europe and the U.S. seem unwilling to even contemplate that we may be infected.

Taking into account the recent increase in travel, immigration, and trade across continents, it is not hard to see how the problem has now become magnified to an alarming level. Parasites, especially the modern "toxified" versions, may well be causing many of the rare diseases now becoming more prevalent, as well as other recently identified or growing problems such as chronic fatigue, fibromyalgia, and arthritis.

The most common verminosis (infestation with or without obvious symptomatology of disease caused by parasitic worms) is intestinal. People who have them not only suffer from a large quantity of lost nutrients (absorbed by the parasites), but also from perforations made by worms in the digestive tract that can open the door to various infections and possible autoimmune deficiencies. Intestinal worm infections are very common and can affect everyone, not only people with poor hygiene habits. Helminths (worms) are transmitted by ingesting the eggs or larvae of parasites, which then hatch in the intestinal tract.

A parasitic infection or reinfection can be acquired through one or more of the following avenues:

▶ From more or less direct contact with an infected person (fecal or sexual).
▶ From self-infection, for example, through anal-hand-mouth contact. By scratching the anal area, eggs can become lodged under the fingernails.
▶ From congenital transmission (mother to fetus).
▶ From commonly contaminated objects.
▶ From soil contaminated by human or animal excrement.
▶ From eating contaminated raw or undercooked meat.
▶ From eating raw fish.

In some countries, raw fish is included in traditional foods. We can avoid the consumption of the larvae or worms by freezing the meat or fish for at least twelve hours, depending on temperature.

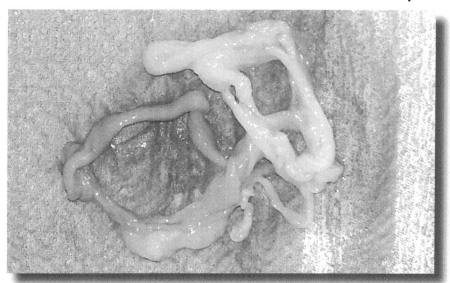

A great photo of a dead parasite, believed to be the Ascaris lumbricoides, or possibly a rope worm in the "seaweed" stage.

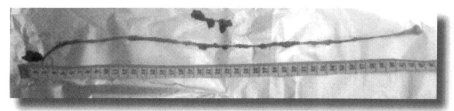

A very good look at how long some helminths are. The more worms the people pass, the healthier they get, and the improvements come faster and faster. This child passed a lot of parasites in the beginning. Then after a few months was no longer passing them and now has an ATEC score of 5. Meaning, he no longer has the diagnosis of autism.

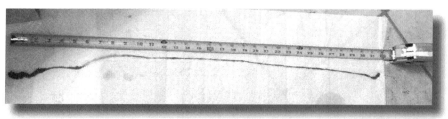

This is the parasite that measured 32 inches.

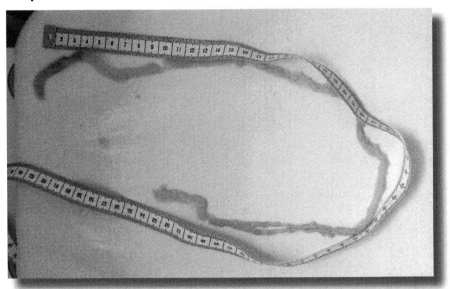

Another long, well washed parasite for the collection. The road to recovery is paved with many dead parasites. Adios Autism...

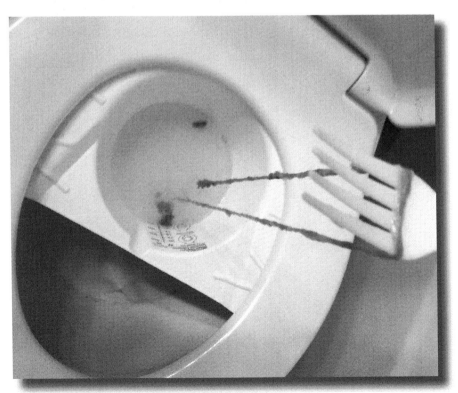

This is a 32-inch parasite that a young boy passed. He went on to have a great day after getting this out.

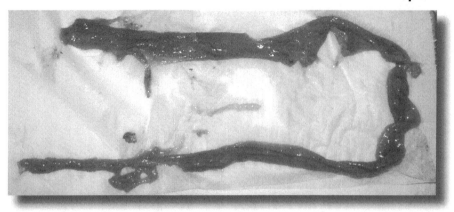

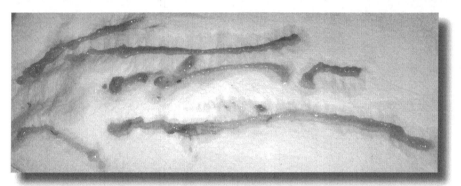

These are rope parasites as confirmed by Dr. Alex Volinsky.

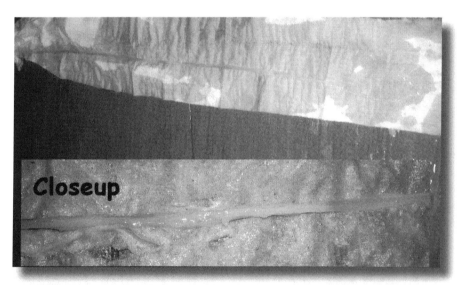

60cm long worm (Oct 1, 2013) from child; 6 months on CD; 2 drops every 1-2hr; no parasite protocol; 1tblsp DE; 2-3 vials of Quinton.

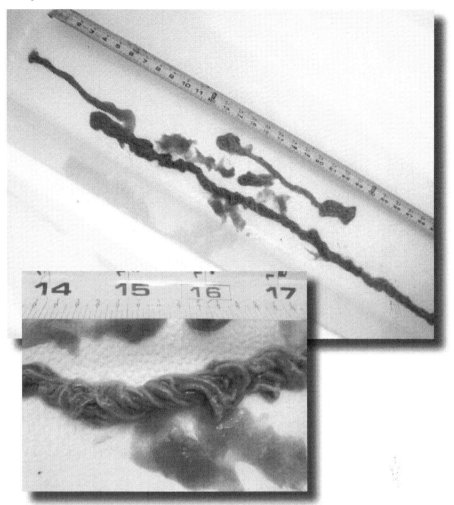

This 33 inch parasite (aka "Chester") was discovered by a woman using the protocol on herself.

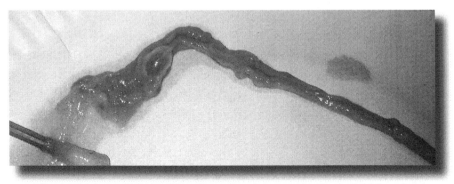

The bubble visible in this photo leads us to believe this is a late stage rope worm.

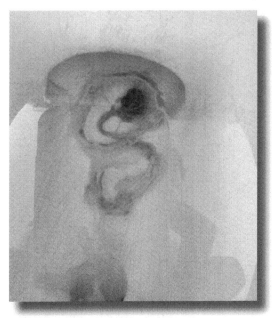

After passing this parasite, the child went on to have a fabulous day at school. It is so great to feel good and healthy.

The FDA recommends freezing and storing [fish] at -4°F (-20°C) or below for seven days (total time), or freezing at -31°F (-35°C) or below until solid and storing at -31°F (-35°C) or below for 15 hours, or freezing at -31°F (-35°C) or below until solid and storing at -4°F (-20°C) or below for 24 hours is sufficient to kill parasites. FDA's Food Code recommends these freezing conditions to retailers who provide fish intended for raw consumption. Note: These conditions may not be suitable for freezing particularly large fish (e.g. thicker than six inches).[2]

▶ From drinking contaminated water.

▶ From consuming contaminated vegetables or fruits. Often we eat poorly washed (parasite infested) vegetables or fruits. There is a common misconception that vegetables from organic farming are free from any problems, pesticides, or chemicals. The danger is that the eggs or larvae of the worms reach the farm soil through animal waste, decomposed forms of natural compost, and manure (fertilizer) added to the field. There are eggs, such as Ascaris lumbricoides, which can survive in soil under extreme temperatures for five years. It is very important to perform a thorough cleaning of fruits and vegetables, and never eat anything raw and straight from the ground, however healthy it may seem.

▶ From parasite infested animals. Parasitic infections are very easy to spread by contact with pets. Veterinarians are quick to insist upon the quarterly deworming of our animals, but there are steps we must take on our own to avoid contamination.

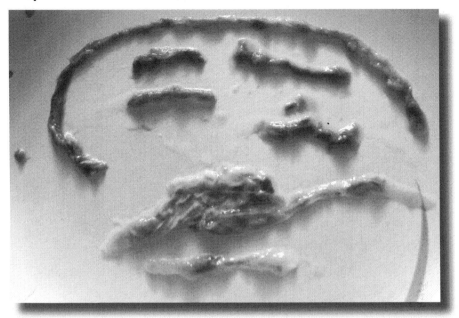

Parasites come in all shapes and sizes. Of course, they can also come out in pieces.

Suggested: Deworm your pet at least every three months for life, as directed by your veterinarian. During the first month, it should be done every week. Prevent pets from eating raw viscera. If animals eat raw meat or raw bones the best option is to freeze the food in advance for at least 12 hours (See citation above). If the deworming treatment is working, the animal will expel the worms in the feces or vomit, which must then be burned or buried, during the eight-day treatment.

Avoid being licked in the mouth by animals as they are in direct contact with feces, soil, and their own anus. When petting an animal, wash your hands with soap and water before eating or handling food, as the eggs of the parasites remain in the animal's hair.

▶ Do not walk barefoot or with open toe shoes in soil or sand.

▶ Avoid Hippotherapy (horseback riding)

Symptoms of Parasitic Infections

The different types of worms and toxic waste produced by parasites in our body may cause the following common problems:

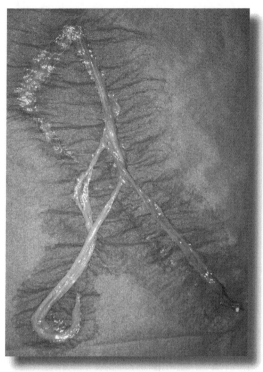

Parasites come in all sizes. Some are very long. These get washed with hot water for photos. This way we get the best look at them.

Blood Disorders & Blood Parasite Diseases

Parasites absorb essential nutrients from the body, such as iron, vitamin B_{12}, and sugars, which may result in certain blood disorders. In addition, some diseases are known to be caused by blood parasites:

Blood disorders:

- Anemia
- Dizziness
- Hypoglycemia
- Weakness

Blood parasite diseases:

- African Sleeping Sickness
- Babesiosis
- Chagas Disease
- Malaria

Fatigue:

The toxic waste produced by the parasites themselves (including ammonia and psychoactive substances), can stress the detox organs and cause disorders of the central nervous system such as:

- Chronic fatigue syndrome (CFS)
- Cold in the extremities
- Dizziness
- Extreme weakness
- Internal cold
- Lethargy
- Low energy
- Night waking
- Restless sleep

Gastrointestinal Symptoms

- Abdominal pain or tenderness
- Blood in stool
- Burning in the stomach
- Chronic constipation
- Chronic diarrhea or diarrhea caused by poor absorption of food
- Colitis
- Cramping
- Cravings for greasy foods and sugary foods, lots of carbs and bread, fruit, fruit juices, alcohol, or vinegar
- Digestive problems
- Distended belly
- Eating more than normal but still feeling hungry
- Excessive bowel movements
- Fever
- Frequent vomiting and nausea
- Gas and bloating (noted after eating)
- Hemorrhoids
- Irritable bowel syndrome (IBS)
- Intestinal irritation
- Intestinal obstruction
- Leaky gut
- Malabsorption syndrome
- Mucous in stool
- Pancreatitis
- Passing a worm in stool

Growth Problems, Weight, & Appetite

Parasites usually live without being detected by the host. They rob the body of many of the essential nutrients in the food consumed. Many overweight people, who are infected with parasites, go hungry for lack of essential nutrients, causing them to eat in excess due to their parasitic infection. Furthermore, depending on the type of infestation, many people are malnourished and cannot gain weight. The following is a list of some possible symptoms:

In children:

- Poor growth
- Poor physical and intellectual development consistent with their biological age

In children and adults:

- Chronic burping
- Craving white flour products; cookies, cakes, pastries, etc.
- Feeling hungry after a meal
- Inability to gain or lose weight
- Long-term obesity
- Loss of appetite
- Obsession and/or compulsion to eat sweets or very specific foods (wheat, sugar, dairy)
- Ravenous appetite
- Uncontrollable hunger to eat more than usual
- Weight gain (specifically around the time of the full moon)
- Weight loss

Mood Problems & Anxiety

Toxins that are released by parasites can irritate the central nervous system. Anxiety and nervousness are often caused by parasites that migrate throughout the body. Some of the problems caused are:

- Anger and irritability
- Anxiety
- Confused thinking (brain fog)
- Depression
- Disorientation
- Forgetfulness
- Lack of coordination
- Mood swings

- Nervousness
- Obsession
- Restlessness
- Slow reflexes

Muscle & Joint Pain

Parasites can travel almost anywhere in the body. When they migrate to the joints and the muscles they can cause cysts and inflammation. These can often be mistaken for arthritis and/or muscle pain.

Toxins from parasites can also accumulate in the joints and muscle tissue causing:

- Chest pains
- Fibromyalgia
- Joint pain
- Muscle cramps
- Muscle spasms
- Numbness of the hands or feet
- Pain in the back, thighs, or shoulders
- Pain in the navel
- Rapid heartbeat
- Restless leg syndrome
- Seizures

Parasites in Children
(including children with ASDs)

Parasites can be found in the body in asymptomatic and symptomatic stages. The former are usually found in adults. Symptomatic stages occur mainly in children, in whom we can often observe the following:

- Anorexia
- Anxiety
- Bruxism (teeth grinding)
- Cramping
- Diarrhea that alternates with periods of constipation
- Excessive Flapping
- Growth retardation
- Headaches
- Inability to gain weight
- Itching/Burning/Picking of the anus
- Nasal itching and/or anal urticaria (hives/rash)
- Nervousness and irritability

- Nose Picking
- OCD (Obsessive Compulsive Disorder)
- Rage
- Smearing feces
- Unexplained laughter or weeping
- Verbal stims
- Weight loss

Tapeworms, and some other parasites, have an affinity for B_{12} and iron. Therefore, lab results that show deficiencies in B_{12} and/or iron can be indicators of parasitic infections.[3,4] Due to its size, the tapeworm consumes enormous amounts of food that it obtains by taking the child's food. This can affect the child's normal development.

Treatment is simple, but it requires that the head of the tapeworm be removed, otherwise it will continue to grow. Tapeworm treatment is separate from this protocol and usually requires niclosamide. However, the only way to be sure the head has been removed is to identify it in the stool.

Respiratory Disease

The passage of larvae through the respiratory system or larval invasion in the lungs may cause symptoms such as:

- Acute bronchitis
- Asthma
- Drowsiness
- Dyspnea (shortness of breath; air hunger)
- Chronic/irritative cough
- Pneumonia
- Shortness of breath or respiratory failure

Sexual & Reproductive Disorders

Immune dysfunction as a result of a parasitic infection can lead to:

- Candida - yeast infections
- Cysts and fibroids
- Erectile dysfunction
- Fluid retention
- Male impotence
- Menstrual problems
- Premenstrual syndrome
- Prostate problems
- Urinary Tract Infections

Skin Disorders & Allergies

External parasites (lice, bedbugs, scabies, etc.) that penetrate the skin can cause itching, redness, and/or rashes etc. However, internal parasites can be responsible for skin disorders as well. Parasites create toxic metabolic waste, and because the skin is the largest organ, the body tries to eliminate them through it, resulting in many skin problems.

Some symptoms may include:

- Allergies (to foods, dust, mold, etc.)
- Anal itching
- Brittle hair
- Crawling sensation under the skin
- Dermatitis
- Dry hair
- Dry skin
- Eczema
- Eruptions
- Hair loss
- Itchy nose
- Itchy skin
- Jaundice
- Psoriasis
- Skin ulcers
- Sores
- Swelling
- Urticaria (hives; skin rash)

Sleep Disorders

The body reacts to parasites during rest periods because at night is when parasites are most active. Nocturnal awakenings are common, especially between 2 and 3am, when the liver tries to rid the body of toxins produced by parasites. This in turn may produce:

- Insomnia
- Teeth grinding
- Bedwetting
- Drooling while sleeping
- Sleep disturbances - multiple awakenings during the night
- Restless sleep

Other Problems Associated with Parasites

- Bad breath

- Blurred vision

- Body odor

- Breathing problems

- Chronic infections: viral or bacterial

- Circulatory problems, numbness in the extremities, difficulty in moving

- Cough or coughing up blood

- Difficulty swallowing

- Excessive salivation

- Fever

- Fluid build-up or retention during the time of the full moon.

- Low immune response

- Peritonitis

- Sensation of a foreign body or discomfort in the throat

- Swollen eyes

- Weight gain during the full moon.

Blood Analysis

The following markers may be present when a person is suffering from a parasitic infection or the resulting allergies:

- Anemia/low iron

- Elevated immunoglobulin (IgE)

- Elevated eosinophils (The eosinophil is a specialized cell of the immune system, more specifically it is a proinflammatory white blood cell. According to the Registry for Eosinophilic Gastrointestinal Disorders (REGID), their known functions include movement to inflamed areas, trapping substances, killing cells, antiparasitic, and bactericidal activity, participating in allergic reactions, and modulating inflammatory responses.)

- High ammonia

- High oxalates

- Low vitamin B_{12}

Measures in the Home Environment
to Prevent Reinfection

It is important to treat all people and pets that live in the same environment to prevent someone from infecting others. Reinfection occurs via underwear, bedding, towels and household items such as children's toys or animals that have been in contact with eggs. It is important to wash all clothing that has contact with intimate body areas at a temperature not below 60°C (140°F).

All bed linen and underwear must be washed daily (or to the extent possible) while performing anti-parasitic therapy. Affected individuals should not share their swimwear with other members of the family, and should use a separate cloth to wash his anal area. It is best to sleep wearing both underwear and pants to avoid involuntary scratching during the night. This will prevent infection through anal-hand-mouth contact because by scratching the anal area, eggs can become lodged under the fingernails. Keep pets away from the place of rest of their owners, such as beds, sofas, blankets, and cushions.

Thoroughly wash fruits and vegetables in water and soak them in CD or CDS solution for a few minutes. Clean the sink with alcohol, as the eggs of many parasites are immune to the pH of normal cleaning products such as soap or bleach. It is important to note that parasites do not leave any kind of immunity behind in the host, therefore, once cured, the person who has suffered can suffer from them again. The only surefire method of killing the eggs of *Ascaris lumbricoides* is in water above 60°C (140°F) or with 96% grain alcohol (Everclear).

Evolutionary Cycles
of Intestinal Parasites

Although there are many more, here is a description of the three most common types of intestinal parasites that can be found in developed countries:

Ascaris Lumbricoides (Roundworm)

Ascaris reproduce quickly, as a single female can lay up to 200,000 eggs each day. This parasite is very common, especially in damp conditions, and when hygiene measures are inadequate. It can affect the entire population, but mostly affects children, seriously disrupting their development and growth. It's so infectious that the WHO estimates that there are about 700,000,000 people infected worldwide, of which around 60,000 cases end in death per year, mainly children.[5]

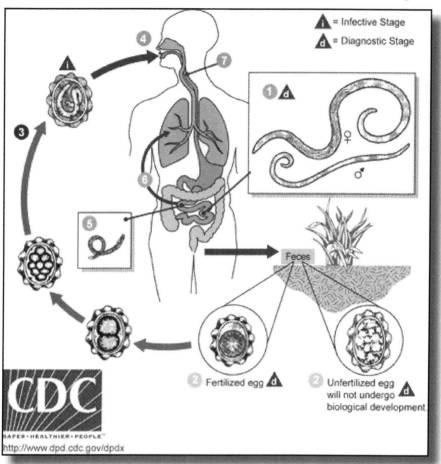

Parasite eggs reach the duodenum through the mouth of the host. Gastric juices rid the eggs of their shells and release the larvae. These larvae, which are highly mobile, penetrate the duodenal mucosa and migrate to the liver. From there, they continue their migration to the heart, reaching the lungs through pulmonary circulation, and finally become trapped in the pulmonary capillaries. Here, the larvae break the thin walls of the capillaries and penetrate the alveoli, bronchioles, and bronchi at which point they are able to travel up through the pharynx. Once the eggs pass the epiglottis (see diagram above), the larvae are swallowed such that they return to the duodenum, where they complete their maturation process. This process takes approximately two to three months to complete; therefore we calculate that to find ourselves completely parasite free, the initial treatment should be done for at least 12-18 months, possibly longer. From there on out, you may only need to follow a routine deworming two to four times a year.

Keep in mind that eggs are expelled through the feces (human or animal) into the environment where they can survive even in harsh conditions, favoring the persistence of the parasite. They are resistant to low temperatures, desiccation, strong acids, soaps, chlorine, formaldehyde (pH between 2 and 11.5), and can live in planted soils for five or more years, creating a "parasite hotbed" that makes them almost indestructible. Once dry, they are transported through the air, fly in air currents like dust that can be inhaled and/or swallowed. We have recovered eggs from nasal mucus, paper currency, potting soil, dust, and in indoor airborne particles, etc.

Taenia Saginata and *Taenia Solium* (Tapeworm)

Taenias reach humans when humans eat their eggs, by the consumption of tissue from infected cattle or pigs. In infected animals, the larvae are encysted in the muscle tissue. If the infected animal is consumed, development may proceed in the human digestive system. Humans are hosts for *T. saginata* (beef tapeworm) and *T. solium* (pork tapeworm). The tapeworm is considered to be solitary, because usually no more than four species are found in any one individual host. The danger of this parasite is that the larvae can migrate to the brain, or other vital organs (cysticercosis). Tapeworms may be detected by identifying segments in the host's stool that the worms discard as they grow. However, tapeworms may go undetected for many years, living asymptomatically within their host.

According to classification, they can vary in size ranging from 2 to 12 meters in length. They consist of a head called the scolex, which attaches to the intestine by means of suction cups, and a body consisting of repeating units called proglottids. A single Taenia can grow from 1,000 to 2,000 proglottids, depending on the type. A tapeworm produces an average of 720,000 eggs per day.

Pinworms (*Enterobius Vermicularis*)

Humans are considered the only host of what are commonly called pinworms (*Enterobius vermicularis*). This type of worm is the most typical in the family because it propagates easily. It is common for children to become reinfected in schools, through contact with others, or through anal-hand-mouth contact. Pinworms have an elongated shape, are whitish in color, and are about 1cm long. They inhabit the large intestine of humans. Female pinworms leave eggs around the anus. Once deposited, the eggs are infectious for a period of up to 20 days. Once in the intestine, it takes between five and eight weeks to develop into adult worms. The most important symptom is intense itching that occurs in the anal area, especially at night. In women, inflammation of the vulvar area is very common.

A pinworm infection is, generally speaking, not very serious. Unlike other parasites, they infect only humans. Transmission from person-to-person happens by handling clothing, bed sheets, towels, and environmental surfaces (such as curtains, carpeting) contaminated with pinworm eggs, which are so light that they are able to become airborne. A small number of eggs can be integrated into air particles that when inhaled follow the same developmental process as ingested eggs. Enemas are extremely useful in removing this parasite from the large intestine.

Graham's method is a simple method of detection. Just after waking and before a bowel movement, press a piece of tape against the anal folds. The tape will catch the remains of eggs and/or parasites that are situated there. With the naked eye we can see small worms no more than an inch long, but with a microscope, many transparent eggs from females and even other species may be seen.

The Importance of Lifelong Deworming

Once we begin the process of deworming, we should recognize that we must maintain this habit of cleaning for the rest of our lives to enjoy good health. It is common among people who have pets, to follow the recommendations of their veterinarians, and deworm their pets every three months. It is interesting to ask why family physicians do not give the same advice to humans. Perhaps some physicians ignore this information, or simply do not consider it important to eliminate these pests, which are just as harmful to people as they are for animals.

It is true that many parasites are not endemic or common outside certain climates, but human migration and global marketing of food products have facilitated the spread of many parasitic pests silently. It is important that we understand the lifecycle of each parasite, from birth to death including reproductive and death stages. This information is crucial for the complete elimination of the parasite. For example, in the case of intestinal parasites treated here with this protocol, some can live in the host for up to ten years, as in the case of a single Taenia, while others may remain in the host for a lifetime, reproducing again and again, as in the case of the pinworms or the well-known Ascaris.

The Kalcker Parasite Protocol & Lunar Cycle Timing

In the modern civilization in which we live, we have lost touch with much of the ancient wisdom of the past. One of the things we have forgotten is how the natural cycle of the moon influences many of nature's routines. This is especially true for the behavior of parasites. They are known to sync their life-cycle with that of the lunar cycle. Your child may demonstrate extreme behaviors on certain lunar cycle days... especially on the full moon and sometimes even the new moon.

Therefore, to maximize effectiveness, this Parasite Protocol is specifically timed to the lunar cycle. Appendix 10, page 477 provides an easy reference for you to look up the days to perform the Parasite Protocol, which is administered over 19 days—numbered 0 to 18—each month; starting three days prior to the full moon and continue during the waning moon. This period of the moon's cycle is very effective for deworming because many nematodes (parasitic worms) travel back into the intestine to mate at this time.

Length of Treatment

This protocol is not a one-time treatment. You should plan for at least 12 to 18 months to insure you have purged multiple parasite life-cycles and continue beyond 12 months if your child is still expelling parasites.

Building on CD

This protocol builds on what you have already learned using CD. During treatment, it is absolutely necessary to continue CD dosing, CD baths and CD enemas.

Tape Worms

This protocol is specifically designed for the deworming of large intestinal parasites, especially round nematodes such as Ascaris. It is effective for most nematodes, but may not be effective against tapeworms. In the case of infestation by Taenias, the recommended treatment is Niclosamide, the preferred medication due to its low toxicity.

Components of the Kalcker Parasite Protocol

This protocol uses some of what you have already learned and should already be doing, along with a set of ingredients you will need to have on hand before you start (shown in bold below). Here is an overview list of the items you will need to have on hand, and the items are described in detail on the pages that follow:

- Meal time (1, 2, 3)
- CD / CDS (4-19)
- CD Baths (20)
- CD Enemas (21, 22)
- Ocean Water (23, 24, 25) (see page 115)
- **Diatomaceous Earth** (26, 27)
- **Lepidium Latifolium Extract (Rompepiedras)** or **Chanca Piedra (Stone Breaker)** (28, 29)
- **Pyrantel Pamoate (Combantrin®)** (30, 31)
- **Mebendazole** (32-36)
- **Castor Oil** (37)
- **Neem** (39, 40)
- **Probiotic (usually THERALAC®)** (41)

Check the following website for the latest information on where to find these products:

www.ProtocolSuppliers.com

You may have noticed one or more numbers in parenthesis following each of the previous items, such as "(40)" for the probiotic. The timing of what to give when, is covered in great detail in the daily charts starting on page 198. These numbers match those found on the daily sample charts to make it easier for you to connect the dots and also be able to identify related notes under each chart. They have nothing to do with the quantity/dosing of any substance. The use of these numbers allows us to comment on specific items and when and where they come into play as shown on the daily sample charts.

We now detail each one of the items on the list above and discuss what you need to know about them and how to acquire them (including their associated numbers on the charts).

Meals (1, 2, 3)

Obviously meals are part of everyone's day. The purpose in mentioning them here is that many of the following steps are related to meal timing. Some actions or ingredients are taken before breakfast, others during or after.

In our example charts, we make some assumptions which include:

- Breakfast (1) is at 7:30am
- Lunch (2) is at 12 noon
- Dinner (3) is at 5pm

CD, CDS or CDH (4-19)

As you learned in Chapter 5, you continue to dose CD (or CDS/CDH) as before during the Parasite Protocol. Nothing changes in that regard with the Parasite Protocol building on top of those steps already in place.

The sample charts assume your child is going to school, and so you may not be able to administer doses of CD during his school day (7-12) unless you are home-schooling, in which case you are encouraged to give hourly CD doses, even if the total exceeds 8 for the day.

CD Baths (Optional) (20)

Our sample charts assume you administer a CD bath just before bedtime. See pages 113 for more information about CD baths.

CD Enemas (21, 22)

Ideally, give your child a CD enema in the morning (21) and another one in the evening (22). However, if your child is going to school, a morning (21) enema may not be a good idea due to the possibility of an "accident." Therefore, consider the morning enema optional, but the night time enema a must do! See page 103 for more information.

Ocean Water (23, 24, 25)

Supplementing ocean water minerals is important to support the body through the detoxification process. See page 115 for more information on ocean water.

Dosing:

(23) A dose of ocean water should be administered upon waking, but five minutes apart from CD dosing.

(24) One dose of ocean water immediately after school (or at lunch time if at home).

(25) One dose of ocean water, 15 minutes before or after dinner.

Diatomaceous Earth (DE) - Food Grade (26, 27)

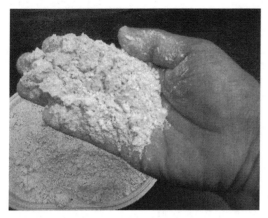

Diatoms are unicellular plants that existed by the trillions in our oceans over 300 million years ago. They are encased by a cell wall that is made of silica. When diatoms die, this microscopic coating deposits at the bottom of oceans. Over time, they pile up in banks forming deposits thousands of meters in size. With the receding of the oceans, these deposits have been uncovered. Through compression, and ultimately fossilization, these silica deposits have given rise to a chalk rock called diatomaceous earth.

DE is an inert, nontoxic compound, which contains a number of minerals such as manganese, magnesium, iron, titanium, calcium silicates, and others. Properly ground, the skeletons of microscopic diatoms become sharp silica needles, harmful to parasites, fungi, yeast, worms, and amoebas. However, these needles are harmless to humans and other warm-blooded animals. Although it is safe to consume diatomaceous earth continuously, the best method (as with everything else) is to allow for periods of rest. During the 18-day treatment, take two teaspoons (5ml) twice a day.

Dosing: ½ to 1 teaspoon twice a day for smaller kids, 1 teaspoon three times a day for adults and bigger kids. Mix with a little water and drink. Given on days 1 through 18. DE mixes well with water but never dissolves. Stir the DE/water slurry vigorously and drink immediately before the DE settles to the bottom. Some people take heaping tablespoons in water, but larger amounts are not necessary. DO NOT take dry!

Note: In rare cases, DE can cause constipation, which can usually be managed by reducing the dosages to 1/2, 1/4 or even 1/8th of a teaspoon. If that doesn't resolve the issue, remove DE from the protocol and continue with all other directions.

Source & Cost: Search online for "Food Grade Diatomaceous Earth." Buy at least 1 pound and expect to pay about $20 more or less. Better yet, buy a five pound bag, which will reduce your cost per pound. DE does not expire or degrade, but should be kept in a dry container. Note: Diatomaceous Earth is often used as non-toxic element in pool filtration systems. You DO NOT want to use this kind of DE since it has been processed. Only get "Food Grade" Diatomaceous Earth!

Lepidium Latifolium Extract
(aka Rompepiedras or Pepperwort) or
Chanca Piedra (aka Stone Breaker) (28, 29)

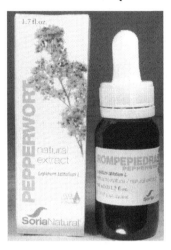
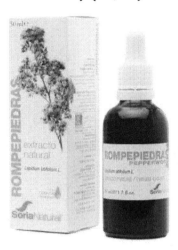
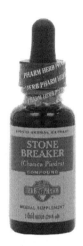

Lepidium Latifolium (Rompepiedras) and Chanca Piedra (Stone Breaker) both break up hard substances in the body. The reason we use it in this protocol is two-fold: It breaks up the protective outer coating of parasites, and annihilates oxalates, which many of our kids have an abundance of because oxalates are produced by parasites.

Note #1: It is often simply referred to as "RP" in our discussion forums.

Note #2: If you are having trouble finding this particular ingredient, don't let its absence stop you from starting the protocol with all other ingredients.

Dosing: 15 drops for a 100 pound child mixed in with the diatomaceous earth/water. Use seven drops for smaller children.

Source & Cost: You have a choice of two herb extracts; Lepidium Latifolium Extract (aka Rompepiedras or Pepperwort) and Chanca Piedra (aka Stone Breaker). One US source is www.mightyguts.com, which sells a 50ml dropper bottle of Pepperwort for about $30. A primary manufacturer in Europe is Soria Natural from Spain that labels their product Rompepiedras, while they also have an English labeled box that says Pepperwort. They both show Lepidium Latifolium on the box.

Pyrantel Pamoate (30, 31)
(Trilombrin/Combantrin®)

Pyrantel pamoate is a broad spectrum anthelmintic, which works by causing a neuromuscular block that produces spastic paralysis of the parasite, and its subsequent expulsion by intestinal peristaltic action, without excitation of the parasites or encouragement of their migration. Pyrantel pamoate acts over a short duration, and tends to be completely eliminated from the body in the feces and urine within three to four days. Pyrantel pamoate is poorly absorbed from the gastrointestinal tract, and approximately 6 to 8% total is found in the urine, with the remainder in the feces. The recommended dose is one daily dose of 10 mg per kilo.

Pyrantel pamoate is incompatible with the use of piperazine, because the two substances neutralize each other. Thus Pyrantel pamoate should not be combined with pumpkin seeds, which contain piperazine, or with antiparasitic drugs that contain piperazine in their formulation.

Dosing: Pyrantel pamoate is given only twice during one cycle of the parasite protocol; once during breakfast on day one (30), and again during breakfast on day five (31). Dose is based on weight and calculated by multiplying your child's weight in kilograms times 10mg of pyrantel pamoate. To make it easy, refer to the following chart:

Pyrantel Pamoate (Trilobrin/Combantrin®) Dosing by Weight		
Pounds	Kilograms	Dose in mg.
20	9	91
40	18	181
60	27	272
80	36	363
100	45	454
120	54	544
140	64	635
160	73	726
180	82	816
200	91	907
220	100	998
240	109	1089

Pyrantel pamoate (often just referred to as Combantrin®) is available in three forms:

- **Liquid:** where each milliliter contains a certain number of milligrams. For example, one available formulation contains 144mg/ml. So a 100lb child would take 3ml.
- **Tablets:** where each usually contains 250mg.
- **Capsules:** where each usually contains 250mg.

You will have to read the label or the particular product you acquire and determine the milligrams to use.

Source: Combantrin® is available by prescription in the US. Most other countries have it available over the counter.

The preferred source of pyrantel pamoate is a compounding pharmacy, as to avoid coloring and flavoring. If you are unable to find it without coloring/flavoring then I would personally use mebendazole for the entire 18 days rather than risk giving your child an ingredient which may cause regression.

Note #1: Some brands of Combantrin® include mebendazole. You want the stand-alone Combantrin®!

Note: #2 Pumpkin seeds should not be consumed with pyrantel pamoate because they neutralize its effects.

Mebendazole (Vermox®/Lomper®) (32-36)

Mebendazole is a drug used in treating diseases caused by helminths (parasites of the gastrointestinal tract). This drug prevents the parasite from using glucose, which results in a decrease in energy and therefore death of the parasite.

Mebendazole is a non-systemic drug which means it is only absorbed, to a limited extent, in the gastrointestinal tract (approximately 5 to 10%). However, if it is consumed with fatty foods then more absorption occurs.

Approximately 2% of the administered mebendazole is excreted in the urine, while the remainder is excreted in the feces. The appropriate dose of mebendazole may be different for each patient as it depends on the type of parasite causing the infection.[6] The most frequently recommended dose is 100mg for children, 200 mg for adults, two times a day for seven of the first nine days of the Protocol.

Adverse effects from mebendazole are generally rare due to its poor absorption. However, it may cause nausea, vomiting, abdominal pain, and diarrhea. Normally these effects are in fact a result of the release of toxins from the very death of the parasite itself. Anti-parasitic drugs can be administered very effectively by diluting them in water, putting the mixture in a small bulb enema, and inserting the anally. This is especially suitable in the case of oxyuriasis (pinworms). Read more about this "implant method" on page 220.

Dosing:

Note: Indicated weights should only be considered a rough guide.

<u>Small Children (20-40lbs.):</u> Days 2, 3, 4, 6, 7, 8 & 9 — Take as little as 25mg of mebendazole with breakfast and dinner, and do NOT do a blitz on Day 9.

<u>Children (41-70lbs.):</u> Days 2, 3, 4, 6, 7, & 8 — 50mg with breakfast and dinner. On Day 9 they can take 50mg, 50mg and 25mg.

<u>Adolescents (71-100lbs.):</u> Days 2, 3, 4, 6, 7, & 8 — 100mg during breakfast and 100mg during dinner. Day 9 is "Mebendazole Blitz Day" where you administer ONE 200mg dose during breakfast; ONE 200mg dose at lunch; and a final 100mg dose at dinner.

<u>Teens & Adults (101 lbs. and up):</u> Days 2, 3, 4, 6, 7, & 8 — 200mg during breakfast and 200mg during dinner. Day 9 is "Mebendazole Blitz Day" where you administer ONE 500mg dose during breakfast and no dose at lunch or dinner for the remainder of the current cycle.

Source: Mebendazole is available by prescription in the US and over the counter in other countries.

Note #1: Some brands combine mebendazole with Combantrin®. You want the stand-alone mebendazole!

Note #2: Mebendazole is mostly sold in tablet form, but it is also available in liquid. DO NOT buy the liquid form—stick with the tablets! I have seen horrible reactions from the "inert" vehicles used in the liquid products.

Castor Oil (37)

Castor oil is extracted from the seed of a plant called Ricinus communis
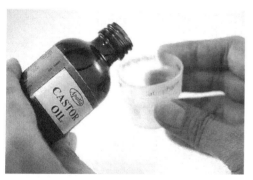
("Higuera del diablo"). Its seeds contain between 50-80% oil, which has a high content of ricinoleic acid, which has excellent laxative and purgative properties. Once you begin anti-parasitic treatments, spastic paralysis may occur in some parasites and many together may form a "knot" of worms that can cause intestinal obstruction. It is important to help your body

purge them by using castor oil. Castor oil should be taken in the morning, two hours after breakfast and other medications. If your child goes to school they take it as soon as they walk in the door from school. A typical dose for a child is 1/2 tsp to 1 tsp, or up to tolerance. The adult dosage is 15 to 30ml (two tablespoons), two hours after breakfast and other medications. If you experience any intestinal distress, mineral purgatives such as Epsom salts, or vegetable purgatives such as senna leaves, can be used.

Castor oil is also available in gelcaps for those who dislike the taste.

Dosing: The amount to administer varies and really depends on the individual's tolerance. A good starting point is ½ teaspoon for smaller children and up to two tablespoons for larger children and adults. Only experimentation will determine the right amount, if castor oil causes diarrhea.

Source & Cost: Readily available in liquid form at most pharmacies in the laxative section. Usually under $10 for 16oz. Also available online.

Neem (Azadirachta indica), Caps or Tea (38, 39)

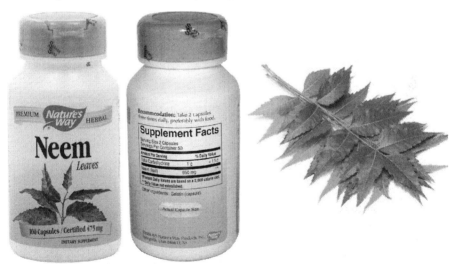

The neem tree is a great natural inheritance of mankind. References in Sanskrit scriptures and ayurvic medicine practices indicate the use of neem since ancient times in Hindu medicine. Even today, Hindus living in rural areas call the neem tree the "village pharmacy" for its ability to alleviate many diseases and is currently endorsed by authorities in India for its use in medicinal preparations. Neem is one of the purifying and detoxifying plants with the greatest potential. Neem has been used to combat all forms of body parasites, external and internal parasites alike. To prepare neem, boil four leaves (normally the contents of an envelope) in one liter of water for five minutes. Drink the tea throughout the day over the course of each parasite protocol.

Dosing: Neem is given each parasite protocol from day 10 through Day 18.

You have a choice of caps or tea. I prefer caps over tea because the taste is strong and unpleasant, so some kids will buck drinking tea.

Caps (assuming 475mg each): An adult takes six in a day, three times two caps at meal times.

Follow the directions on the bottle. Give a full dose for teens and adults 100 lbs. and over. Small children receive ¼ to ½ dose.

If using caps, give one dose during breakfast and one dose at dinner.

Tea: Give four doses throughout the day. Prepare a tea from the leaves, one tea bag in one liter of water (add stevia if needed to cover some of the bitter taste). One tea bag usually contains approximately four leaves. If using loose leaves, then make one liter of tea with four neem leaves. If using crushed leaves, then use approximately one slightly heaping teaspoon.

Neem Tea Dosing	
Weight of Person	**Total Daily Amount (To be split into 4 doses)**
20-34 lbs	100 ml
35-49 lbs	200 ml
50-64	300 ml
65-84	400 ml
85-109	500 ml
110 and over	600 ml

Source & Cost: Neem capsules cost about $8 for 100x 475mg caps. Look in your local health food store. One popular brand in the US is Nature's Way®. BioPure™ sells a product called *Neem Synergy* which contains a few additional herbs that do not affect the neem.

Neem tea can be purchased in bags or as dried leaves.

THERALAC® (Probiotic) (40)

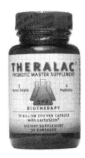

THERALAC® is a probiotic that should be given during the parasite protocol to help reestablish good gut flora. Ideally, it is rotated every other month with THERALAC® TruFlora®.

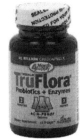

The key reason for recommending THERALAC® over other probiotics is explained in this paragraph excerpted from their website:

THERALAC® probiotics survive transit through the harsh acidity of the stomach and arrive alive in the intestinal tract. THERALAC's ACID PROOF™ technology utilizes sodium alginate from seaweed in a unique formulation that assures survival at pH 1.6 for 90 minutes, the most severe stomach acid conditions normally experienced. Other probiotics that claim acid resistance are tested at pH 2.5 – 3.0, or >10 times less acidic than pH 1.6 – not a fair test. THERALAC's ACID PROOF® technology is protected by US Patents 7,122,370 and 7,229,818. This technology goes beyond resisting stomach acid and involves keeping the probiotic cells together in a viscous alginate-gel moving in group-force, not as separate individual cells like other probiotics, deep into the intestinal tract while retaining key formula ingredients, LactoStim® and Sodium Alginate in close proximity.

Dosing: One capsule of THERALAC® is given each and every night at bedtime, irrelevent of age/weight. This probiotic is also to be given outside of the 19 Parasite Protocol days.

THERALAC® can be given at the same time as CD if your child swallows capsules. However, if you are using the THERALAC® powder form then give it at least five to ten minutes after the last CD dose of the night. See their website for more information about the powder form.

Special exception: Some people do not tolerate probiotics, in which case we have no choice but to leave them out. In some of these cases, sauerkraut and fermented veggies may help to cultivate beneficial bacteria.

Source & Cost: Amazon carries "THERALAC® 30 caps by Master Supplements Inc." for $37.

Sample Parasite Protocol Daily Calendar

To assist you in understanding the Parasite Protocol and how it changes from day to day, we have prepared the following visual set of daily charts showing how all the pieces fit together. To prepare this set of charts, we made up the following times for example purposes only:

- Your child's awake time is between 6am and 10pm.
- Breakfast is at 7:30am
- Your child goes to school, which starts at about 9am
- School is out at about 2:30pm
- Dinner is at 5pm

As stated earlier, each dose or activity is labeled with a unique number. Those numbers relate to notes below each chart AND they match longer descriptive notes in the previous pages.

You are encouraged to copy/enlarge the blank chart in Appendix 9 (page 475) and workout your real-life schedule based on these example charts.

Refer to the lunar calendar (Appendix 10, page 477) for the exact days the protocol should be followed, as well as to get an idea of behaviors related to parasites around the full and new moon.

After four years of biomed and no major gains, we decided to try mms/cd protocol. We started in April and are currently on our second parasite protocol. Initially, we were really intimidated by the enema part but realized if we were apprehensive our 7 yr old daughter would pick up on that. We told her that what we were about to do would help her feel better we gave her the iPad right before the procedure and a new fav toy (beanie boos) and she was game. After it was over she said "no more booboo in my tummy". We all cried. To make a three-month adventure short and sweet, her team at school cannot figure out how her fragmented speech has gone from 2-3 word utterances to long, drawn out sentences. Her expressive language and receptive have increased. Her auditory processing speed has quadrupled. The most amazing part thus far has been the increase in social skills. Or just the fact that she is interested in engaging. Socially she was nonexistent and is now at a four year old level. We just spent a week with family and she was saying hi and engaging without being prompted!!! She now has a million questions, wants to know when and where we are going and the sequence in which events will take place. All this from a girl who never asked questions before mms! STOP thinking about trying! Just Do It!! For the first time in seven years, I can hear the bells of freedom ringing!!!! Thank you Kerri Rivera !!!!

Day 0 (3 days before Full-Moon)

Time	Meal Time	CD / CDS / CDH	CD / CDS / CDH Bath	CD / CDS / CDH Enema	Ocean Water	Diatomaceous Earth	Lepidium Latifolium Extract (Rompepiedras / RP)	Pyrantel Pamoate (Combantrin)	Mebendazole	Castor Oil	Neem	Probiotic
6:00 AM		4		21	23							
6:30 AM												
7:00 AM		5										
7:30 AM	1											
8:00 AM		6										
8:30 AM												
9:00 AM		7										
9:30 AM												
10:00 AM		8										
10:30 AM												
11:00 AM		9										
11:30 AM												
12:00 PM	2											
12:30 PM												
1:00 PM		11										
1:30 PM												
2:00 PM		12										
2:30 PM												
3:00 PM		13			24							
3:30 PM												
4:00 PM		14										
4:30 PM												
5:00 PM	3											
5:30 PM												
6:00 PM		16		22								
6:30 PM												
7:00 PM		17			25							
7:30 PM												
8:00 PM		18										
8:30 PM												
9:00 PM		19	20									
9:30 PM												40

Day 0 - Notes:	
1, 2, 3	Breakfast, Lunch & Dinner
4 - 19	At least 8 CD doses throughout the day, preferably more, at least 30 to 60 minutes away from food.
20	CD Bath at the end of the day.
21, 22	Enema in the morning (optional) and in the evening (mandatory).
23 - 25	3 doses of ocean water at least 5 minutes away from CD.
40	Probiotic at the end of the day

Day 1 (2 days before Full-Moon)

Time	Meal Time	CD / CDS / CDH	CD / CDS / CDH Bath	CD / CDS / CDH Enema	Ocean Water	Diatomaceous Earth	Lepidium Latifolium Extract (Rompepiedras / RP)	Pyrantel Pamoate (Combantrin)	Mebendazole	Castor Oil	Neem	Probiotic
6:00 AM		4		21	23							
6:30 AM												
7:00 AM		5										
7:30 AM	1					26	28	30				
8:00 AM		6										
8:30 AM										*		
9:00 AM		7										
9:30 AM												
10:00 AM		8										
10:30 AM												
11:00 AM		9										
11:30 AM												
12:00 PM	2											
12:30 PM												
1:00 PM		11										
1:30 PM												
2:00 PM		12										
2:30 PM												
3:00 PM		13			24					37		
3:30 PM												
4:00 PM		14										
4:30 PM												
5:00 PM	3					27	29					
5:30 PM												
6:00 PM		16		22								
6:30 PM												
7:00 PM		17		25								
7:30 PM												
8:00 PM		18										
8:30 PM												
9:00 PM		19	20									
9:30 PM												40

Day 1 - Notes:	
1, 2, 3	Breakfast, Lunch & Dinner
4 - 19	At least 8 CD doses throughout the day, preferably more, at least 30 to 60 minutes away from food.
20	CD Bath at the end of the day.
21, 22	Enema in the morning (optional) and in the evening (mandatory).
23 - 25	3 doses of ocean water at least 5 minutes away from CD.
26 - 29	Diatomaceous Earth and Lepidium Latifolium with breakfast and dinner.
30	Dose of Combantrin with breakfast
* 37	Castor oil 1 hour after breakfast or immediately upon return from school.
40	Probiotic at the end of the day

Day 2 (1 day before Full-Moon)

Time	Meal Time	CD / CDS / CDH	CD / CDS / CDH Bath	CD / CDS / CDH Enema	Ocean Water	Diatomaceous Earth	Lepidium Latifolium Extract (Rompepiedras / RP)	Pyrantel Pamoate (Combantrin)	Mebendazole	Castor Oil	Neem	Probiotic
6:00 AM		4		21	23							
6:30 AM												
7:00 AM		5										
7:30 AM	1					26	28		32			
8:00 AM		6										
8:30 AM												
9:00 AM		7										
9:30 AM												
10:00 AM		8										
10:30 AM												
11:00 AM		9										
11:30 AM												
12:00 PM	2											
12:30 PM												
1:00 PM		11										
1:30 PM												
2:00 PM		12										
2:30 PM												
3:00 PM		13		24								
3:30 PM												
4:00 PM		14										
4:30 PM												
5:00 PM	3					27	29		33			
5:30 PM												
6:00 PM		16		22								
6:30 PM												
7:00 PM		17		25								
7:30 PM												
8:00 PM		18										
8:30 PM												
9:00 PM		19	20									
9:30 PM												40

Day 2 - Notes:	
1, 2, 3	Breakfast, Lunch & Dinner
4 - 19	At least 8 CD doses throughout the day, preferably more, at least 30 to 60 minutes away from food.
20	CD Bath at the end of the day.
21, 22	Enema in the morning (optional) and in the evening (mandatory).
23 - 25	3 doses of ocean water at least 5 minutes away from CD.
26 - 29	Diatomaceous Earth and Lepidium Latifolium with breakfast and dinner.
32, 33	Small Child Dose: 100mg Mebendazole with breakfast and dinner. Teen/Adult Dose: 200mg Mebendazole with breakfast and dinner.
40	Probiotic at the end of the day

Day 3 (Full-Moon)

Time	Meal Time	CD / CDS / CDH	CD / CDS / CDH Bath	CD / CDS / CDH Enema	Ocean Water	Diatomaceous Earth	Lepidium Latifolium Extract (Rompepiedras / RP)	Pyrantel Pamoate (Combantrin)	Mebendazole	Castor Oil	Neem	Probiotic
6:00 AM		4		21	23							
6:30 AM												
7:00 AM		5										
7:30 AM	1					26	28		32			
8:00 AM		6										
8:30 AM										*		
9:00 AM		7										
9:30 AM												
10:00 AM		8										
10:30 AM												
11:00 AM		9										
11:30 AM												
12:00 PM	2											
12:30 PM												
1:00 PM		11										
1:30 PM												
2:00 PM		12										
2:30 PM												
3:00 PM		13		24						37		
3:30 PM												
4:00 PM		14										
4:30 PM												
5:00 PM	3					27	29		33			
5:30 PM												
6:00 PM		16		22								
6:30 PM												
7:00 PM		17		25								
7:30 PM												
8:00 PM		18										
8:30 PM												
9:00 PM		19	20									
9:30 PM												40

Day 3 - Notes:	
1, 2, 3	Breakfast, Lunch & Dinner
4 - 19	At least 8 CD doses throughout the day, preferably more, at least 30 to 60 minutes away from food.
20	CD Bath at the end of the day.
21, 22	Enema in the morning (optional) and in the evening (mandatory).
23 - 25	3 doses of ocean water at least 5 minutes away from CD.
26 - 29	Diatomaceous Earth and Lepidium Latifolium with breakfast and dinner.
32, 33	Small Child Dose: 100mg Mebendazole with breakfast and dinner. Teen/Adult Dose: 200mg Mebendazole with breakfast and dinner.
* 37	Castor oil 1 hour after breakfast or immediately upon return from school.
40	Probiotic at the end of the day

Day 4

Time	Meal Time	CD / CDS / CDH	CD / CDS / CDH Bath	CD / CDS / CDH Enema	Ocean Water	Diatomaceous Earth	Lepidium Latifolium Extract (Rompepiedras / RP)	Pyrantel Pamoate (Combantrin)	Mebendazole	Castor Oil	Neem	Probiotic
6:00 AM		4		21	23							
6:30 AM												
7:00 AM		5										
7:30 AM	1					26	28		32			
8:00 AM		6										
8:30 AM												
9:00 AM		7										
9:30 AM												
10:00 AM		8										
10:30 AM												
11:00 AM		9										
11:30 AM												
12:00 PM	2											
12:30 PM												
1:00 PM		11										
1:30 PM												
2:00 PM		12										
2:30 PM												
3:00 PM		13			24							
3:30 PM												
4:00 PM		14										
4:30 PM												
5:00 PM	3					27	29		33			
5:30 PM												
6:00 PM		16		22								
6:30 PM												
7:00 PM		17			25							
7:30 PM												
8:00 PM		18										
8:30 PM												
9:00 PM		19	20									
9:30 PM												40

Day 4 - Notes:	
1, 2, 3	Breakfast, Lunch & Dinner
4 - 19	At least 8 CD doses throughout the day, preferably more, at least 30 to 60 minutes away from food.
20	CD Bath at the end of the day.
21, 22	Enema in the morning (optional) and in the evening (mandatory).
23 - 25	3 doses of ocean water at least 5 minutes away from CD.
26 - 29	Diatomaceous Earth and Lepidium Latifolium with breakfast and dinner.
32, 33	Small Child Dose: 100mg Mebendazole with breakfast and dinner. Teen/Adult Dose: 200mg Mebendazole with breakfast and dinner.
40	Probiotic at the end of the day

Day 5

Time	Meal Time	CD / CDS / CDH	CD / CDS / CDH Bath	CD / CDS / CDH Enema	Ocean Water	Diatomaceous Earth	Lepidium Latifolium Extract (Rompepiedras / RP)	Pyrantel Pamoate (Combantrin)	Mebendazole	Castor Oil	Neem	Probiotic
6:00 AM		4		21	23							
6:30 AM												
7:00 AM		5										
7:30 AM	1					26	28	31				
8:00 AM		6										
8:30 AM										*		
9:00 AM		7										
9:30 AM												
10:00 AM		8										
10:30 AM												
11:00 AM		9										
11:30 AM												
12:00 PM	2											
12:30 PM												
1:00 PM		11										
1:30 PM												
2:00 PM		12										
2:30 PM												
3:00 PM		13			24					37		
3:30 PM												
4:00 PM		14										
4:30 PM												
5:00 PM	3					27	29					
5:30 PM												
6:00 PM		16		22								
6:30 PM												
7:00 PM		17		25								
7:30 PM												
8:00 PM		18										
8:30 PM												
9:00 PM		19	20									
9:30 PM												40

Day 5 - Notes:	
1, 2, 3	Breakfast, Lunch & Dinner
4 - 19	At least 8 CD doses throughout the day, preferably more, at least 30 to 60 minutes away from food.
20	CD Bath at the end of the day.
21, 22	Enema in the morning (optional) and in the evening (mandatory).
23 - 25	3 doses of ocean water at least 5 minutes away from CD.
26 - 29	Diatomaceous Earth and Lepidium Latifolium with breakfast and dinner.
31	Dose of Combantrin with breakfast (NO Mebendazole today!)
* 37	Castor oil 1 hour after breakfast or immediately upon return from school.
40	Probiotic at the end of the day

Day 6

Time	Meal Time	CD / CDS / CDH	CD / CDS / CDH Bath	CD / CDS / CDH Enema	Ocean Water	Diatomaceous Earth	Lepidium Latifolium Extract (Rompepiedras / RP)	Pyrantel Pamoate (Combantrin)	Mebendazole	Castor Oil	Neem	Probiotic
6:00 AM		4		21	23							
6:30 AM												
7:00 AM		5										
7:30 AM	1					26	28		32			
8:00 AM		6										
8:30 AM												
9:00 AM		7										
9:30 AM												
10:00 AM		8										
10:30 AM												
11:00 AM		9										
11:30 AM												
12:00 PM	2											
12:30 PM												
1:00 PM		11										
1:30 PM												
2:00 PM		12										
2:30 PM												
3:00 PM		13			24							
3:30 PM												
4:00 PM		14										
4:30 PM												
5:00 PM	3					27	29		33			
5:30 PM												
6:00 PM		16		22								
6:30 PM												
7:00 PM		17			25							
7:30 PM												
8:00 PM		18										
8:30 PM												
9:00 PM		19	20									
9:30 PM												40

Day 6 - Notes:	
1, 2, 3	Breakfast, Lunch & Dinner
4 - 19	At least 8 CD doses throughout the day, preferably more, at least 30 to 60 minutes away from food.
20	CD Bath at the end of the day.
21, 22	Enema in the morning (optional) and in the evening (mandatory).
23 - 25	3 doses of ocean water at least 5 minutes away from CD.
26 - 29	Diatomaceous Earth and Lepidium Latifolium with breakfast and dinner.
32, 33	Small Child Dose: 100mg Mebendazole with breakfast and dinner. Teen/Adult Dose: 200mg Mebendazole with breakfast and dinner.
40	Probiotic at the end of the day

Day 7

Time	Meal Time	CD / CDS / CDH	CD / CDS / CDH Bath	CD / CDS / CDH Enema	Ocean Water	Diatomaceous Earth	Lepidium Latifolium Extract (Rompepiedras / RP)	Pyrantel Pamoate (Combantrin)	Mebendazole	Castor Oil	Neem	Probiotic
6:00 AM		4		21	23							
6:30 AM												
7:00 AM		5										
7:30 AM	1					26	28		32			
8:00 AM		6										
8:30 AM										*		
9:00 AM		7										
9:30 AM												
10:00 AM		8										
10:30 AM												
11:00 AM		9										
11:30 AM												
12:00 PM	2											
12:30 PM												
1:00 PM		11										
1:30 PM												
2:00 PM		12										
2:30 PM												
3:00 PM		13		24						37		
3:30 PM												
4:00 PM		14										
4:30 PM												
5:00 PM	3					27	29		33			
5:30 PM												
6:00 PM		16		22								
6:30 PM												
7:00 PM		17		25								
7:30 PM												
8:00 PM		18										
8:30 PM												
9:00 PM		19	20									
9:30 PM												40

Day 7 - Notes:	
1, 2, 3	Breakfast, Lunch & Dinner
4 - 19	At least 8 CD doses throughout the day, preferably more, at least 30 to 60 minutes away from food.
20	CD Bath at the end of the day.
21, 22	Enema in the morning (optional) and in the evening (mandatory).
23 - 25	3 doses of ocean water at least 5 minutes away from CD.
26 - 29	Diatomaceous Earth and Lepidium Latifolium with breakfast and dinner.
32, 33	Small Child Dose: 100mg Mebendazole with breakfast and dinner. Teen/Adult Dose: 200mg Mebendazole with breakfast and dinner.
* 37	Castor oil 1 hour after breakfast or immediately upon return from school.
40	Probiotic at the end of the day

Day 8

Time	Meal Time	CD / CDS / CDH	CD / CDS / CDH Bath	CD / CDS / CDH Enema	Ocean Water	Diatomaceous Earth	Lepidium Latifolium Extract (Rompepiedras / RP)	Pyrantel Pamoate (Combantrin)	Mebendazole	Castor Oil	Neem	Probiotic
6:00 AM		4		21	23							
6:30 AM												
7:00 AM		5										
7:30 AM	1					26	28		32			
8:00 AM		6										
8:30 AM												
9:00 AM		7										
9:30 AM												
10:00 AM		8										
10:30 AM												
11:00 AM		9										
11:30 AM												
12:00 PM	2											
12:30 PM												
1:00 PM		11										
1:30 PM												
2:00 PM		12										
2:30 PM												
3:00 PM		13			24							
3:30 PM												
4:00 PM		14										
4:30 PM												
5:00 PM	3					27	29		33			
5:30 PM												
6:00 PM		16		22								
6:30 PM												
7:00 PM		17			25							
7:30 PM												
8:00 PM		18										
8:30 PM												
9:00 PM		19	20									
9:30 PM												40

Day 8 - Notes:	
1, 2, 3	Breakfast, Lunch & Dinner
4 - 19	At least 8 CD doses throughout the day, preferably more, at least 30 to 60 minutes away from food.
20	CD Bath at the end of the day.
21, 22	Enema in the morning (optional) and in the evening (mandatory).
23 - 25	3 doses of ocean water at least 5 minutes away from CD.
26 - 29	Diatomaceous Earth and Lepidium Latifolium with breakfast and dinner.
32, 33	Small Child Dose: 100mg Mebendazole with breakfast and dinner. Teen/Adult Dose: 200mg Mebendazole with breakfast and dinner.
40	Probiotic at the end of the day

Day 9 (Mebendazole Blitz Day)

Time	Meal Time	CD / CDS / CDH	CD / CDS / CDH Bath	CD / CDS / CDH Enema	Ocean Water	Diatomaceous Earth	Lepidium Latifolium Extract (Rompepiedras / RP)	Pyrantel Pamoate (Combantrin)	Mebendazole	Castor Oil	Neem	Probiotic
6:00 AM		4		21	23							
6:30 AM												
7:00 AM		5										
7:30 AM	1					26	28		34			
8:00 AM		6										
8:30 AM										*		
9:00 AM		7										
9:30 AM												
10:00 AM		8										
10:30 AM												
11:00 AM		9										
11:30 AM												
12:00 PM	2											
12:30 PM												
1:00 PM		11										
1:30 PM												
2:00 PM		12										
2:30 PM									35			
3:00 PM		13			24					37		
3:30 PM												
4:00 PM		14										
4:30 PM												
5:00 PM	3					27	29		36			
5:30 PM												
6:00 PM		16		22								
6:30 PM												
7:00 PM		17			25							
7:30 PM												
8:00 PM		18										
8:30 PM												
9:00 PM		19	20									
9:30 PM												40

Day 9 - Notes:	
1, 2, 3	Breakfast, Lunch & Dinner
4 - 19	At least 8 CD doses throughout the day, preferably more, at least 30 to 60 minutes away from food.
20	CD Bath at the end of the day.
21, 22	Enema in the morning (optional) and in the evening (mandatory).
23 - 25	3 doses of ocean water at least 5 minutes away from CD.
26 - 29	Diatomaceous Earth and Lepidium Latifolium with breakfast and dinner.
34	Blitz Day - Small Child Dose 1: 200mg Mebendazole with breakfast. Teen/Adult Dose: 500mg Mebendazole with breakfast ONLY!
35	Blitz Day - Dose 2: 200mg Mebendazole with lunch (or right after school) Teen/Adult Dose: N/A
36	Blitz Day - Dose 3: 100mg Mebendazole with dinner. Teen/Adult Dose: N/A
* 37	Castor oil 1 hour after breakfast or immediately upon return from school.
40	Probiotic at the end of the day

Day 10

Time	Meal Time	CD / CDS / CDH	CD / CDS / CDH Bath	CD / CDS / CDH Enema	Ocean Water	Diatomaceous Earth	Lepidium Latifolium Extract (Rompepiedras / RP)	Pyrantel Pamoate (Combantrin)	Mebendazole	Castor Oil	Neem	Probiotic
6:00 AM		4		21	23							
6:30 AM												
7:00 AM		5										
7:30 AM	1					26	28				38	
8:00 AM		6										
8:30 AM												
9:00 AM		7										
9:30 AM												
10:00 AM		8										
10:30 AM												
11:00 AM		9										
11:30 AM												
12:00 PM	2											
12:30 PM												
1:00 PM		11										
1:30 PM												
2:00 PM		12										
2:30 PM												
3:00 PM		13			24							
3:30 PM												
4:00 PM		14										
4:30 PM												
5:00 PM	3					27	29				39	
5:30 PM												
6:00 PM		16		22								
6:30 PM												
7:00 PM		17			25							
7:30 PM												
8:00 PM		18										
8:30 PM												
9:00 PM		19	20									
9:30 PM												40

Day 10 - Notes:	
1, 2, 3	Breakfast, Lunch & Dinner
4 - 19	At least 8 CD doses throughout the day, preferably more, at least 30 to 60 minutes away from food.
20	CD Bath at the end of the day.
21, 22	Enema in the morning (optional) and in the evening (mandatory).
23 - 25	3 doses of ocean water at least 5 minutes away from CD.
26 - 29	Diatomaceous Earth and Lepidium Latifolium with breakfast and dinner.
38, 39	Start dosing Neem Caps with breakfast and dinner. If using tea, 4 doses throughout the day.
40	Probiotic at the end of the day

Day 11

Time	Meal Time	CD / CDS / CDH	CD / CDS / CDH Bath	CD / CDS / CDH Enema	Ocean Water	Diatomaceous Earth	Lepidium Latifolium Extract (Rompepiedras / RP)	Pyrantel Pamoate (Combantrin)	Mebendazole	Castor Oil	Neem	Probiotic
6:00 AM		4		21	23							
6:30 AM												
7:00 AM		5										
7:30 AM	1					26	28				38	
8:00 AM		6										
8:30 AM												
9:00 AM		7										
9:30 AM												
10:00 AM		8										
10:30 AM												
11:00 AM		9										
11:30 AM												
12:00 PM	2											
12:30 PM												
1:00 PM		11										
1:30 PM												
2:00 PM		12										
2:30 PM												
3:00 PM		13			24							
3:30 PM												
4:00 PM		14										
4:30 PM												
5:00 PM	3					27	29				39	
5:30 PM												
6:00 PM		16		22								
6:30 PM												
7:00 PM		17			25							
7:30 PM												
8:00 PM		18										
8:30 PM												
9:00 PM		19	20									
9:30 PM												40

Day 11 - Notes:	
1, 2, 3	Breakfast, Lunch & Dinner
4 - 19	At least 8 CD doses throughout the day, preferably more, at least 30 to 60 minutes away from food.
20	CD Bath at the end of the day.
21, 22	Enema in the morning (optional) and in the evening (mandatory).
23 - 25	3 doses of ocean water at least 5 minutes away from CD.
26 - 29	Diatomaceous Earth and Lepidium Latifolium with breakfast and dinner.
38, 39	Neem Caps with breakfast and dinner. If using tea, 4 doses throughout the day.
40	Probiotic at the end of the day

Day 12

Time	Meal Time	CD / CDS / CDH	CD / CDS / CDH Bath	CD / CDS / CDH Enema	Ocean Water	Diatomaceous Earth	Lepidium Latifolium Extract (Rompepiedras / RP)	Pyrantel Pamoate (Combantrin)	Mebendazole	Castor Oil	Neem	Probiotic
6:00 AM		4		21	23							
6:30 AM												
7:00 AM		5										
7:30 AM	1					26	28				38	
8:00 AM		6										
8:30 AM										*		
9:00 AM		7										
9:30 AM												
10:00 AM		8										
10:30 AM												
11:00 AM		9										
11:30 AM												
12:00 PM	2											
12:30 PM												
1:00 PM		11										
1:30 PM												
2:00 PM		12										
2:30 PM												
3:00 PM		13			24					37		
3:30 PM												
4:00 PM		14										
4:30 PM												
5:00 PM	3					27	29				39	
5:30 PM												
6:00 PM		16		22								
6:30 PM												
7:00 PM		17		25								
7:30 PM												
8:00 PM		18										
8:30 PM												
9:00 PM		19	20									
9:30 PM												40

Day 12 - Notes:	
1, 2, 3	Breakfast, Lunch & Dinner
4 - 19	At least 8 CD doses throughout the day, preferably more, at least 30 to 60 minutes away from food.
20	CD Bath at the end of the day.
21, 22	Enema in the morning (optional) and in the evening (mandatory).
23 - 25	3 doses of ocean water at least 5 minutes away from CD.
26 - 29	Diatomaceous Earth and Lepidium Latifolium with breakfast and dinner.
* 37	Castor oil 1 hour after breakfast or immediately upon return from school.
38, 39	Neem Caps with breakfast and dinner. If using tea, 4 doses throughout the day.
40	Probiotic at the end of the day

Day 13

Time	Meal Time	CD / CDS / CDH	CD / CDS / CDH Bath	CD / CDS / CDH Enema	Ocean Water	Diatomaceous Earth	Lepidium Latifolium Extract (Rompepiedras / RP)	Pyrantel Pamoate (Combantrin)	Mebendazole	Castor Oil	Neem	Probiotic			
6:00 AM		4		21	23										
6:30 AM															
7:00 AM		5													
7:30 AM	1					26	28				38				
8:00 AM		6													
8:30 AM															
9:00 AM		7													
9:30 AM															
10:00 AM		8													
10:30 AM															
11:00 AM		9													
11:30 AM															
12:00 PM	2														
12:30 PM															
1:00 PM		11													
1:30 PM															
2:00 PM		12													
2:30 PM															
3:00 PM		13			24										
3:30 PM															
4:00 PM		14													
4:30 PM															
5:00 PM	3					27	29				39				
5:30 PM															
6:00 PM		16		22											
6:30 PM															
7:00 PM		17			25										
7:30 PM															
8:00 PM		18													
8:30 PM															
9:00 PM		19	20												
9:30 PM													40		

Day 13 - Notes:	
1, 2, 3	Breakfast, Lunch & Dinner
4 - 19	At least 8 CD doses throughout the day, preferably more, at least 30 to 60 minutes away from food.
20	CD Bath at the end of the day.
21, 22	Enema in the morning (optional) and in the evening (mandatory).
23 - 25	3 doses of ocean water at least 5 minutes away from CD.
26 - 29	Diatomaceous Earth and Lepidium Latifolium with breakfast and dinner.
38, 39	Neem Caps with breakfast and dinner. If using tea, 4 doses throughout the day.
40	Probiotic at the end of the day

Day 14

Time	Meal Time	CD / CDS / CDH	CD / CDS / CDH Bath	CD / CDS / CDH Enema	Ocean Water	Diatomaceous Earth	Lepidium Latifolium Extract (Rompepiedras / RP)	Pyrantel Pamoate (Combantrin)	Mebendazole	Castor Oil	Neem	Probiotic
6:00 AM		4		21	23							
6:30 AM												
7:00 AM		5										
7:30 AM	1					26	28				38	
8:00 AM		6										
8:30 AM												
9:00 AM		7										
9:30 AM												
10:00 AM		8										
10:30 AM												
11:00 AM		9										
11:30 AM												
12:00 PM	2											
12:30 PM												
1:00 PM		11										
1:30 PM												
2:00 PM		12										
2:30 PM												
3:00 PM		13			24							
3:30 PM												
4:00 PM		14										
4:30 PM												
5:00 PM	3					27	29				39	
5:30 PM												
6:00 PM		16		22								
6:30 PM												
7:00 PM		17			25							
7:30 PM												
8:00 PM		18										
8:30 PM												
9:00 PM		19	20									
9:30 PM												40

Day 14 - Notes:	
1, 2, 3	Breakfast, Lunch & Dinner
4 - 19	At least 8 CD doses throughout the day, preferably more, at least 30 to 60 minutes away from food.
20	CD Bath at the end of the day.
21, 22	Enema in the morning (optional) and in the evening (mandatory).
23 - 25	3 doses of ocean water at least 5 minutes away from CD.
26 - 29	Diatomaceous Earth and Lepidium Latifolium with breakfast and dinner.
38, 39	Neem Caps with breakfast and dinner. If using tea, 4 doses throughout the day.
40	Probiotic at the end of the day

Day 15

Time	Meal Time	CD / CDS / CDH	CD / CDS / CDH Bath	CD / CDS / CDH Enema	Ocean Water	Diatomaceous Earth	Lepidium Latifolium Extract (Rompepiedras / RP)	Pyrantel Pamoate (Combantrin)	Mebendazole	Castor Oil	Neem	Probiotic
6:00 AM		4		21	23							
6:30 AM												
7:00 AM		5										
7:30 AM	1					26	28				38	
8:00 AM		6										
8:30 AM										*		
9:00 AM		7										
9:30 AM												
10:00 AM		8										
10:30 AM												
11:00 AM		9										
11:30 AM												
12:00 PM	2											
12:30 PM												
1:00 PM		11										
1:30 PM												
2:00 PM		12										
2:30 PM												
3:00 PM		13			24					37		
3:30 PM												
4:00 PM		14										
4:30 PM												
5:00 PM	3					27	29				39	
5:30 PM												
6:00 PM		16		22								
6:30 PM												
7:00 PM		17			25							
7:30 PM												
8:00 PM		18										
8:30 PM												
9:00 PM		19	20									
9:30 PM												40

Day 15 - Notes:	
1, 2, 3	Breakfast, Lunch & Dinner
4 - 19	At least 8 CD doses throughout the day, preferably more, at least 30 to 60 minutes away from food.
20	CD Bath at the end of the day.
21, 22	Enema in the morning (optional) and in the evening (mandatory).
23 - 25	3 doses of ocean water at least 5 minutes away from CD.
26 - 29	Diatomaceous Earth and Lepidium Latifolium with breakfast and dinner.
* 37	Castor oil 1 hour after breakfast or immediately upon return from school.
38, 39	Neem Caps with breakfast and dinner. If using tea, 4 doses throughout the day.
40	Probiotic at the end of the day

Day 16

Time	Meal Time	CD / CDS / CDH	CD / CDS / CDH Bath	CD / CDS / CDH Enema	Ocean Water	Diatomaceous Earth	Lepidium Latifolium Extract (Rompepiedras / RP)	Pyrantel Pamoate (Combantrin)	Mebendazole	Castor Oil	Neem	Probiotic
6:00 AM		4		21	23							
6:30 AM												
7:00 AM		5										
7:30 AM	1					26	28				38	
8:00 AM		6										
8:30 AM												
9:00 AM		7										
9:30 AM												
10:00 AM		8										
10:30 AM												
11:00 AM		9										
11:30 AM												
12:00 PM	2											
12:30 PM												
1:00 PM		11										
1:30 PM												
2:00 PM		12										
2:30 PM												
3:00 PM		13		24								
3:30 PM												
4:00 PM		14										
4:30 PM												
5:00 PM	3					27	29				39	
5:30 PM												
6:00 PM		16		22								
6:30 PM												
7:00 PM		17		25								
7:30 PM												
8:00 PM		18										
8:30 PM												
9:00 PM		19	20									
9:30 PM												40

Day 16 - Notes:	
1, 2, 3	Breakfast, Lunch & Dinner
4 - 19	At least 8 CD doses throughout the day, preferably more, at least 30 to 60 minutes away from food.
20	CD Bath at the end of the day.
21, 22	Enema in the morning (optional) and in the evening (mandatory).
23 - 25	3 doses of ocean water at least 5 minutes away from CD.
26 - 29	Diatomaceous Earth and Lepidium Latifolium with breakfast and dinner.
38, 39	Neem Caps with breakfast and dinner. If using tea, 4 doses throughout the day.
40	Probiotic at the end of the day

Day 17

Time	Meal Time	CD / CDS / CDH	CD / CDS / CDH Bath	CD / CDS / CDH Enema	Ocean Water	Diatomaceous Earth	Lepidium Latifolium Extract (Rompepiedras / RP)	Pyrantel Pamoate (Combantrin)	Mebendazole	Castor Oil	Neem	Probiotic
6:00 AM		4		21	23							
6:30 AM												
7:00 AM		5										
7:30 AM	1					26	28				38	
8:00 AM		6										
8:30 AM												
9:00 AM		7										
9:30 AM												
10:00 AM		8										
10:30 AM												
11:00 AM		9										
11:30 AM												
12:00 PM	2											
12:30 PM												
1:00 PM		11										
1:30 PM												
2:00 PM		12										
2:30 PM												
3:00 PM		13			24							
3:30 PM												
4:00 PM		14										
4:30 PM												
5:00 PM	3					27	29				39	
5:30 PM												
6:00 PM		16		22								
6:30 PM												
7:00 PM		17			25							
7:30 PM												
8:00 PM		18										
8:30 PM												
9:00 PM		19	20									
9:30 PM												40

Day 17 - Notes:	
1, 2, 3	Breakfast, Lunch & Dinner
4 - 19	At least 8 CD doses throughout the day, preferably more, at least 30 to 60 minutes away from food.
20	CD Bath at the end of the day.
21, 22	Enema in the morning (optional) and in the evening (mandatory).
23 - 25	3 doses of ocean water at least 5 minutes away from CD.
26 - 29	Diatomaceous Earth and Lepidium Latifolium with breakfast and dinner.
38, 39	Neem Caps with breakfast and dinner. If using tea, 4 doses throughout the day.
40	Probiotic at the end of the day

Day 18

Time	Meal Time	CD / CDS / CDH	CD / CDS / CDH Bath	CD / CDS / CDH Enema	Ocean Water	Diatomaceous Earth	Lepidium Latifolium Extract (Rompepiedras / RP)	Pyrantel Pamoate (Combantrin)	Mebendazole	Castor Oil	Neem	Probiotic
6:00 AM		4		21	23							
6:30 AM												
7:00 AM		5										
7:30 AM	1					26	28				38	
8:00 AM		6										
8:30 AM										*		
9:00 AM		7										
9:30 AM												
10:00 AM		8										
10:30 AM												
11:00 AM		9										
11:30 AM												
12:00 PM	2											
12:30 PM												
1:00 PM		11										
1:30 PM												
2:00 PM		12										
2:30 PM												
3:00 PM		13			24					37		
3:30 PM												
4:00 PM		14										
4:30 PM												
5:00 PM	3					27	29				39	
5:30 PM												
6:00 PM		16		22								
6:30 PM												
7:00 PM		17			25							
7:30 PM												
8:00 PM		18										
8:30 PM												
9:00 PM		19	20									
9:30 PM												40

Day 18 (Last Day!) - Notes:	
1, 2, 3	Breakfast, Lunch & Dinner
4 - 19	At least 8 CD doses throughout the day, preferably more, at least 30 to 60 minutes away from food.
20	CD Bath at the end of the day.
21, 22	Enema in the morning (optional) and in the evening (mandatory).
23 - 25	3 doses of ocean water at least 5 minutes away from CD.
26 - 29	Diatomaceous Earth and Lepidium Latifolium with breakfast and dinner.
* 37	Castor oil 1 hour after breakfast or immediately upon return from school.
38, 39	Neem Caps with breakfast and dinner. If using tea, 4 doses throughout the day.
40	Probiotic at the end of the day

Parasite Protocol *Off Days*

Days "19" through to the next "Day 0" are "Off Days" where you discontinue parasite meds and herbs. Here's a simple chart showing what to continue doing and what to stop during this *off* time:

Continue with these:	Stop these:
CD / CDS / CDH Dosing	Diatomaceous Earth
CD / CDS / CDH Baths	Lepidium Latifolium
CD / CDS / CDH Enemas	Pyrantel Pamoate (Combantrin®)
Ocean Water	Mebendazol
Probiotic	Neem
	Castor Oil

Of course this represents a hypothetical case and your situation may call for taking other meds or supplements.

Detection of Parasites in Stool

It is necessary to detect the parasites by observing the stool carefully. For that we use a small plastic basin, and a plastic stick or fork for examination.

Author's Note: One of the moms who is a part of our forum came up with some guidelines for processing your child's stool for parasite identification. She calls it, "Everything You Wanted to Know About Sorting Through Poop." Here are her suggestions:

Supplies:
- rubber gloves
- paper plates
- plastic forks (plastic sticks, chop sticks, or plastic back scratcher)
- a pen
- a coin
- toilet hat

I like to use a plastic "toilet hat" also known as a specimen collector or a specimen collection unit, which goes under the toilet seat and collects the stool before it sinks into the bottom of the toilet (available on Amazon.com).

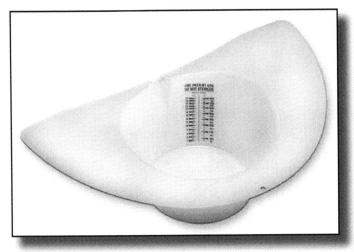

The Collection:

When your child poops, it is collected in the toilet hat (specimen collector). After I get my child cleaned up and taken care of, I remove the toilet hat from the toilet and put the specimen on a paper plate with my plastic fork. I have a look for anything interesting and then transfer that part to a clean plate using my trusty plastic fork. I discard the remainder of the specimen into the toilet, flush and put that dirty paper plate in the bathroom garbage. (We now line with kitchen garbage bags, and I change it after each of these poops.) On the clean plate with the suspected worm, I may add a bit of water and swish it around to get the worm cleaner. I then may transfer the worm to a third plastic plate to get a clear picture. On the clean plate with the washed worm, I write the date, and the initials of the person the worm came from. If you need help identifying the worm, place a penny next to the worm (for size context), snap a picture, and mail the image to kerri@cdautism.org, (Kerri collects the photos for documentation purposes, so send those worm pictures). Then flush the worm and put all paper plates, gloves, and fork in garbage and take it outside. Now, you can go find out what your child has gotten into while you were doing all this.

Clean Up:

Use HOT water (60°C/140°F), and sterilize with 96% (180 proof) grain alcohol (Everclear).

Microscope

It is very useful to have a microscope for diagnosis because it enables you to see both the small parasites that may appear in the blood, as well as eggs or larvae in the feces. This way we are more accurately able to determine if the number of parasites decreases. A simple microscope that costs about $100 is suitable for this kind of identification. The easiest method to determine what you see is to compare your sample to images you find on Google. This way you can enlarge the images, see various samples from different angles, and get a much wider variety of samples than if you were comparing a sample with many textbooks.

Bulb Enemas (aka "Implant")

To prevent anal itching from pinworms, night wakings, etc., you can use a bulb enema or small catheter/syringe with a dilution of 50mg of mebendazole in 10 to 15ml of water for small children, or 100mg of mebendazole in 15 to 20ml of water for larger children/teens/adults. The best way to do this is to introduce the medication together with the water in the rectum immediately before bedtime and hold overnight. If you are using the "implant," a morning enema is mandatory.

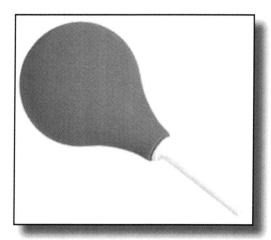

So we did the 100mg of Mebendazole with 20ml of water. He kept it in and we did it right before bed... Next day a ton of worms came out!!! Better yet he started singing songs with a tune - 3 different songs over the last 2 days and counting on his fingers very purposefully! His aide at school said he did amazing today - no behaviors, very focused, better articulation and better social interest.

The Worm Whisperer

The following words of wisdom are from a mom who has earned the nickname *The Worm Whisperer* (although her ability to destroy parasites may make the *Worm Ninja* more apropos). Her dedication and diligence have not only made the difference in the life of her son, but countless other children who are what she calls "extreme cases." The information presented here may be the difference between an older/aggressive child living with their family or going to a group home for the care that their family is no longer able to provide them. Thank you Robin, for being a pioneer and for never giving up. Thank you for having the guts, the know-how, and the generosity to share what you have learned with those who need it most.

Extreme Cases by Robin Goffe

This section is for older children who may be violent, self-injurious, destructive, physically aggressive, high risk and/or bedridden.

Some families have children who are older when they first start treatment. My son was 18 years old. We call ourselves the "last chance" group. We say this because our children have lived their whole lives infested, unbeknownst to us. Our children lived as happy, relatively easily manageable, learning-disabled children: perhaps slightly annoying with their routines of movie dialogue scripting or attachment to Disney movies, maps, or little known facts. They were mostly friendless but pretty easy to take care of. However, during the hormonal teen years, things took a grave turn. We may have chalked up their newfound solitude to just giving up socially for lack of friends. They did not fit in. We had no idea that something else was brewing. The hormones within them began to have a bitter war with the parasites living inside them, and a war would soon break out. Their mental state would diminish considerably. What we are faced with are grown, strong children who are mentally ill and violent, self-injurious, and destructive. Some have even become so ill that they had to stay in bed.

This "last chance" is an opportunity to try ONE MORE THING before putting them in a group home; to give them away—for their own safety and the safety of their families.

These things that I am going to share with you are unique to the standard treatment outlined in the book. It is a more aggressive treatment because it is needed. Our children are so highly infested that it is shocking to tell you what we have found. There is a lot to do, but there is a method. It is time

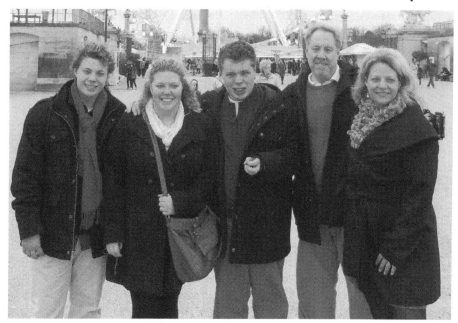

The Goffe family.

consuming and it is a lot of work. But here I will outline what we did to get our son from an aggressive, self-injurious, destructive young man to one who has regained patience, language, understanding, and reasoning; but best of all, the opportunity to remain in our home. With continued treatments, he has the hope for a future: a job perhaps, and maybe even a family of his own.

Beginning treatment for the older child and especially one who is aggressive, self-injurious, violent, and destructive is one done starting low and slow.

Day one = one drop.

I kept a very detailed journal, and I will simply tell you what we did. I will tell you what worked for us and what did not. I will also tell you what I shared with others that worked for them as well. I am not a physician. I am not a chemist. I am a mother in love with my son and his utmost comfort was my main concern. My only goal was to clear his parasites. I had no idea that the things I learned by digging through his stool for 9 months would eventually give me the nickname, "The Worm Whisperer." Although intestinal parasites have been around longer than man, and they are smart enough to live within a human being lifelong, they can go completely undetected. I was ready to plot out a war against them. By the beginning of our 9th month of treatment, I estimate that I had cleaned and examined 35 pounds (16 KG) of solid parasites. Hard to believe? I have 80% of them photographed. The last two months in jars total seven pounds and a running total of the combined length will be at over 200 feet (61 meters), at the publishing of this book. There is not a classroom in the world that can teach what I learned in my bathroom day after day in latex gloves and a hospital mask. There was a fan blowing on me to manage the stench and by the third week my gag reflex was under control.

I examined the parasites, the pieces, how did it die? What was my son feeling at the time? Was he violent? Sweating? Slapping his legs from the pain of the parasites moving around and torturing him from the inside? I needed to eliminate these worms without allowing them to cause my son pain as they were killed. I had no idea the monsters I was to face.

In March of 2013, we started our son on one drop of chlorine dioxide. One of the most feared things that the parents of adult sized children face is the dreaded enema. It is just not something that most of us grew up with as standard care. But even so, my husband and I knew it was something that made sense. There are toxins inside these kids. They must be flushed out. The bowel is the way out. So on the very first day and the very first drop, we also explained to our severely autistic child that we were going to help his belly feel better. Our son, by this time, was so severe in regression that I can only best explain him as non-human. He was no longer speaking, unable to react to us, had stopped answering to his name, and could no longer contain the saliva in his mouth. He walked with a 12-inch drool hanging from his mouth. He ate like an animal, glaring at us. He was frequently violent: jumping on cars and denting them in, kicking down fences and destroying property.

This was the child that we were going to start giving enemas to. If we could do it, anyone can.

Each day we went up a drop; two drops on day two, three drops on day three, and so on. He was edgy and tired. We went for walks, as per usual, to deal with his aggression, but by day seven he began to have a runny nose and had a great deal of fatigue. We were so happy since we knew this was a sign to look for; that the immune system was kicking in. He slept for about 15 hours as we woke him and dosed him every hour and by the next morning there were about 25 white, hairy, thin looking objects in his stool. We knew these were worms and that we had our answer. After three weeks we began to see 4-6 inch parasites in all shapes and sizes, yet the aggression continued. It was here that I learned that what we were experiencing was POWS (Pissed Off Worm Syndrome). By this point we were at 13 drops, and while we were killing the smaller parasites, we were only pissing off the larger ones. The parasites do not like their environment disturbed, and subsequently they cause distress to the host. Parasites excrete ammonia, (possibly, leading to hyperammonemia and possibly seizures), morphine, and a meth-like substance. As these toxins enter the body, they can also cause aggression and anger. We had many possessions broken during these tantrums. We stopped valuing material objects.

It was here that we were told about—double dosing. So even though our son was getting about the equivalent of two drops an hour, if we saw increased aggression, OCD or self-injurious behavior we would give him four (see page 103 for an explanation of double dosing). If he did not calm down, we gave him another four drop dose. This was the perfect return attack for the parasites. Within a few moments the aggression settled. His red face and wild eyes diminished, and we had made it past another hurdle.

We used the double dose method dozens and dozens of times over the following months, and this helped tremendously to curtail the aggression caused by the parasites.

By the third week of treatment, we were concerned about the time during the night that our son would not be getting doses. So for the next six months our family had a dosing schedule, dosing additionally at midnight, 2am, 4am and picking back up to hourly doses from 6am to 10pm. This schedule was shared by not only my husband and I, but also our son's siblings, who would also set their alarms and take their turns, while we all rotated lack of sleep.

By the second month we found that our son's behavior not only changed around the full moon but the new moon as well. The standard protocol uses mebendazole over the full moon. However, with the older, more aggressive children we have had success with including mebendazole over the new moon cycle as well. These mini mebendazole courses feature shorter bursts of 5-6 days each, over the new and full moons beginning four days before each. We also deemed it necessary to start earlier in the moon phase than with the younger kids, since the infestation was greater, and the parasite movement occurred earlier, causing behaviors sooner.

For the child that has aggression, every parent must remember that the behavior is parasite related. During treatment you will see a variety of behaviors stemming from the parasites attempting to control their environment aka— the host. We found that increasing the frequency of the dose dampened the violence and aggression. It can be difficult to trust your child who is lost in a rage. You feel deceived and hurt. Those were our frequent emotions as well. It does pass. It took about 4-5 months for the rages to stop. They happened everywhere and were happening even on the toilet while trying to expel the parasites. Have a plan. Music worked very well for us. So did reading books. Find something to distract, and always give soothing, comforting tones. We frequently told our son how much we loved him and we rubbed his head and back. These herxing behaviors may be avoided through the use of a new method of preparing CD called CDH (see Chapter 7, page 155 for more info on CDH).

CDH: This new preparation method has really been a huge asset for the older kids that need to go higher in drops. At around 20 drops, the volume of the regular CD became unpleasant, making some children nauseous. My son was one of them. With the CDH preparation, I firmly believe that the older, tough-nut children will have more success with getting to the appropriate levels needed to start expelling the larger parasites. It is my personal belief that the amount needed in many of the non-seizure older kids with aggression, violence, self-injury, and destruction to be between 75-100ml of CDH daily. This amount may have a connection to the voltage needed in order for the mitochondria in the white blood cells to be given the power to not only kill the parasites, but to also destroy the bacteria. The job is two-fold, and must be done quickly as once the parasite is dead, the bacteria want to devour them immediately. I say these things because I have seen the condition of the parasites every day. I found that if I can kill the parasite with the least amount of disturbance or preparedness by the parasite, then there is no time for them to fight back and cause herxing. The bacteria also come into play and must be dealt with. Higher amounts of CDH kill both, without so much as a frown or a concern on the face of my son.

Stevia: I found that by adding the sweetener stevia to the CDH, the process can be more pleasant and does not affect the properties or effectiveness of the dose. As proven by Lamotte ClO_2 test strips (see page 467 for information on using the test strips).

Humidifier: In the beginning months, the infestation level is so high that nightly doses may have to be sacrificed in order to start breaking down the will of the parasites. It is not about seeing them every day, but slowly and consistently breaking their will. The constant aggressive irritation of the CDH will kill parasites, stopping them from making gains. There is another layer of nighttime treatments, and that is the humidifier. We fill a cool air humidifier that holds one gallon of water, and put 35 drops of activated CD (NOT CDH) and let it run all night near our son's head. This too was a method we used for maximum parasite elimination.

Spices and Herbs: It is urgent that we work constantly with our older kids to rid the body of parasites and pathogens. We have found that for kids that can easily swallow pills, filling empty gel capsules with the recommended herbs and spices in this chapter under Other Medicinal Plants (page 231) helpful. We have found great results by filling the gelcaps with the variety mentioned there: black walnut, ginger, rue, wormwood, and yarrow and giving two to four different ones with each meal as a toxic feast to the parasites. Don't narrow your selection to those mentioned here—get them all. There is no plan or pattern. Use any combination.

Colonics: Professional colonics have been an important addition to healing and cleansing parasites in our older kids. We started these a few months after our son was accustomed to the routine enemas. This has been a wonderful addition, and we try to do at least one weekly. Some places will allow you to do inserts, and we have taken our CDH there working up to 50-100ml CDH with great success.

Limiting Undesirable Behaviors

Probiotics: If you are using probiotics and your child is aggressive or becomes aggressive after restarting the probiotics, consider removing them as a first step. There could be such a high infestation rate that the child's system does not distinguish between good bacteria and bad bacteria.

Enemas: CD enemas should start on day one of treatment for the aggressive/older child. Since they have such a high rate of infestation, it is necessary to clear the pathogens on a continuing cycle from the very beginning. Please follow instructions for enemas starting on page 103.

Diatomaceous Earth (DE): In some children, the DE may shred the larger parasites to death, causing them to spew additional toxins into the child's body, which results in herx symptoms. Discontinuing DE for a few months may help to ease the distress, and give a cleaner kill.

Salt Baths: There are times that the body is unable to pull out the toxins fast enough. Be careful about killing too fast (dosing without or not enough enemas). If you have done enemas, and there still seems to be distress, you can buy a 40-pound bag of plain pool salt, take 9 pounds of salt and put it into a hot bath. Allow the salt to dissolve and have the child soak for one hour. If the child sweats during the bath, this is a good sign, as it shows toxins are being pulled out. Do not use Epsom salts. They contain magnesium. Magnesium feeds parasites as well as biofilm. Plain pool salt is cheap, and helps to remove toxins.

Dandelion Tea: This is an incredible detoxing source as well. There have been times that our son was in and out of a salt bath all day drinking dandelion tea to get the built-up toxins out. This is a tea ready made by Traditional Medicinals® (traditionalmedicinals.com).

Tips on What to Expect During the Parasite Elimination

Intestinal parasites have been on Earth longer than humans. Their plan is to find a host, and to continue to create life. They have the home advantage by living inside of your child. There are many things that I have learned while at war with them. They have a plan and so should you.

Situations We Have Come Across

Peetox: As you kill the parasites, they are alerted that you have taken away their joyful life. As a result, they do things to the host to show their displeasure. One of the things the parasites do is to spew toxins, including a morphine-like substance that can cause your child to not feel that he needs to urinate or that he is urinating. Naturally, this can lead to accidents. This is not the child's fault, but only a part of the parasite elimination process. One of the most difficult things we did was to put our 18-year-old son in adult diapers. It was heart breaking because it felt that we were moving backwards instead for forwards. However, this was only temporary, and for his own dignity. Especially if they go to school; perhaps being in diapers for a while is the answer. Our son was in and out of them for about two months. This does end.

Sleepytox: As you are going higher in drops, the CD is assisting the immune system to get the parasites out. It will take a lot of energy to do this. Remember, your child is the host and there is a war going on! Sometimes, your child may be tired for days. Our son slept for nearly the entire summer at the beginning of his treatment. Allow the rest they seek. Now our son gets higher doses of CD on the weekends, and he is very tired and sleeps then, too. By Monday morning, we can usually get a big fat rope worm after our efforts. Sleepytox is great because you can get a lot done on your home "to do" list.

Behaviors/OCD/Tics: Some may become alarmed because their child starts having behaviors that they did not have before treatments, or they feel that the behaviors have gotten worse. Parasites have a plan. It is to stay alive and to procreate. They want their eggs to return back into a host to repeat the cycle. So, you may see behaviors of playing with feces, touching their anus to their mouth, trying to put their fingers into your mouth or another person. There are finger and nail chewing, and spitting. These are all parasite controlled behaviors. We have found that eliminating parasites helps to minimize this behavior and it will eventually subside. There may also be a mineral deficiency attached as well. We have found that giving PLENTY of ocean water can help to tame these behaviors. Our 19-year-old son gets over 200ml OW mixed with 400ml spring water per day.

POWS (Pissed-Off Worm Syndrome): POWS presents itself when you have been dosing, and your child seems weepy, is pacing, and/or unhappy. Sometimes it is really that you have pissed off the worms, but are not killing them. Always check with Kerri regarding your concerns. But many times the answer is to go up in drops not down. You need to kill them—not piss them off, or they will fight back.

Clear Zone: This time period can be about five to seven days before the full moon; once infestation is brought down after six months or more of treatment. You may be able to start seeing glimpses of your child being lucid. This is a good time for an ATEC test.

High Volume Eating: Often times, the kids reach a point where they realize that they have been starving. The parasites have been taking a bulk of their nutrients, causing their mental deficiencies. They may even be eating non-stop all day. It is tough to juggle the timing and effectiveness of the CD with the continued eating. Allowing the child to eat high volumes of food while dosing with CD will still kill the parasites, but the CD levels may not be high enough to avoid a herx. Though the parasites may be killed the CD level may not be high enough to also kill off the bacteria eating the dead parasite. One solution we found was to give our son homemade bone broth with ocean water many times a day. This will help to replace the lack of nutrients, meanwhile reducing the overeating enough to continue the CD without risking a herx reaction.

Weight Loss: Our son lost 50 pounds during the first seven months of treatment. He was very over weight at 5'9" and 200 pounds. The weight loss brought concern to people who had not seen him for long periods. During this time I estimate that 35 pounds was solid parasites. His stomach was very bloated, as was his face. Our children are full of parasites and pathogens (i.e., yeast, bacteria, etc.), and all of these things can make them gain weight or be bloated. Our son is now in the normal weight range for his height, and has a flat stomach.

Night Terrors: During the night you may see that your child has trouble settling down, or they may wake in the night screaming your name. They may even do night walking, possibly leaving out the front door in a sleepwalk state. We saw these behaviors years ago, as our son was heading into a higher infestation level. Now that we are on the healing end, many of the behaviors return as sort of a rewind. The behaviors that came into play going down the ladder are sometimes repeated heading back up the ladder to wellness. We feel that our son was experiencing separation anxiety, and the recognition that he had total control again. This new gained independence may be frightening. At a point, our son entered the peetox stage (see above). He had no feeling or sensation to urinate, so he was put into adult diapers. As our son's infestation rate decreased, the normal behaviors like waking in the night and feeling the urge to urinate returned. Then, as he would get up to go to the bathroom, he would suddenly stop, and feel perhaps lost and afraid to continue this task alone. He would scream out or wander around whimpering. Although night wakings were disturbing, we found them to be a necessary passage for bringing our son to reality. In order to give comfort, at night we continued the CD humidifier, as well as CD ear and nose drops. Many times a CD bath before bed was calming as well.

Emotional Blindness: Because the toxins that the parasites excrete are substances that have the effects of morphine, ammonia, and histamine, these toxins can cause emotional confusion in your child. They may be confused by your laughter, smiles, and affection. Your positive and loving encounter may be perceived as threatening or challenging. Your smile may bring a rage. Any spoken words by you no matter how soothing they may be, could be perceived as a confrontation. This is difficult on both parent and child, as the child may see you as a threat and perhaps even as mocking them; while you as the parent feel rejected in your affections. Many times the child's behaviors evolve into a stoned-out loss of reality and presence. These are all related to the toxic build up and defense of the parasites. Their motivation is to remain in the host; they show their displeasure to the discomforts we have given them in our elimination attempts. Many times during these episodes, we have found it best to avoid words or eye contact, but rather to offer double doses as outlined by Kerri, and keep a calm environment. We have found that these toxic levels can be lowered through salt baths and dandelion tea.

Despite the behaviors that may be brought on by a parasite protocol, the results are amazing. In our family we are finally getting our son back. I would recommend staying the course. As we know, these kinds of parasitic infestations in immune-comprised children will not go away on their own. Children do not "grow out of" worms. In fact, the worms will continue to grow inside of them. The following parasites were expelled by my older son, by making the aggressive modifications aimed at older children. By removing these parasites we are seeing the first stages of recovery. The jars on the following page represent seven pounds of worms in less than two months.

Yours in healing,
Robin

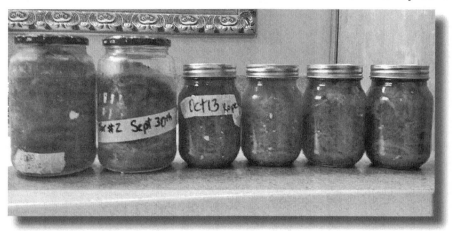

7 lbs. of 35 lbs. (total) of the parasites extracted in 9 months (160 feet in total above).

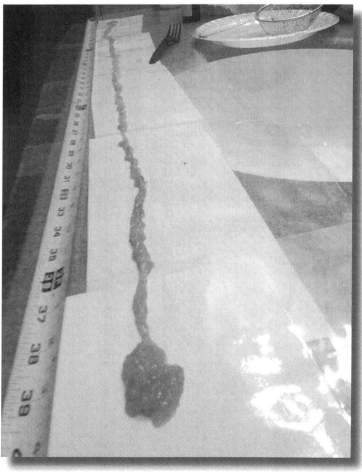

39+ inch long worm.

Other Medicinal Plants

Author's Note: The following information is extremely powerful for our continued health and well-being. However, these plants and foods ALONE have NOT been proven to heal autism. Rather, follow the 18-day deworming protocol presented starting on page 187. When this is done for 12-18 months it has proven to be an important part of the protocols that have led to the recovery of many children. With that in mind, some parents of older children, and aggressive/self-injurious children have started to implement a few of the plants and foods listed below, in addition to the aforementioned 18-day protocol. In many cases, these additions have led their children to increased gains through increased parasite elimination.

A number of other plants are also effective for deworming. If, after three months of treatment, the problem persists we can change the type of plant, or repeat any plant that was effective in previous months. We can use them in combinations, mixing several plants at once, or take them individually. Plant formulations that should be considered are alcoholic extracts, in oil or by infusion, and include the following plants:

- Clove (*Syzygium aromaticum*)
- Common Rue (*Ruta graveolens*)
- Dandelion (*Taraxacum officinale*)
- Gentian Root (*Gentiana lutea*)
- Mint (*Mentha sativa*)
- Mugwart/Common Wormwood (*Artemisia vulgaris*)
- Pomegranate Root Bark (*Punica granatum L.*)
- Southernwood (*Artemisia abrotanum*)
- Sweet Wormwood (*Artemisia annua*)
- Sweetflag/Calamus Root (*Acorus calamus*)
- Tansy (*Tanacetum vulgare*)
- Walnut shell (*Juglans*)
- White Fraxinella (*Dictamnus albus*)
- Yarrow (*Achillea millefolium*)

Preventative Food & Diet

There are groups of foods that should be avoided if you have a parasitic infection. For example, dairy products in general, refined sugars (sucrose, fructose, corn syrup), flour (especially refined), and overly sweet foods in general. The list of foods and plants below promote good internal balance of the body, hence becoming our allies. With good production of stomach acid, a normal level of healthy bacteria, and proper bile production, it is impossible for parasites to survive for long. Worms need an acidic environment that comes from the breakdown of sugars and putrefaction from the ingestion of unhealthy or processed foods. It is very important to eat raw vegetables and fruit juices, which provide us with enzymes and other elements necessary to protect us.

Choucroute/sauerkraut (fermented cabbage in salt).

Many people have low levels of stomach acid, which is the cause of many intestinal problems, because the body is unable to defend itself against intruders. Sauerkraut juice or cabbage/sauerkraut is one of the most powerful stimulants for your body to produce stomach acid. The use of unpasteurized fermented foods (water kefir, soy sauce, miso, etc.) is highly recommended for its stimulation of the beneficial bacterial flora that is responsible for generating control over parasites. Take a few spoonfuls of cabbage juice before meals, or better yet sauerkraut juice, because it will do wonders to improve your digestion.

Author's note: I do not recommend soy, in any form, for anyone with an ASD.

Garlic

Garlic, eaten regularly, turns the stomach and intestine into a lethal environment for parasites, providing constant protection. Garlic is the quintessential home remedy to eliminate intestinal parasites naturally. It has been used by many different cultures such as Chinese, Greek, Roman, Indian, and Babylonian.

Garlic is still in use today by practitioners of modern medicine. It is used both fresh and as an oil. The simplest treatment is to eat three cloves of garlic every morning, or take a teaspoon of garlic oil. Alternatively, mix crushed garlic in a little cold water and drink the mixture immediately. Another recipe is to cut and crush four cloves of garlic, place them in milk, and allow the mixture to sit overnight. Take the liquid while fasting the next day.

Pumpkin Seed

Pumpkin seeds contain a substance called piperazine. It acts by paralyzing the parasites, which allows them to be removed easily.

We can find piperazine commercially in pharmacy drug formulations or naturally, as we said, in the seeds of the pumpkin. This traditional method of deworming has been used around the world since man can remember. There are several effective traditional formulas, below we describe one of them:

Use one cup of peeled and mashed pumpkin seeds (about 80 seeds). Mix them with coconut water and two tablespoons of honey. Take the mixture over three hours on an empty stomach. Do not eat during this three-hour period. At the end of the three hours, take castor oil in order to quickly eliminate the parasites.

Papaya and Papaya Seeds

Papain is a digestive enzyme contained in papaya that is capable of breaking down the outer layer of adult parasites. The milky juice of unripe papaya is a powerful agent for destroying roundworms. The adult dose is one tablespoon of fresh green papaya juice, an equal amount of honey, and three or four tablespoons of hot water. Two hours later, administer a dose of castor oil mixed with warm milk. This treatment should be repeated for two days if necessary. For children seven to ten years of age, half of this dose should be administered. For children under three years of age, one teaspoon (5ml) of the mixture is sufficient.

Papaya seeds are also useful for this purpose as they are rich in papain and caricin. For every tablespoon of crushed, fresh seeds, add an equal amount of honey. Take the dose of one teaspoon (5ml) daily in the morning or at night on an empty stomach for ten days, rest five days and repeat the cycle three times. We recommend the use of a purgative.

Ginger

Ginger not only helps to combat intestinal parasites but also reduces nausea and can help calm nerves. For hundreds of years, fresh ginger has proven to be highly successful in destroying intestinal worms. The most common way to consume ginger is raw or by infusion. Ginger extract may also be sprinkled on a variety of foods.

Propolis

Propolis is a resin like substance gathered by bees from the bark and leaf buds of trees, to help disinfect, build and maintain their hives. Propolis has been used for at least 3,000 years. Its use dates back to the Egyptians and the Romans, and remains in use today. To the Greeks we owe the name pro, meaning "before" and polis, meaning "city." This translates as "defenses before the city," or "defender of the city." Thanks to the antibiotic action of propolis, which protects against the activity of viruses and bacteria, the hive is one of the most sterile places known to nature.

Many scientific studies have proven the antiparasitic activity of propolis, therefore it is recommended for treatment of: *Giardia*, amoebas and roundworms, and also for intestinal infections caused by gram-positive bacteria.

Take propolis, diluted in water or fruit juice, for treatment of parasites, for seven days, on an empty stomach. Use Propolis standardized at 30% in either propolis tincture or capsules. Take three drops per kilo of weight, or three capsules one half-hour before each meal. A seven-day treatment cycle should include seven days on, followed by seven days off; repeat three to five times to ensure complete elimination of parasites or bacteria. Repetition of the treatment is essential to halt bacterial reproductive cycles. By repeating the treatment at least three times, the effective elimination of parasites is ensured. The benefits of propolis are that it has no side effects, is well tolerated, and is highly effective.

Pomegranate Bark

Pomegranate bark contains an alkaloid known as punicine, which is highly toxic to earthworms. It is used by decoction of the root bark, stem, or fruit. The root bark is preferable because it contains a greater quantity of the alkaloid than the bark of the trunk. This alkaloid is also highly toxic to tapeworms. A cold decoction of root bark, preferably fresh, should be given in quantities of 90ml to 180ml three times per day (for adults), with one-hour intervals between cups. A purgative should be taken after the last glass. For children, a dose of 20ml to 60ml is appropriate. A decoction is preferably used to eliminate solitaires (tapeworm, *Taenia Solium*).

Carrots

Carrots are another effective home remedy for eliminating intestinal parasites in children. The chemical constituents of carrots attack pests by preventing their development. It is one of the most effective natural treatments for children, when given a small cup of grated carrots each morning until the problem desists.

Condiments

Seasoning plants are also powerful weapons to keep in mind in our everyday cooking. Since time immemorial, mankind has used them to control parasitic diseases. The following are most interesting because of their effects:

- Cayenne
- Cinnamon
- Cloves
- Paprika
- Pepper
- Tarragon
- Thyme
- Turmeric

Thank you Andreas and Miriam for sharing what I know will be very enlightening, not only to the families of children with autism, but to people all over the world suffering from mysterious symptoms consistent with parasitic infections. I want to share one interesting tidbit about parasite infections before we get into the FAQs on parasites and the parasite protocol.

"We have a tremendous parasite problem right here in the U.S. It is just not being addressed."[5] - Dr. Peter Wina, Chief of Patho-Biology in the Walter Reed Army Institute of Research in 1991. (The problem existed in 1991, and with modern globalization parasites are more prevalent than ever, yet they still not being addressed.

Parasite Protocol FAQs

I showed my family practitioner pictures of the worms we have found. He thinks they are not a parasite, but just mucous. How can I be certain?

It can be difficult to identify parasites, and most general practitioners are not trained to do so. Some parents have success with a local vet, who analyzes samples in their office. As a crude test, you can pour boiling hot water onto your specimen. If it falls apart, it is probably biofilm or mucous. If it withstands the wash, it is probably a parasite. Unfortunately, most stool analyses are notorious for false negatives. If you put hot water on parasites, they do not dissolve. Mucous dissolves in any water—hot or cold.

Is it ok to do the Kalcker Parasite Protocol during pregnancy?

No. Don't do any kind of detox or parasite protocol while you are pregnant or nursing. Any detox will release toxins into the blood stream that could potentially negatively impact the developing fetus or nursing baby. If you are planning on getting pregnant, it would be advisable to do whatever detox or deworming procedure before pregnancy.

When is it appropriate to stop the parasite protocol? In other words, does every child on this protocol need both the CD and the other parts of the Parasite Protocol or are there some that only need CD? This is a critical question since these are two protocols joined together and not every child may need both. We have done the Parasite Protocol and have never passed parasites so I am uncertain about my child.

Usually the Parasite Protocol is repeated for 12-18 months, sometimes less. The most important thing is to make sure that there are no fertilized eggs left that could hatch at a later date. As it is very difficult to know if there are remaining eggs, it is important to complete the 12-18 month treatment. The Parasite Protocol is a complete protocol heavily researched to achieve the best results. The Parasite Protocol in conjunction with CD has been shown to be one of the most effective methods to heal regressive autism. Parasites are cyclical and need to be treated as such. You continue with the parasite protocol until no more parasites are seen—be that in behavior or actually in the stool.

What does the process of worms toxifying the brain look like?

Ascaris lumbricoides (roundworm), for example, produces at least five different toxins: Malondialdehyde, ammonia, histamine, formaldehyde, and morphine. Malondialdehyde is responsible for oxidative stress, and is mutagenic.[7] Ammonia, which can lead to hyperammonemia, can be responsible for seizures, tremors, flapping, poor coordination, growth retardation, combativeness, lethargy, and other symptoms. Comparing hyperammonemia with the symptoms known as regressive autism yields overwhelming similarities. Formaldehyde has been shown in some laboratory studies to affect the lymphatic and hematopoietic systems. Morphine inhibits nerve reactions and slows intestinal peristalsis. It also keeps the immune system from finding parasites, and from doing anything about them. This is a reason we often can't identify parasites. We only find parasites when the infection is acute, not chronic. This is because IgE or IgM reactions are altered by morphine. Histamine can lead to chronic inflammation in the body.

As a family, we expect to be doing the CD and parasite protocols for some time. How do we know when to stop? Should we wait until we have a few months of no symptoms?

We do it until full recovery is reached.

We have been doing full oral dose CD and the Parasite Protocol. We are seeing some amazing changes, but we don't see worms. Are we doing something wrong?

CD affects parasites of different sizes. You may be clearing parasites that would be undetectable to the naked eye, or nematodes that are very small and therefore hard to detect in the stool.

Why is my child so deficient in vitamins?

As a general rule, most children with autism are deficient in vitamins. In the first place many pathogens feed off of vitamins intended for the host, and helminthes especially love B12 and iron. Since many of us, especially those of us living in cold climates, do not receive enough sun, we are deficient in vitamin D. Calcium is used by the body as an antagonist for acid inflammation; all acidity in the body is compensated by calcium, and therefore it is usually low with the kids on the spectrum. As our children heal, these deficiencies fade and homeostasis returns.

I just gave mebendazole, Not pyrantel this AM. What should I do?

Don't stress. Tomorrow is a new day, and you can begin again. Give mebendazole tomorrow as that is tomorrow's scheduled dose.

Aren't there some parasites that are good for us and help our immunity and gut healing?

A parasite is defined as a living being that is dependent on a host for survival, to the detriment of that host.

For those of you that continue the parasite protocol thru the new moon, how many days do you stay on it? We are now 3 days past the new moon.

Some people treat month long. The Kalcker protocol itself is 18 days long. Each family has to find a protocol that suits them. Some folks use mebendazole 3 days before the new moon, the day of, and three days after. Other families use herbal remedies on the off days. If you consult with a healthcare provider, this would be a question to ask them. Each child is unique and has different needs when it comes to treating parasites.

Why are live worms not digested? Poisons?

Live helminths are protected by a glucosoid mucous with positively charged ions, making them resistant to stomach acid, or digestive fluids. When they die, the mucous separates from the helminth, leaving them open to digestive enzymes. We often see the mucous, as well as semi-digested helminths, in the stool of people using the protocol.

Does everyone in the family need to do the parasite protocol at the same time? With or without CD, enemas, diatomaceous earth, Rompepiedras/stone breakers, and castor oil? My (neurotypical) daughter will take the anti-parasitic drugs, mebendazole, and pyrantel pamoate, but not these other parasite protocol ingredients, which is why I ask.

Your entire family needs to do the protocol at the same time, or you risk reinfection. Neurotypical family members should do as much of the protocol as possible. If someone will only take the meds, so be it. However, I feel the more the better.

Do I need to separate the neem from CD?

Yes, I give neem with food, and would separate from CD by at least an hour.

If I don't see any worms, does that mean my child doesn't have parasites, or are we just missing the eggs?

Just because you don't see parasites doesn't necessarily mean you don't have any. For example, *Toxocara canis* or *Toxocara cati*, which are very common in our pets (and can infect humans as *Toxocariasis*), are not expelled in fecal matter. Some families on the protocol did not see actual worms until month seven.

To what extent do the rest of us need to do the CD protocol? Is it the same as our ASD children? And, is it necessary to do the whole nine yards with the full Parasite Protocol for the whole 12 months? Are there any shortcuts for healthier individuals?

All of the family members, including pets, need to be on anti-parasite treatment for a year and thereafter lifetime maintenance is best. As mentioned before, with neurotypical family members, you do as much as you can, but the anti-parasitic medications are crucial to preventing reinfection.

Is diatomaceous earth a binder and therefore must it be given apart from food, medication, and supplements?

No. It is not a binder. It is fine to give with or without food, and does not affect medication or supplements.

Do you have to do the Protocol forever if you are fully recovered or is there a maintenance plan?

When the child gets to where you want him, you can start to pull things. Then, we do maintenance dosing of CD; one dose on Monday and one on Thursday. We do the Parasite Protocol for a week every three months since we live in a world of parasites. It is good preventative medicine for all. Ocean water is also good for all of us. See Chapter 13 (page 319) for the complete maintenance plan.

Does CD kill parasites?

Yes. CD kills amoebas, *Giardia lamblia*, and other smaller parasites. CD does not kill the larger macroparasites due to their higher oxidative stress resistance.

When is it ok to start the parasite protocol prior to reaching full dose of CD?

Healing autism is a marathon not a sprint. The point is to heal with the least amount of aggravation. Therefore, you should be at a full dose of CD before starting, and have added in enemas and baths. If you are seeing Herxheimer reactions then don't start yet. Obviously, everyone must make his or her own decisions.

Where in the gut do helminths live? Do CD enemas (300 ml) reach them?

It depends on the type of helminth. There are more than 300 different helminths so they could be in many different places. However, most live in the small intestine. Some lay their eggs in the rectum. The size of the person will dictate how high an enema will reach.

Do you tell your kids that they have worms? Do you show them? Are they scared? My son is very interested about everything in the world and asks 4,000 questions a day. What do I tell him?

How to handle this situation is unique to each and every family. There is no right or wrong answer here. The following are some suggestions we have received from families on the protocol:

Nope. My husband was just telling me a story from when he was a kid about another kid who got teased all the time about having worms. He still remembers it. So, no I will not tell my kids.

My kids (ages 10 & 7) know about worms because we have talked about their Lyme disease and other symptoms for a long time. I think it helps them understand why they feel grumpy or sick and why the enemas help. But, I think every child is different. The risk is that they might tell their friends. I tell them that it is private information and that pretty much everyone has worms but some people have more and get sick from them. And, I told them that even most doctors don't know this but slowly people are learning and getting smarter about this and a good diet, etc... My boys like to see the big ones, and try for new records. They like to show their brother the records. I think that's a boy thing.

I have a 10 year-old, and I tell him that we have parasites. I have not showed him anything, I ask him to leave the room before I start to sort the poo. ;)

My son had another bowel movement FULL of worms, pinworms— and I mean hundreds. This is only our second day on CD (1/2 drop in 8 fl. oz.) so a bit thrown to the deep end. Has anyone else had a start like this? How did everything go from there on?

I have seen it a handful of times. I get VERY excited about this. Everyone has autism a bit differently. But, if we see worms early, in many cases the recovery begins early too. That may be the case for your child.

I understand that even organic produce needs to be washed properly. What is the best way to wash my fruits and vegetables?

The Ascaris eggs are resistant to UV, and can withstand a pH from 2 to 11.5. Eggs are killed by heating to approximately 60°C (140°F). Spray your fruits and veggies with CD spray. 10 drops per 1 fl. oz., of water, no need to rinse off.

Anyone notice a huge growth spurt after starting the parasite protocol?

Many parents have reported their children resumed growth as well as weight gain. No real surprise considering they are getting back what the parasites were taking from them.

Do we need to treat our pets if they are taking heartworm medication?

> Yes, heartworm medication does not address intestinal parasites, which can infect us and our children. We need to deparasitize our pets, as well as ourselves.

We put "cascara sagrada" in place of castor oil because for my son and me, it is difficult to take the oil. Is it ok?

> Cascara sagrada is not the same thing as castor oil and is not part of the protocol. An alternative solution to liquid castor oil is to buy castor oil in softgels. You will need many but it does solve the taste problem.

My son is very high in Trichinella spiralis, which is a roundworm from undercooked meat or pork. It's supposed to be rare in the US, so I'm wondering how my child would have picked this up. Any ideas? No undercooked meat here for the kids, and we don't eat pork.

> At this moment we have not seen a relationship between *Trichinella spiralis* and autism. It may be a multi-parasitic infection, or a misdiagnosis. Apart from the standard protocol, your child might need something else. I would consult the practitioner for the appropriate dosage, and only if your child has a definite Trichinella spiralis diagnosis.

How do we know if there are parasites in the brain, and what can we do about it?

> Parasites in the brain are very rare. (According to the CDC, *Cysticercosis* is a parasitic tissue infection caused by larval cysts of the pork *tapeworm*. These larval cysts infect brain, muscle, or other tissue, and are a major cause of adult onset seizures in most low-income countries. An individual acquires cysticercosis from ingesting eggs excreted by a person who has an intestinal tapeworm.)[6] Larvae can be seen on a scan. Many people assume that the problem causing behavioral issues, or mental issues, must be located in the brain. However, the problem likely exists elsewhere. If the blood contains toxins, this will affect the brain. For example, if you ingest too much alcohol, your brain, nervous system, etc. will be affected, but the problem is not in the brain itself. We can think the same way about parasites. The chemicals that they produce will have effects on the brain, however, rarely will the parasites be located there.

Do parasites cause autism? If so, why doesn't every child with parasites have autism?

> Regressive autism has been called parasitological vaccinosis by Dr. Andreas Kalcker. This is a cross reaction between a child with parasites that receives certain vaccines. Further research is needed for a definitive answer.

Why don't normal lab tests find parasites?

Generally speaking, lab tests need to find living creatures or eggs. The eggs are only present certain days of the month, and even on those days they won't necessarily be present in a particular stool sample. Living worms are extremely rare in stool because they are generally passed only once they die. They are very good at avoiding being excreted in stool. Furthermore, if they die internally, they can be partially or fully digested within our bodies before being expelled.

Are some labs better than others? Is it worth taking a stool sample to a vet if they send it out, or only if they look under a microscope?

We haven't found a lab that consistently finds parasites. Metametrix™ has identified parasites, but in our experience and the experience of the families I have helped, we have not found a lab that is consistent. It is only worth sending a sample to a vet if they are identifying parasites with a microscope.

Combantrin® is available in tablet and liquid form. Which is better?

I hate the liquid and never use it. It may have added colors and flavors. If you absolutely can't find it without additives, I would use only mebendazole instead of using pyrantel with additives.

Why are there no systemic drugs in the protocol?

They are not needed with this Protocol. Treating parasites without systemic drugs is much safer and easier on the body. The suggested treatments using mebendazole and pyrantel pamoato are nearly unabsorbed by the body, meaning that we do not add more toxins to an already overloaded body.

When does a child need systemic drugs?

This is necessary only for certain parasites like cysticercosis, which is caused by tapeworms, hookworms, Trichinella spiralis (from pork), or other hard to kill helminths. These may be identified by a blood test. The practitioner may prescribe systemics depending on the situation.

Should I start on the new moon if my child's behavior declines then?

The full 18-day Kalcker Parasite Protocol always starts before the full moon. However, some parents have found that by treating parasites for 3 days over new moon that they are able to get through the new moon as well as the full moon with limited issues if any.

Is there a time in the moon calendar, where it is normal that there are no worms in the stool? (We don't have any at new moon.)

Further research is necessary to determine this definitively.

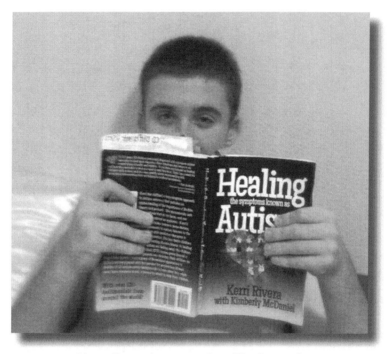

Hero Guy taking a peek at *The Protocol*.

Chapter 9

Step 4 - Other Supplements

*"One of the first duties of the physician is to educate
the masses not to take medicine."*
~ ***William Osler***

Most of the families that followed this Protocol, and recovered their children, used a combination of these additional supplements along with CD. Each supplement combination is completely unique, depending on the symptoms of the child, and how the child reacts to each intervention. If after *The Diet*, full *CD Protocol*, and three *Kalcker Parasite Protocols* we are still dealing with an autism diagnosis, then families start adding in supplements. This section is about "unfinished business." I like to do three Kalcker Parasite Protocols before adding back in supplements because parasites love supplements, especially vitamin B_{12} and iron.

I feel when we supplement deficiencies in children with underlying parasitic infections, it can result in resistant parasites. We aren't making the child healthier; we're making the parasites healthier and stronger. If significant supplementation does little or nothing to change lab values in subsequent blood, urine, and stool tests, then it's fair to say that we have a flaw in our approach. Pathogens and parasites can cause vitamin/mineral deficiencies. By killing them, instead of feeding them with additional supplementation, we are focusing on the root cause of the symptoms that we call autism.

When I came back from our first *Defeat Autism Now!* doctor visit, I had thousands of dollars in supplements that I did not know how to use. We kept going to different doctors hoping to find the one that had the answer. At one point, Patrick was on a protocol, given to me and supervised by a doctor, which called for 70+ different supplements a day. He looked worse during the entire nine-month period that we followed that protocol. In hindsight, all those years of supplementation made it harder to eliminate Patrick's pathogens.

That is why this protocol focuses on the excesses instead of the deficiencies for children with an autism diagnosis. If by eliminating the excesses of viruses, bacteria, candida, parasites and heavy metals, we can see a reduction in the symptoms known as autism, then eventually we can reach full healing.

Commonly, when a new family contacts me, they send me a list of all the supplements their child is taking. I frequently see lists of 30+ supplements that may be combined in ways that negate their effects. For example, probiotics are given in the morning with breakfast, or GABA with food. Both are incorrect, probiotics go alone at night right before bed, and GABA is always taken without food. If there is a legitimate reason for a certain supplement, then it absolutely must be given correctly or it's just excess noise in the body, and more stress on the detox organs.

The following list of supplements can be considered after *The Diet*, ocean water, CD, and three months of the *Kalcker Parasite Protocol* (except probiotics and enzymes which may start day one). This chapter is to be used as a starting point for your own research on these supplements. This list contains references and the websites used in this research with some of the more pertinent information about products.

Probiotics

The vast majority of the families who have recovered their children with this Protocol have used THERALAC® brand probiotic. It is a prebiotic plus probiotic in a capsule that can withstand stomach acid, which allows it to pass to the small intestine, where the beneficial bacteria are needed. THERALAC® contains three *lactobacillus* and two *bifidobacterium* strains.

The paragraph below was slightly modified from www.theralac.com where you can find more information. Please visit their site for details on references contained within the text.[1] The following two paragraphs were taken from different sources, and help explain benefits of THERALAC®, specifically for children on the spectrum.

> Probiotics are defined as: "Live microorganisms that when administered in adequate amounts confer a health benefit to the host" (World Health Organization 2001). According to the International Probiotics Association (IPA), the benefits of probiotics can include reduction in diarrhea caused by antibiotics and rotavirus, alleviation of symptoms of lactose intolerance, alleviation of symptoms of food and skin allergies in children, reduction of recurrent ear and bladder infections, and other positive indications.

How Does THERALAC® Benefit My Immune System?

THERALAC®'s five probiotic strains work in unison to support the mucosal immune system on the intestinal surface; activation signals are then sent to the body's systemic immune system. This is a gentle and controlled process because THERALAC®'s strains are beneficial. Essentially, the immune system is put on alert so that it is ready to act quickly if there is an appearance of pathogenic microorganisms.[2]

Many children with autism have chronic digestive problems. In fact, gastrointestinal symptoms in autistic children often first appear in conjunction with initial changes in emotion and behavior during the onset of autism, leading researchers to suspect a gut-brain connection.[3]

Normally, proteins are digested in stages by enzymes; first to peptides, and then to smaller amino acid components, which are absorbed into blood capillaries in the gut mucosa. The larger peptides are generally unable to cross this mucous membrane barrier; if they do, however, they can act as opioids affecting neurotransmitters in the brain causing abnormal behaviors and/or activity. These incompletely digested peptides—known as exorphins, casomorphins, and gluteomorphins usually come from milk proteins such as casein, or from wheat (gluten), and are structurally similar to morphine. The formation of excess peptides in the gut is possibly associated with sub-optimal enzyme activity, or an insufficient supply of enzymes required to breakdown these peptides. So if we repair the imbalance of beneficial bacterial organisms in the gut and the gut lining, while killing the pathogens causing the dysbiosis, we have the opportunity to heal children with autism. Probiotics can be used to improve the quality of the gut mucosa.[2]

In addition to aiding in the repair of the gut lining and improving digestion, there is also evidence that probiotics can help with detoxification of heavy metals such as toxic mercury.

The paragraph below was taken from the presentation "Gut biology and Treatment" by Dr. Anju Usman:

Emerging literature is showing the beneficial effect of oral probiotics on mood and anxiety symptoms. In a double-blind, placebo controlled randomized parallel group study, daily use of probiotics reduced psychological distress.[5] A number of studies have shown the anti-anxiety effects of probiotic use in patients with medical conditions.[6]

Dr. Vincent Young, University of Michigan (2009): "the gut ecosystem needs to be preserved and that changing the ecosystem through stresses such as antibiotics could irreversibly change the ecosystem, with deleterious effects." Dr. Young has studied the effects of antibiotics on the microbes in our gut. He found that mice when given particularly strong antibiotics completely wiped out all their normal gut microbes. Even more striking, clostridium species and fungal species are then able to overgrow without the bacteria there to fend them off.

There is no doubt in my mind that probiotics helped get my son's gut back in order, helped improve my own health, and that of thousands of families of children on the spectrum. Probiotics should be given without food, directly before bedtime. This way, they have the entire night to proliferate in the small intestine where they are needed.

Special note for those with PANDAS/PANS: We have received some reports where some PANDAS/PANS and/or older children were becoming violent and having more SIBs while on probiotics. Be observant and watch for behavior changes when adding probiotics. In addition, know that we may need to remove them for a period of time!

Omega-3 & Omega-6 Fatty Acids

Omega-3 and omega-6 fatty acids are polyunsaturated fatty acids and are considered essential fatty acids. Essential fatty acids must be consumed because your body cannot produce them. They are important for brain development, immune system and cardiovascular function, and normal metabolism. Omega-3 and omega-6 fatty acids are commonly found in marine and plant oils. While a healthy diet often provides adequate supplies of both, supplementation is sometimes necessary.

Omega-3 fatty acids also help to regulate energy levels, as well as normalizes blood sugar levels. They help improve concentration as well as mental vividness. Using omega-3 fatty acid supplements helps with anxiety, mood swings, and depression. They are especially significant in the treatment of autism. The entire body benefits from ingesting omega-3 fatty acids; from physical development, to relaxation from anxiety and jitteriness, to developing brain cells; all of these aspects can aide in the treatment of autism.[6]

Omega-6 fatty acids promote healthy brain function and assists with skin and hair growth, bone development, and metabolism. A healthy balance of omega-3 and omega-6 fatty acids promotes heart health and minimizes inflammation. Omega-6 may also be used to treat allergies, eczema, osteoporosis and premenstrual syndrome.[7]

Unlike omega-3 fatty acids, excessive consumption of omega-6 fatty acids can have negative effects. Therefore, their consumption must be monitored. Omega-6 fatty acids, in large quantities, can promote inflammation in the body that may lead to flare-ups of eczema, acne, and the aches and pains associated with arthritis. It is recommended that you maintain about a 4:1 ratio of omega-6 to omega-3 fatty acids.

Some research has been done that suggests improvements in overall health, cognition, sleep patterns, social interactions, and eye contact when children on the spectrum were given an EFA (Essential Fatty Acid) supplement.[8]

Furthermore, another study showed the positive effects of EFA's on dyspraxia (a motor disorder frequently associated with cognitive, behavioral, and social challenges). The participants showed improvements in reading, spelling and behavior during the treatment period.[9]

I have personally found that I really like omegas from YES™ Supplements. Dr. Brian Peskin has some very informative videos on YouTube discussing the merits of vegan versus animal based omega sources. I highly recommend you have a look for yourself. My own son, and many other children have built up to taking one tablespoon, two times a day.

L-carnitine

L-carnitine is a vital amino acid that promotes healthy neural levels of acetylcholine, an important neurotransmitter that aids memory and proper brain function. Research suggests that an L-carnitine deficiency may be implicated in a number of conditions, including ME/CFS (chronic fatigue syndrome), diabetes, Alzheimer's, dementia, and autism.

L-carnitine is composed of two essential amino acids, lysine and methionine. It is produced in the liver and kidneys and is contained in most cells of the body. It is required for the proper metabolism of fat and helps with mental concentration, and energy production. It transports long-chain fatty acids across the mitochondrial membrane so that they can be burned to produce energy.

A clinical trial studying the use of L-carnitine as a potential therapy for autism demonstrated the children taking L-carnitine showed improvements in their ability to relate to people, body use, adaptation to change, listening response, verbal communication, sociability, sensory/cognitive awareness, and health/physical behavior. There are a few articles that may be helpful for a better understanding of the importance of this amino acid. Check out an article by Henke Schultz, "L-carnitine helps kids with autism, study finds" and another by Emily Singer, "Defects in carnitine metabolism may underlie autism."

The average dose for L-carnitine is anywhere from 250-1000 mg per day with food, depending on weight and reactions.

GABA

GABA (gamma-aminobutyric acid) is an amino acid and a neurotransmitter (a type of chemical responsible for carrying information from one cell to another). It is produced naturally in the body, but is also widely available in supplement form. Manufacturers claim that GABA supplements can help boost the brain's GABA levels and, in turn, treat anxiety, stress, depression, and sleep problems.

The GABA system acts as something of an information filter to prevent the nerves from becoming over stimulated. It has long been suspected that this filtering process is compromised in many autistic children. Impairment of the GABA system could overwhelm the brain with sensory information, leading to many of the behavior traits associated with autism. GABA is also believed to play a key role in the early development of the brain.[10]

GABA is also involved with the production of endorphins in our brain, which make us feel positive and upbeat. GABA can reduce stress, relieve anxiety, and increase alertness. GABA can be helpful for behavior, language, and possibly even seizures.

GABA is used for control of seizure activity and works on the same receptors as the drug Keppra®. GABA is also useful for speech, helps facilitate language in nonverbal children, and improves language in children that are beginning to speak.

If you are going to give GABA to your child, the max is 5,000 mg per day, divided into two doses, one in morning and one at night, always on an empty stomach. In the evening, GABA can be given 15 minutes after your last dose of Chlorine Dioxide, with your probiotic. I start at 250 mg two times a day, one in the morning and one at night. I then titrate up the dose daily or every other day if everything looks good. If you observe sleepiness or irritability it is a good idea to back down.

5-HTP (5-Hydroxytryptophan)

5-HTP, also known as oxitriptan, is a naturally occurring amino acid. It is a chemical precursor to the neurotransmitters, serotonin and melatonin from tryptophan. 5-HTP works in the brain and central nervous system by increasing the production of the chemical serotonin. Serotonin can affect sleep, appetite, temperature, sexual behavior, and pain sensation.

From *Saving Eli: One Family's Struggle* - Vitamin Research Products website:

> While not clearly understood, researchers know that serotonin pathways are disturbed in autism, contributing to sleep disorders and mood. Tryptophan has been shown to help but has been banned by the FDA since 1989. We found that 5-HTP helped immensely, calming tantrums and increasing communication with our son.[11]

5-HTP is used between 50 mg and 200 mg, divided into two doses, morning and evening with food. I have seen it help children with autism for attention, focus, sleep, and cravings.

L-theanine

L-theanine or gamma-glutamylethylamide or 5-N-ethyl-glutamine, is an amino acid commonly found in tea. Theanine is able to cross the blood–brain barrier, and is reported to have positive effects on mood, stress, and cognition.

The following is excerpted from the L-Theanine website:[12]

> Many people experience stress on a daily basis and are looking for natural and safe ways to manage it. For thousands of years, it has been suggested that drinking green tea will make one relaxed. Recently this relaxation effect was found to be true and works because of an amino acid called L-Theanine which is found in the tea. Clinical research will show that ingesting up to 200mg of L-Theanine will promote the creation of the very important "anti-stress" neurotransmitter in the brain called GABA or gamma-aminobutyric acid. This results in a relaxed, clear and alert mental state.

> When used in the correct amounts in supplemental form, L-Theanine may:

- Reduce Stress
- Reduce Occasional, Simple Nervous Tension
- Promote Relaxation without Drowsiness
- Promote Mental Clarity and Focus
- Promote Positive Mood
- Promote Alertness
- Promote Learning and Memory
- Help Prevent Jitters Caused By Caffeine

I have found that when we can reduce these symptoms in individuals with ASDs we can get an increase in speech, learning, focus, concentration, and attention. L-Theanine is given with GABA upon waking, and can also be given at bedtime if needed, always without food. You can work up to 200 or 250mg/day.

Pycnogenol®

Pycnogenol® (pic-noj-en-all) French maritime pine bark extract acts as a potent blend of antioxidants, it is a natural anti-inflammatory, stimulates generation of collagen and hyaluronic acid and help with natural dilation of blood vessels by supporting production of nitric oxide.[13]

Pycnogenol® is not a supplement I tend to use very often, because it is an antioxidant, and therefore cannot be combined with chlorine dioxide. However, in some people it has proved necessary and helpful for speech and reduction of seizures. It should be given in the morning with food at a dose between 25 and 400 mg/day depending on need. Pycnogenol® may not be suitable for children who are sensitive to phenols.

L-Carnosine

L-Carnosine is a dipeptide of the amino acids beta-alanine and histidine. It is highly concentrated in muscle and brain tissues.

L-Carnosine is believed to stimulate the frontal areas of the brain, resulting in overall improved levels of functioning. More and more research shows that the frontal lobes and temporal lobes in the brain control emotion, epileptic activity, cognitive, expressive speech, and abstract thinking. Studies have shown Carnosine to improve language, socialization, and overall level of functioning in individuals within the autism spectrum. It has also been shown in studies to have anti-seizure properties without the side-effects of prescription anti-seizure medications.

Research indicates it prevents the formation of the beta amyloid plaque that is found not only in neurological conditions such as Alzheimer's, Parkinson's and autism, but also in the eyes in degenerative eye conditions and in the pancreas in diabetes. It is a neuroprotectant, with a study indicating it reduced severity of damage in stroke patients.[14]

Chez and coworkers found that after eight weeks on L-carnosine, children showed statistically significant improvements on the Gilliam Autism Rating Scale (GARS). They relate this to the likely ability of L-Carnosine to enhance neurological function, perhaps, in the enterorhinal or temporal cortex.[15] This enhancement in neurological function has led to speech in many of the families that I have worked with.

I have also seen L-Carnosine help reduce seizures in some children and increase language in others. It is given twice a day with breakfast and dinner at a dose of 200 to 400mg, 2 times a day. If you note hyperactivity, remove it.

Taurine

Taurine is an amino acid, a chemical that is a required building block of proteins. Taurine is found in large amounts in the brain, retina, heart, and in blood cells called platelets. It can be consumed through eating meat and fish.

Autism and Low Taurine

"Are You Dangerously Deficient in Taurine"[16] explores possible problems associated with a taurine deficiency. Among the problems noted in the article is autism and low taurine levels. In the article, Leonard Smith MD writes about the benefits of taurine, some of which can be of interest to people dealing with autism spectrum disorders:

- Brain and nervous system function
- Helps eliminate toxins
- Stabilizing the brain (can be effective in treating seizure disorders)

Taurine, like all amino acids, must be given without food. The maximum dose is between 500 and 1,500 mg.

DMG

DMG, or dimethylglycine, is an amino acid that can be found in many common food items like meats (especially liver), various grains, and beans. It has been classified as a type of amino acid that is closely linked to vitamin B.

There have also been interesting developments in the use of a DMG supplement for children with autism. Because many children who have autism are unable to tolerate eye contact, and some have problems forming complete sentences and thoughts studies investigated whether an increase in DMG consumption could help to alleviate many of these problems. In fact, the study found that when children with autism were given supplemental DMG they appeared less frustrated and showed a marked increase in their speaking and cognitive abilities.[17] At present, this research remains novel and therefore further investigation is necessary to determine what the long-term effects of DMG supplementation might have on children on the spectrum.

The following paragraphs were excerpted from *Defeat Autism Now!*[18]

Dimethylglycine (DMG) for Autism

For over 20 years ARI has been hearing from parents who have tried DMG on their autistic children. In many cases remarkably good results have been seen, especially in enhancing speech. In some cases, drug-resistant seizures have been stopped by DMG. (See New England Journal of Medicine, 10-21-82, pgs 1081-82).

There is an extensive research literature on the safety and health benefits of DMG. Many studies have shown that DMG enhances the effectiveness of the immune system, improves the physical and athletic performance of humans and other animals (e.g. race horses) and has, all in all, a very wide range of beneficial effects. It is very safe. I have seen no evidence of any toxic or significant adverse effects.

Many parents have reported that, within a few days of starting DMG, the child's behavior improved noticeably, better eye contact was seen, frustration tolerance increased, the child's speech improved, or more interest and ability in speaking was observed.

A full dose of DMG is 900 mg per day, taken without food upon waking. However, it is best to start at a lower dose and slowly work up to 900 mg over a week or so. If you see an increase of hyperactivity (which is rare), reduce the dose. If no improvement is seen within a month I would switch to TMG.

TMG - Trimethylglycine (Betaine Anhydrous)

TMG (Betaine anhydrous} is a chemical that occurs naturally in the body, and can also be found in foods such as beets, spinach, cereals, seafood, and wine.

How does it work?

A form of betaine called betaine anhydrous helps in the metabolism of homocysteine, a chemical involved in the normal function of many different parts of the body, including blood, bones, eyes, heart, nerves, and the brain. Betaine anhydrous prevents the buildup of homocysteine seen in people who have problems with its metabolism from birth.[19]

The following is excerpted from the *Autism Canada Foundation*.[20]   Please visit their site...

www.autism.org

...for full references contained within the text.

The benefits of taking DMG or TMG range from behavioral changes, reduction of seizures, and decreased obsessive-compulsive behaviours to improved language. DMG and TMG have been reported from thousands of families to be quite beneficial to many individuals with autism.

Research on humans and laboratory animals has shown that DMG and TMG enhance the effectiveness of the immune system. Some children and adults with autism have seizures, and there are published reports of decreases in seizure activity as a result of DMG. A double-blind placebo-controlled study by Drs. Shin-siung Jung, Bernard Rimland, and Stephen M. Edelson involving 84 participants documented a significant decrease in behavioral problems.

It should be noted that some kids tolerate DMG but not TMG. TMG is given upon waking without food, in a dose of 500mg. If DMG didn't yield improvements in language, then we switch to TMG.

FAQ's

There are times when I do see undigested food in my son's stools. I am particularly concerned. He never complains of stomach pains. But I do see some at times, especially cashews. Should I bother with an enzyme? Or is it better without one. If so, which brand?

I love enzymes. Kirkman has one with Isogest®, 851/180 is the number, and it's broad spectrum. Also, Biofilm Defense® is great for dissolving the biofilm. A number of the parents online have used Ness® enzymes Gastric comfort formula #601 very successfully.

How should I administer THERALAC®?

The best time to administer probiotics is at bedtime. Children's THERALAC® is a granular formula so you can sprinkle it on yogurt or mix it into a smoothie and still obtain the same benefits! So how do you take it? We recommend that you take a level 1/4 teaspoon and fold it into yogurt, applesauce, or food of a similar consistency and let it sit for a minute. This is to keep the granules as close together as possible, thus allowing our acid proof gel matrix to form around the product. Visit the THERALAC® website for more info:

www.theralac.com/childrens-theralac.aspx

Supplement Dosing Overview

Supplement	Dose	Time of Day	Empty Stomach (ES) or With Food (WF)
Probiotics	1 cap	Before Bed	ES
Omega-3/ Omega-6	1 Tbsp	With any meal 1-3x / day	WF
L-Carnitine	250-1000mg/day	With any meal 1-3x / day	WF
GABA	Up to 2,500mg 2x/day	Upon waking & at bedtime	ES
5-HTP	50-200mg	Morning & Evening	WF
L-Theanine	Work up to 200-250mg/day	Mornings or Mornings & Nights	ES
Pycnogenol	25-40mg a day/as needed	Morning	WF
L-Carnosine	200-400mg 2x / day	Morning & Evening	WF
Taurine	500-1500mg/day	Morning, Noon & Night	ES
DMG	900mg/day	Morning	ES
TMG	500mg/day	Morning	ES
Enzymes	1 cap w/meals	Morning, Noon & Night	WF

Chapter 10

<u>Step 5 - Chelation</u>

So, let's say we're clipping along; full Diet, CD, Kalcker Parasite Protocol, and we've added in whatever supplements the child specifically needs and the child still has autism. Recovery is still not a reality... yet! At this point, it's time to look at chelation.

Why use Chelation for Autism?

Chelation became very popular in the world of autism about a decade ago, when things were heating up around the Thimerosal/Autism connection. Today, many of our children are still metal toxic. Metal challenges (testing that shows metals in urine) from any of the thousands of children whose families I have helped show the same thing—extremely high levels of mercury, lead, aluminum, as well as sometimes tin, cadmium, and other metals.

These heavy metals can come from various sources such as:

- Coal burning power plants. According to the EPA, coal-fired power plants in the United States emit about 48 tons of mercury into the air every year, where more than half of this mercury falls within five miles of the plant itself. When it reaches the water, microorganisms consume it and convert it into a substance called methyl mercury.
- Drinking water
- Our food supply
- Cookware
- Deodorant
- Beauty products
- Dental amalgams
- Vaccines, etc.

Heavy metals are known to accumulate in different parts of the body including organs, bones, joints, and the brain, etc. Metal toxicity can provoke inflammation, kill neurons, cause behavioral changes, affect the thyroid and other master glands, lower T-cell counts, and cause a myriad of other symptoms. Furthermore, new research shows that fluoride in drinking water makes the aluminum that we ingest more bio-available. As was reported in the journal *Brain Research*, the combination of aluminum and fluoride causes the same pathological changes in brain tissue found in Alzheimer's patients.[1]

Many children with autism also have impaired methylation cycles. The result of this impairment is an inability of the body to rid itself of excess metals, thereby prolonging chronic illness.

What exactly is methylation?

Methylation reactions are those that involve the transfer of a methyl group from one compound to another. The methylation cycle is the name given to a biochemical pathway that contributes to a range of crucial bodily functions, including:

- Detoxification
- Immune function
- Maintaining DNA
- Energy production
- Mood balancing
- Controlling inflammation

Impairments or mutations on the methylation cycle can lead to problems with:

- ASD's
- Alzheimer's
- Diabetes
- Allergies and Asthma

An overload of toxins (including heavy metals), can contribute to the impairment of the methylation cycle, and if the methylation cycle is impaired the body is unable to detoxify as needed, therefore creating a vicious catch 22.

We need to help our children's bodies rid themselves of their excess metals as part of the healing process. Dr. Usman has shown us that heavy metals are present in the biofilm, and Dr. Klinghardt has shown that removing mercury can be directly related to a reduction in chronic infections.[2]

Let's get those metals out!

What exactly is Chelation?

Chelation is a process used to rid the body of heavy metals. It is described as a chemical process in which a substance (chelator) is used to bind molecules, such as metals or minerals, and hold them so that they can be removed from the body.

Some of the most common chelators used in the world of autism are:

EDTA

This is an amino acid that attracts lead, other heavy metals, and some minerals from the bloodstream and expels these toxic elements in the urine. EDTA works to remove excess lead from the body, but it is not specific to mercury or methyl mercury as are DMSA or DMPS. It can be taken orally, by rectal suppository, or IV.

DMSA

This is an FDA approved drug that can be used in children when lead toxicity is suspected, however it can also be effective at removing other heavy metals including mercury and arsenic. It can be taken orally, transdermally, or given as a suppository.

DMPS

DMPS is given to remove mercury from the body. It can be given IV, intramuscularly, subcutaneously, transdermally, or by suppository.

Patrick has been prescribed all of these at different points of his life, and I can't say that I saw miraculous results during the time that I used them. However, some families have seen results, and this is something you may want to discuss with your doctor. After years of using chelators, and seeing other families use chelators, I have opted for a gentle approach. I like to use two products: bentonite clay baths and Bio-Chelat™. These products are strong enough to help the body rid itself of heavy metals, but have not been shown to stress the liver or provoke undesirable detox symptoms.

Knowing now that metals are in the biofilm, I feel it is short sighted to focus solely on metals or heavy metals rather than all the pathogens in the biofilm.

Bentonite Clay Baths

Bentonite clay is sedimentary clay composed of weathered and aged volcanic ash. Bentonites are more widely known as healing clays used for detoxing, cleansing, and drawing out impurities. They are used in many everyday products such as toothpaste, antacids, and cosmetics.

Indigenous people have used bentonite clay for centuries; Dr. Weston A. Price in his book, "Nutrition and Physical Degeneration,"[3] stated that when studying the diets of native tribes he examined their knapsacks. Among the tribes examined in the High Andes, in Central Africa and the Aborigines of Australia, Dr. Price reported that some knapsacks contained balls of volcanic ash clay, a little of which was dissolved in water.

Bentonite is known as "swelling clay." When bentonite clay absorbs water and swells up, it is stretched like a sponge. Toxins are drawn into these spaces through electrical attraction and bound. In fact, according to the Canadian Journal of Microbiology, bentonite clay can reportedly absorb pathogenic viruses, as well as herbicides and pesticides.[5]

One of my personal favorites has been *Even Better Now*®'s product available at:

www.evenbetternow.com

"EBN® Cleansing Clay is 100% pure sodium bentonite clay which has the highest cation exchange capacity (CEC of 98-107 meq/100g) of any bathing clay that we tested on the market. This clay is high purity air-classified sodium bentonite, selectively mined, consisting of micronized particles, which is a free-flowing powder. EBN® Cleansing Clay is 100% pure, hypoallergenic, and free of viruses, bacteria, yeast, and mold, as well as having a high cation exchange capacity."

There are other quality clays on the market, but EBN® tests every batch for heavy metals when it comes in. No, I do not receive financial gain from the company.

Bio-Chelat™

Another product I really like for gentle (low and slow) chelation is Bio-Chelat™. This is a German product containing a minimal amount of EDTA, which is FDA approved as a food substance. According to a clinical trial carried out in Germany:

The therapeutic value of the Bio-Chelat™ in the context of other chelators that are currently on the market is seen as follows: Chelators work relatively fast, but they are also very strong with a relative high washout of important trace elements and a high degree of specific side effects. Bio-Chelat™ works much gentler than most common chelators.

Although during the treatment a significant decrease of the body's heavy metal ion load was seen, this is accomplished without greatly disturbing the mineral and trace element relationships. The reduction of zinc should be looked at with caution and may easily be corrected throughout the treatment.[5]

I have seen very positive changes in many of the children who added in either bentonite clay baths, Bio-Chelate™, or both. As with any other intervention, add them separately while closely observing your child. Keep a log to record any changes, progress, or reactions you observe. Even if you don't see anything right away, I would keep using the products for a minimum of three months. Again, since they work LOW and SLOW changes may not be apparent at the outset, but that doesn't mean they are not helping to heal your child's body.

I use the CD baths every other day and then two times a week I do bentonite clay baths. I don't do the CD bath and the bentonite clay bath on the same day. I do them at opposite ends of the week.

Three days or so later, we'll add in the Bio-Chelat™. Again, follow the instructions on the package, and you can always start low and work your way up. Since Bio-Chelat™ doesn't alter the CD, the drops can be added to a single dose of CD. In addition, since the drops have no flavor, it is suitable to add them to water or any other drink your child might consume throughout the day.

Common Errors in Chelation:

Urine analysis without provocation:

Many families will do urine analysis to see if there are heavy metals present. If you have not done any chelation (oral or intravenous) you really don't get a good picture of what kinds of metals are actually in the body. Simply because the metals don't show up in urine, doesn't mean they are not present in the bones, the intestinal tract, the brain, and organs, etc. If we don't do any sort of provocation, we may end up with a false negative, leading a family to believe that their child is not metal toxic, when in fact they are. Bentonite clay baths and Bio-Chelat™ are gentle enough that they will not cause any harm to a child (metal toxic or no) but can greatly help reduce the heavy metal load, as well as other toxins in the body.

Healing the gut before starting chelation:

A doctor once told me that we had to heal the gut before we could start the chelation process. However, in the children that I have seen recover, probably up to the last month before they recover, their gut might still not yet be perfect. For example, one of the little girls that recovered continued to suffer from constipation at 30 days before she lost her autism diagnosis. However, at this stage something seemed to switch, she started having regular bowel movements and within 30 days she lost her diagnosis.

Basically we're healing the intestines as we're chelating, as we're healing everything else. They are all parts of the puzzle. I would never put chelation before the CD or parasite protocols. However, it's definitely something that's part of our road when, after these other approaches, children have not yet recovered. At some point after we have the CD, ocean water, parasite protocol and some supplements is when we can add in chelators. It's not like I'm saying, "Oh we'll talk about that in a couple of years." We want our children recovered in less time. It's like a marathon, we keep the pace, never lose our heads, or break into a sprint.

Do not chelate with constipation:

If the child suffers from constipation, it's really important that we start moving the intestines when we're using chelators. There are a few options open to us for moving the intestines. I have found that the most effective is through the use of CD enemas. If your child isn't having a daily bowel movement, I would do an enema once a day. If you absolutely can't do enemas, get that child in a CD bath. We're finding that 50 to 100 drops in a bathtub is allowing children who previously had constipation to have bowel movements.

There are a few children/adults on the protocol that will not do enemas, or the parent will not. Whatever their situation may be, we have to get the bowels moving again. In this case, we do 50 to 100 drops in their bath water along with their max oral dose every day. The result has been that they're having regular bowel movements. That's one way we can move it along and then you can keep chelating. It's really important to have a daily bowel movement with any kind of chelation because otherwise the toxins are simply reabsorbed through the intestinal wall, whether they're heavy metals or other pathogens.

IV chelation is not the only means by which to cure autism:

I think at one point between 2006-2008, we were all focused on the problem in the world of autism being the heavy metals, because there was mercury/Thimerosal in the vaccines. We had to get the mercury out of our children. Well, part of the problem is they're not detoxing. As mentioned before, methylation cycles are impaired in children on the spectrum. I met a young girl whose parents were both allopathic doctors and they really believed at that point, as most of us did, that heavy metals were the problem with autism. If we could get the heavy metals out then they would recover. The parents did 122 IV chelations and their child never improved. At this point I have lost touch with them, but these are things that we have to learn along the way. I know now that it is NOT just about chelation, and why metals are NOT the only important piece. All of the pieces play a role and likely interact to cause autism in our children. There is a symbiotic relationship between the viruses, bacteria, candida, and parasites that exist in the biofilm. Since CD can break down biofilm and kill the pathogens living in it, as well as neutralize heavy metals, it has been a very powerful tool for us.

Doing a blood test to look for heavy metals:

Generally speaking, within three days of heavy metals entering the bloodstream, the body will deposit the heavy metals into tissues, organs, and eventually bones. For this reason, a blood test is not the best place to look for heavy metals in children with autism. Unless the child has very recently been exposed to heavy metals, we are unlikely to see elevated levels of heavy metals through a blood analysis.

The articles at the end of this book (Appendices 13 & 14) will provide further insight as to why chelation can be so important for our children on the spectrum.

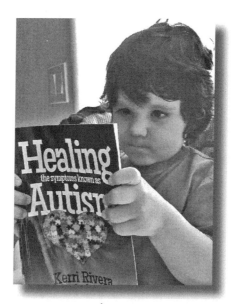

Luca

Chapter 11

Step 6 - Hyperbarics

by Bob Sands (Introduction by Dr. Beatrice Golomb)

"What Oxygen is to the lungs, such is hope to the meaning of life."
~ Emil Brunner

We were fortunate enough to have the amazing Bob Sands write this chapter on hyperbarics explaining its importance in healing ASD's.

Note: Throughout this section of the book, the author, Robert Lyne-Sands uses the actual names of the people with whom he came in contact with. In some instances it is with their permission, in others it is not. The accuracy of quotations, opinions expressed within this chapter, and the names used are solely the responsibility of Robert Lyne-Sands. Great care has been taken to remain within the bounds of current journalistic integrity and practice.

Robert Lyne-Sands new book, *OXYGEN: The First Medicine, Volume 1 CANCER*, is expected to be released January 2014.

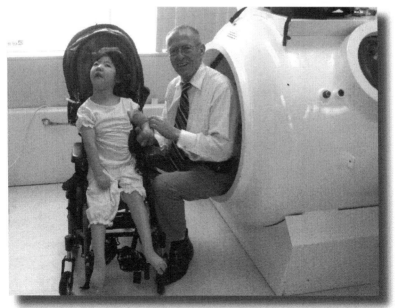

Robert Lyne-Sands author of the Hyperbaric section of the book, with one of his young patients, getting ready for a session.

> **Robert Sands** is one of only about five licensed manufacturers of hyperbaric oxygen therapy (HBOT) machines in the US, with extensive experience in clinical hyperbaric treatment, whose expertise will be an exceptional asset to this project. He has designed and manufactured HBOT machines for the US, Australia, Britain, Thailand, and many other nations, for naval/military use, civilian diving use, and medical use. He has the theoretical understanding of HBOT therapy that derives from intimate involvement in the process of designing and manufacturing these machines. He has the practical experience that derives from running a set of HBOT centers, and personally overseeing greater than 20,000 hours of HBOT sessions over 35 years.
> ~ Dr. Beatrice Golomb, MD, PhD.
> Professor of Medicine. UCSD 2011.
>
> *Beatrice Alexandra Golomb, MD, PhD (PI) is singularly qualified to lead this study. She has expertise in GWI including authorship of four RAND reports related to GWI29-31, and work in the scientific literature. She has been a member, since its inception, of the Department of Veterans Affairs Research Advisory Committee on Gulf War Veterans' Illnesses, and served as Scientific Director of this Committee. As a licensed internist, she is a primary care physician for a panel of ~280 veterans, including GWV, at the VA San Diego Healthcare Center.*

Recently, I sought the answer to something that was puzzling me. My friend, Dr. Bernard Gunter, is a revered and renowned psychologist in his eighties and, if anyone would know the answer, Bernard would.

"Does God, Great Spirit in the Sky, The Universe or whatever unseen deity you worship give you freedom for personal choices or is everything predestined?"

Bernard's eyes twinkled. He was never in a hurry to answer a question. In my mind, Dr. Bernard Gunter is sort of the American version of the Dali Lama.

He thought for a moment, selecting his words carefully, and then replied, "Funny you should ask that—just the other day I was talking with Eckhart Tolle and asked him that very same question. Tolle replied, 'God allows you to think that you have free will and free choice—and you do, by and large. However the roadmap is laid out for you beforehand.'"

Just as I suspected.

Dr. Bernard Rimland, Kerri Rivera, and the Hand of God.

On January 20th, 2006, a tall, glamorous woman walked into my San Diego clinic; her name was Kerri Rivera. She had brought her small five-and-a-half-year-old son, Patrick all the way from Mexico for hyperbaric oxygen therapy. The little fellow was absolutely gorgeous, but had a vacant stare and made no eye contact with any adult, rarely even with his mother. Day after day Patrick spent time in the chamber.

Kerri explained to me that Patrick developed normally for almost the first two years of his life. Then, to comply with vaccine regulations, Patrick received the DPT, HepB, and Influenza B (Pentavalente) vaccines in one day. Patrick fell into a complete zombie-like state after the injections. By the time Kerri arrived in San Diego, she had already done her homework. She blamed the vaccinations and had already undertaken the task of healing her son.

After her own experience with autism, Kerri wanted to help people and she was already doing the DAN! Protocol, etc., as Dr. Rimland has done so much for the children and she had a lot of respect and admiration for him and his work.

One day, I walked into the clinic and told her, "We're having lunch with Bernie tomorrow. Get a babysitter." At that point, totally shocked, she said, "Oh my God, yes, but I don't have anything to wear!"

"Trust me, what you have on would be just fine." A flustered Kerri rushed off to purchase some dressy clothes—she was, after all, a woman originally from Chicago. The very next day, we were sitting with Bernie and his wife Gloria in a quaint little restaurant, *The Green Tomato*. If the reader wishes to see that day, just go to your computer and look up Bernie on Wikipedia and there you will see Kerri in her black business suit (http://en.wikipedia.org/wiki/Bernard_Rimland).

Over lunch, Bernie and Kerri bonded immediately. None of us at the table realized that Bernie was suffering from cancer and had less than a year to live. Driving the short distance back to my clinic I made the observation to Kerri that I suspected she was about to become a scientist, and no longer just a trophy wife. "Be careful," I warned her, "Bernie Rimland's mantle will be heavy on your shoulders."

Kerri turned her face toward me and said, "I will carry that mantle willingly and with honor."

After a few days, Bernie told me that he thought Kerri had what it takes to carry the torch and help families heal their children with autism. I saw a lot of Bernie in the next nine months. He would come down to the clinic for regular hyperbaric treatments because it eased the pain of his cancer. Just before his death, he told me, "I will not die before I have found the reason for and defeated autism." But die he did on November 21, 2006, at the age of 78.

As I drove to Bernie's grave, I anticipated many, many people lining the way with some hundreds even thousands thronging the memorial park, similar to Giuseppe Verdi's funeral, in 1901, where 200,000 people gathered. At his graveside, the thousands of mourners spontaneously burst into the "Slaves Chorus" from his Opera, Nabucco.

I was stunned upon arriving. Probably less than thirty or so weeping caregivers of children with autism were present at the burial, along with Gloria and Bernie's three children. WHERE WERE ALL THE PEOPLE, THE MOTHERS AND FATHERS, THE RESEARCHERS AND SCIENTISTS? I asked myself. It was my first Jewish funeral and I think that the booming sound of the shovel full of earth that I threw down onto his plain casket made me look heavenward and ask, "God, where are you now?"

I drove home, eyes unfocused with tears, and stone eggs of the birds of unhappiness in my heart, stopping only to purchase two fine bottles of wine to toast Bernie. I knew one would not be enough. Arriving at my house, I found the fine crystal goblet my Mom had left me, filled it, and played Neil Diamond's, Morningside over and over, with each playing, another glass, held high to Bernie...

Morningside
The old man died
And no one cried
They simply turned away

And when he died
He left a table made of nails and pride
And with his hands,
He carved these words inside
'For my children'

Morning light
Morning bright
I spent the night
With dreams that make you weep
Morning time
Wash away the sadness
From these eyes of mine
For I recall the words an old man signed
'For my children'

And the legs were shaped with his hands
And the top made of oaken wood
And the children
That sat around this great table
Touched it with their laughter
Ah, and that was good

Morningside
An old man died
And no one cried
He surely died alone
And truth is sad
For not a child would claim the gift he had
The words he carved became his epitaph
'For my children'

In fact, as I sit here writing this, I play Diamond's melody and listening to the words makes my heart swell and my eyes become damp.

The morning after Bernie's funeral, hung-over and miserable, I pondered: Did my beloved friend Bernie die feeling that he failed? I now doubt it for he had passed his mantle to carry on his search for the cure without fear, without the need for accolades and rewards and to do so with integrity. I did not know it, but before his passing, Bernie and Kerri had been in communication. Bernie had given her permission to translate his *Defeat Autism Now!* Protocol into Spanish, Kerri's other language, as well as other tasks.

In review, I now see God's Hand at work—and it started one afternoon at the Green Tomato. Thus, my question to my friend on free will versus predestination right at the start of my notes on this section.

Brain overload and frozen fingers.

At the time, when Kerri asked me to write this section of her book about hyperbaric oxygen therapy and the treatment of challenged children, my mind went into overload. Why? Kerri was (in my view and that of others) the most efficient and effective health scientist with a high normalization rate of challenged children (autism, etc.). With her own hospital-quality hyperbaric oxygen center, Kerri had first-hand knowledge that to normalize such an afflicted person required a lot more than some trips in a oxygen chamber or some Silver Bullet response from a pharmaceutical company.

My brain whistled like an express train rushing through a tunnel. I thought of the dozens of children that hyperbaric oxygen therapy has helped at my different centers. Some of the little guys were so badly damaged they would repeatedly punch at their own head, or chewed on their own wrists. I'm thinking of Marco as I write this. Ten years later, he still punches. A clearly defined casualty of a hotshot thimerosal vaccination, normal until three, his parents won a multimillion-dollar lawsuit against Big PHARMA. There has been some progress over the years; but it will be a matter of unrelenting attention to Marco.

I remember another little guy; a handsome, articulate smiling boy of about 12 years of age named Chase. Meeting him and his parents, you would never know he had autism or ADHD. Chase was a "runner." When his treatment in the chamber was over, he would promptly disappear out of the clinic doors. Eventually, Chase would be carted back down by one of the upstairs nurses. "Chase" by name and chased by nature.

After one such session in the chamber, he rocketed out and into the restroom of the clinic. I was sitting at the controls when he came back. Chase climbed up onto my knee and said, "I love you Bob," and he rubbed his hands across my face. From the terrible odor I knew in an instant what was all over my face and my lips. Chase had used his hands instead of toilet paper and bypassed the washbasin on the way out.

"Oh goodness," came from his horrified mother. "He got you. I am so sorry. It is one of his favorite jokes."

"Not to worry," I said, "I have eaten and tasted this in a variety of forms most my life." So, whenever I hear somebody say, "Sands is not a Doctor so he doesn't know s—t from Shinola," I think of Chase.

Normalizing kids is so rewarding, but you have to take a chance on s**t.

My fingers were not ready for the keyboard as I tried to wade through dozens of experiences with these children, my own personal experiences, and finally adding input from experts in the field of pediatric abnormalities. (Many of these experts became my close, personal friends as the years went by.)

For any parent or caregiver to delve into all of the opinions and conclusions of the so-called experts, it is a bewildering journey through a lot of contradictory and self-serving educated guesses and erroneous assumptions. To arrive at something that the reader will identify with, and believe in, I have to go way back. After 70 years on the face of this planet, I have reached certain conclusions about the treatment of children that enables me to write this section. Mind you, I'm not stuck in my ways and I am open to change my thoughts and conclusions as the science improves on treating children with autism.

Little Patrick Rivera, Little Bobby Sands
Something in Common?

Here is something that I doubt my adult children even know about. In 1947, polio was raging throughout Australia. I was seven years of age and had developed a sore throat and fever. My father, a wealthy man, called the very best doctor to my bedside—yes physicians did make house calls in those days. I can even remember the doctor's name, Dr. Bradfield. His father had been the engineer that designed the Sydney Harbor Bridge. My dad, with all of his money drew a lot of water in those days and could get almost anything he wanted. Bradfield came in and examined me briefly; after all he had other house calls that night.

Bradfield told my Mom and Dad that he did not think I had polio, but perhaps diphtheria and that I should spend time in isolation in the infectious disease hospital overlooking Botany Bay, "just in case." The next morning an ambulance came and, in spite of my fear, pleading, misery, and tears they carted me away. The three-hour journey became a six-hour journey. The ambulance broke down outside the Sydney airport. I remember looking out of the rain spattered window and seeing the aircraft clearly visible over the fence. We sat on the side of the road for almost two hours before the replacement ambulance came to transport me, and my journey continued to a huge colonial building complex, built by convicts and perched on rolling, green lawns that looked down onto the Pacific. The complex was known as, The Coast Infectious Disease Hospital, which later became Prince Henry Hospital. I was terrified and clutched my teddy bear, *Threadbare*, under the blankets. Threadbare became my only friend for the next four months, and a glimpse of airplanes over the fence became an enduring memory of the trip.

My parents were already there and had obviously filled out all of paperwork. I never got to say goodbye to them since it was an infectious disease hospital. As they walked past a big hopper window, they paused momentarily and Mum waved through the window. I saw them maybe three times in the next four months when the nurses wheeled my bed up against the window that looked out into the hall. They would tap on the glass and smile at me but because my father was quickly bored, after about five minutes they would wave and be gone for another couple of weeks. It was a long way for them to travel.

The night of my arrival, a team of doctors and nurses arrived and they rolled me onto my side. Full syringes lay on a tray; in those days they were glass with little thumb and finger holes on each side and each needle was reused and supposedly resharpened before their next use. This meant that the needles were thick and long. One-by-one these needles were inserted into my upper thigh on the left-hand side. The pain was agonizing and I'm sure I screamed and screamed. I remember at least three nurses holding me down. At seven, I was just a little fellow. There had to be at least 20 of these very large syringes. Checking the history books, I believe that they were mostly penicillin and sulfa drugs. I might add, it was already known to Doctor Bradfield that I was highly allergic to sulfa and remained so for my entire life.

The next morning, when I awoke, I found that I was paralyzed from the feet up to just under my arms. Threadbare was my only friend for the next four months. The days all blurred together. One thing I do remember vividly is that I used to deliberately wet the bed. I did so only when a lovely red-haired nurse with a band of freckles across her nose was on duty. This nurse was kind and gentle, probably in her twenties. After she had changed the sheets, she would stroke my cheek and tell me that everything was going to be okay and not to worry about wetting the bed. The other older nurses scolded any of the other pediatric patients if they had an accident. At some point later, my gentle nurse told me that I really did not need to wet the bed to get her attention. I soon stopped and I still got a cuddle from her. Such a display of care and affection was unknown to me from my parents back at home.

After that stay in the hospital, I was never the same. I know that there was constant discussion amongst my family members that I should be placed in some sort of an institution because my behavior was "contrary and stubborn." I was either talking my head off, trying to make my family love me, or distant, and as such, I was said to be "uncooperative." Soon after, I was placed in a Hogwarts-style boarding school.

Could that childhood experience have made me what I am today, forever alone, but rarely lonely? As the years ticked by, to my surprise (and I think everybody else's), the school counselors found that I had a genius IQ. Amongst the 1,200 boys, I was second from the top.

After seventeen years of treating so-called challenged children, I have yet to find one that was not as smart as a whip in something.

I managed to burn every social bridge at the boarding school, thrown out of every special social club at Newington. On Saturday afternoon, after mandatory sports such as Cricket or Rugby, the other boarders would get to do things they wanted like billiards, photography, or gardening (these were clubs that you had to apply for and join). However, I had been expelled from each of them so I wandered alone each Saturday afternoon and finally picked the lock on a large room-sized cage full of Sulfur-Crested Cockatoos and other Australian parrots. I would sit alone with them and be jeered at by the boys in the garden club that were planting and weeding. Within weeks, these birds would happily climb all over me, enjoying my company. The birds loved me, but the boys and masters did not. To me, it was a two-way street. Animals made better friends than people. Eventually some of the other boys would come and beg to be allowed to accompany me into the cage so they too could have that same privilege.

Do not get the wrong impression of my beloved Newington College in Sydney Australia; even today I dream of the sanctuary of that place. It was better than what I had with my family back home.

The really curious thing is that my mind had blotted my hospital stay out, or had hidden it in some black cabinet in my brain where the really bad things are kept to allow me to get on with the reality of NOW. I remembered the illness and isolation only when Kerri asked me to write this. The details have returned with clarity: the old iron beds, the smiling face and freckles of my favorite nurse, being cold at night, the colors on the wall, the distant sight of the ocean through a window on the other side of the big ward, the frame of the window so far away that it looked like a painting hanging there. If I close my eyes as I write I can see it now.

I now ask myself, "Is this the way children with autism feel?"

I don't know. What I do know is that my old friend and confidant, teddy bear, is sitting on the desk as I write this. I reach out to rub Threadbare's head and a great calmness washes over me. The little fellow is 64-years-old now and there is a great competition amongst my adult children to see who gets him after I die.

Botched diagnosis
The incorrect pharmaceutical response.

With almost 40 years of working in medicine behind me, and now in my retirement, I do know that neither diphtheria nor polio were the problem. The suffocating "Bull Neck" or the "Strangling Angel of Children," diphtheria, had not happened to me, nor did the withered limbs of poliomyelitis set in after paralysis.

Simply put, Dr. Bradfield cocked it all up in a big way by guessing, not taking enough time and arriving at the wrong medical response on his visit. The relentless attack on me with sulfa drugs caused paralysis, which was probably what is commonly known today as Guillain–Barré Syndrome, a disorder affecting the peripheral nervous system. Ascending paralysis, weakness beginning in the feet and hands and migrating towards the trunk, is the most typical symptom; the disease is usually triggered by an infection.

It sure sounds similar to what happened to little Patrick, and probably to the reader's challenged child as well.

Migrating to America in 1990 with my tribe of offspring.

I arrived in the United States over twenty years ago. If the reader is interested enough, a quick look at a funny but classy "roast" presentation is on YouTube. You can find it by searching "Robert Lyne-Sands" on YouTube.

After completing the United States Navy transportable chamber development project, I arrived in swank, Pacific Palisades, on the outskirts of Los Angeles; living amongst all of the Hollywood greats. I was going nuts with boredom and became the "Bob Clampett" of the area; jogging down the leafy streets I always said Gudday to any celebrity. I rarely remembered their names but knew their faces. They never replied on the first go past, but then I would jog backwards, keeping pace with them (big stars like Madonna always ran with a group of minders) and I would yell out "I said Gudday. My goodness, your manners are appalling." I might add, it was not just me; they never ever nodded to each other when their paths crossed either.

Around this time, I opened the very first freestanding hyperbaric oxygen therapy center. It was more or less hidden away in Santa Monica on 6th Street. Tucked away in what used to be an old motel, you could almost refer to it as a "speakeasy" center, akin to something from the days of prohibition, where you had to knock on the door three times before being let in. I would only treat people who had been referred by another patient. Most of these people were from the entertainment industry in Hollywood, many with the HIV virus, and lots of folks with chronic fatigue syndrome.

The kiss of death in Hollywood is to be known to be ill. Hyperbaric oxygen therapy works so well that the word soon got around, and I was inundated with patients, some famous and well-known, and others just hardworking folk in the movie industry. Thus, I ended up being known for some years as "Mr. Oxygen," and because of the remarkable effects of HBOT, I befriended many of these celebrities, who subsequently invited me as their guest to many of the big Hollywood functions (the only one that I missed was the Academy Awards).

One of the first of these talented people that became my close friend was Harold Michelson. Harold was an award-winning art director working out of DreamWorks. He was suffering the aftermath of a mild stroke. His wife Lillian had told me that her Harold loved crossword puzzles, but since his stroke he would put the across answer in the down column. This caused him immense frustration since his answer was usually correct, just in the wrong place. Five treatments in the little chamber were all it took for Harold to get his verticals and horizontals in the right place. The big thing that he noticed was that his blood pressure stabilized, his lung problems normalized, and he needed less medication for his diabetes.

Harold still stood well over 6-feet–tall, though stooped with old age. We hit it off immediately because Harold had a quick wit and loved a good laugh. The stories and banter between us were constant. Harold was extremely talented yet self-effacing. He really was a hero in the truest sense of the word. As young man, he made over 40 flights across the English Channel to bomb Germany. As navigator, Harold sat in the nosecone of the B-17 and either froze with the cold on the trip or froze with fear when making the lower-level bombing run. "Bob, I was so frightened of the flak from the antiaircraft fire from the Germans on the ground. As the puffs of smoke would erupt around the front of the aircraft, shrapnel would pierce plexi-glass windows in front of me. I would hold the navigational map in front of me and try to believe that the thin paper would stop the lethal fragments."

The first challenged child to be treated in a hyperbaric chamber—Emily.

I need to jump forward in time for a moment before getting back to Harold Michelson and his wife, Lillian. I went back into production of hyperbaric chambers after I realized the great need for hospital-grade dispensing of oxygen to the public. There were no rules preventing me from doing this even though I'm not a physician. All my patients needed was a prescription from a registered physician; that was the easy part. My first center was in San Diego.

In the first few months of patient treatments we received a call from a father in Canada. His daughter, Emily, had cerebral palsy. The father had read that hyperbaric oxygen therapy would perhaps help his little girl normalize, and so when he asked me what I thought I gave him my usual answer, "I do not know, I am not a physician." And then I added, "I would hate for you to waste your money on a trip from Canada to San Diego if it doesn't work."

The father replied, "I have two choices. I can go to England where there is snow on the ground or I can come to San Diego. It is an easy choice to make."

So father and daughter duly arrived. Emily was the most delightful child. When she walked through the door she had a crash helmet on, knee guards, and wrist-guards to prevent serious injury when she would crash, face first, into the floor. We learned a lot in the first ten days of treating Emily. One of the first things was the fact that fathers can never properly do a good job on their daughter's hair. I felt for the father since Emily had lots and lots of hair and was never still for a moment (I have a few daughters myself). Emily would arrive looking like a rag doll; her little blonde head would have pins, bits of string and ribbon through it. So the very first task of our nurses would be to grab Emily (usually tearing around the clinic), and comb her hair out to make her more presentable.

Now, the really big thing that we noticed was that on day ten she arrived at the clinic without any of her body armor. Yes, she still "toe-walked" because her heels did not touch the floor. To compensate, she would park her little fists against her chest, push her elbows out to keep a center of gravity, and rush around the clinic. On day 11, father and daughter spent five hours at the San Diego Zoo without the usual body protection. Emily never lost balance or tumbled even once. Follow-up visits over the last 17 years find that Emily is living a normal life. Yes, she still has some walking problems, but never needed to undergo the mutilating surgery that was recommended to her by her Canadian doctors. During 20 days of hyperbaric oxygen treatments in San Diego, something had changed in Emily's brain.

Likely the most important introduction in my life...
The Great-Spirit-in-the Sky's (God's) hand at work.

Listening to the improvements that little Emily had made, Harold Michelson was both enchanted and excited.

"Did you know that Lillian and I have an autistic son? We need to introduce you to a couple of people in San Diego. Dr. Eric Courchesne, who runs the autism research center for the University of San Diego, known as the Autism Center of Excellence or ACE."

Lillian chimed in and said, "I really must call them about you. Eric is a gem and his wife Rachel is also a research doctor. They work side-by-side and will be so helpful."

With Emily's positive results, and more children making gains at the center, I called the Courchesne couple at the ACE and offered to provide them with the use of a $150,000 hospital-grade hyperbaric chamber for one full year. There was no response to my offer.

While you may imagine that the UCSD-ACE Research Center is located in some lofty center of learning, it is in fact to be found in a delightful millionaire's village known as La Jolla in Southern California, a block or so from the Pacific Ocean. On the top floor of a three-story building, an elegant balcony ran across the front of the building, while red and white umbrellas and tables make it look more like a posh restaurant than a research center.

I waited about a month and called again and repeated my offer of a hyperbaric chamber, operated by trained technicians for a year, or whatever time it took to make a decision on efficacy, at zero cost to the ACE. About an hour after making the second call, my secretary told me that a Dr. Rachel Courchesne was on the line and needed to speak to me on an urgent matter. I picked up the telephone, anticipating a good conversation but this is the way that it went, all one-way at me. Dr. Rachel was in fine fury and, looking back, the only way I could have put a word into that conversation would have been to fold the word flat and slip it into the tirade, sideways. She told me that it was amateurs such as myself that muddied the scientific waters of autism research and that, essentially, I should crawl back into whatever hole I came out of.

She made it clear to me that the mission of the ACE was to perform research to find a cure with pharmaceuticals. In fact, the ACE receives funding from drug companies, and that I should not bother them again. I was taken aback, to say the least.

A decade later, Dr. Eric is apparently doing fine work. For example, in his recent research, quoted widely in the media, he has found that the frontal lobes of an autistic child's brain is abnormally large. This is an observation, perhaps useful in the future, but only time will tell. But does it matter to you the reader whether this is so? Maybe yes, maybe no, so let's hold off on that sort of thing until we get into the scientific part of the book.

Let's get back to Dr. Rachel's harangue of me. In my mind, there is no doubt about the fact that for her, at least, it was all about the money and the potential for a patented silver bullet for Big PHARMA. If successful, a drug company could charge you a huge amount of money to heal your child with autism. At worst, there would be the ability to raise more money for research despite scant evidence of clinical results on children.

An example of this ability to raise money on a potential medical marketplace is the fact that in the year 2012, the National Institute of Health (NIH) allocated $100 million over a five-year period to a bunch of ACE research across the United States. So much for Lillian's glowing endorsement of Dr. Rachel.

However, the Michelson's other introduction proved to be a link in the chain.

Autism research with integrity—Dr. Bernie Rimland.

"A dear friend of ours, Dr. Bernard Rimland, also has a research center in San Diego which he calls Defeat Autism Now!, or DAN! for short. Bernie's son, Marc, is a true autistic savant. The movie with Dustin Hoffman and Tom Cruise, Rain Man, was modeled around Bernie and Gloria's son. Bernie was the technical advisor for the film. You must meet Bernie."

Lillian was especially grateful and fond of Bernie and his wife, Gloria. Back in the early 1950s, autistic children were attributed to cold, hard, heartless mothers. Many psychologists and psychiatrists agreed with the "Emotional frigidity" hypothesis, which suggested that the mothers were the cause of what we now know as autism. A lot of children in the United States were taken by force from their parents, and placed in isolated institutions to "protect" them from their parents. Bernie Rimland alone stood against this hypothesis; after all Bernie did have degrees in psychology, including a PhD. In fact, it was Bernie that took away the shame, the blame, and the guilt of many loving parents who were bullied into believing labels put upon them by the so-called "learned."

Driving forces behind autism research centers.

Unlike the La Jolla location for the ACE, Bernie's Autism Research Institute (ARI) was about five minutes drive from my San Diego hyperbaric oxygen dispensary; two minutes of freeway, a quick turn into Adams Avenue, and I had arrived. Again with an erroneous assumption, I had thought that Bernie's ARI would be similar to the ACE La Jolla location. In fact, I drove past Bernie's place three times before I found it. An unassuming, clay-colored, converted storefront, with a little sign on the front door that said, "Autism Research Institute." I knocked on the door and walked in. Instantly, the smell of antiquity and old books overwhelmed me and beguiled me, like something out of a Harry Potter movie. Stacks of papers were high on the floor almost in a willy-nilly fashion. A gentleman dressed in a checkered shirt came towards me. "Bob Sands? The Michelson's said to expect you." He peered over his glasses and gray whiskers at me. In that one glance, we created a bond of friendship that lasted for more than a decade. At least once or twice a month we would lunch together along with his wife, Gloria; always two blocks from his Center, at the *Bleu Boheme*. Bernie and Gloria would carefully examine the menu and then they would both look out and recommend, "Let's all order the fried green tomatoes."

Bernie was interested in clinical results. He would turn over any stone that would perhaps unlock the mystery of autism. When I first met Bernie, 1 in 850 children born in the United States was afflicted with this mysterious and terrifying disorder. As I write, autism spectrum disorders have spiked to 1 child in every 88. So when the phone rang at the ARI, Bernie would often answer it and ask many questions, if the person believed that they had found a cure or a clue. He never discarded anything, in stark contrast to my encounter with Dr. Rachel at the ACE in La Jolla. I once listened in when he spoke with a lady who believed that you could cure autism by filling crystal glasses to different levels and rubbing your fingers around the edges to create pure tones.

Bernie put the telephone down and said to me, "It could be worth looking into. Music does create new neuronal wiring in small children, for example, or a mother singing to a child." I had already mentioned to him that when a child with autism was in the chamber, if you played unfamiliar sounds such as whale songs, or bagpipes, the unresponsive child would often brighten up and look around.

"Maybe new neuronal connections are being established," Bernie pondered as he rubbed his whiskers.

In those days, I worked on weekends. If I wanted to chat with Bernie, Sunday was the best day. No staff to answer the telephone, so he always did. I once asked him whether he took a day off and his response was succinct:

"When autism takes a day off so will I."

Bernie, a $2.6 million donation and his ARI.

Now, here is the most interesting of Bernie Rimland's driving forces—to me at least. It was not about dollars or ego, not in the slightest.

At that time, I was also friends with another Bernie, the renowned anthropologist, Dr. Bernard Aginsky. To avoid confusion between the two Bernie's I will refer to him as Dr. Aginsky. He was in his late 90s at the time, as rich as Croesus. For many years, he had leased the penthouse of the La Jolla Shores Hotel, right on the beach of one of the most desired parts of Southern California. Again, like most of my friends, Dr. Aginsky was a humble man and thought nothing of his wealth other than as a means of accomplishment. Out of the blue, one day in my office, Dr. Aginsky looked at me thoughtfully and then asked, "I have $2.6 million and I want to give it to somebody that would make a difference. Can I give it to you?"

I immediately thought of Bernie and the children with autism and the nonprofit status of the Autistic Research Institute. "Hold that thought Dr. Aginsky. I will give you an answer in a couple of days."

A couple of days later, Bernie and I were traveling to take part in a medical internal review board. I was wearing a shirt with French cuffs and a silk tie. Bernie had on his usual checkered shirt. He confided in me once that he had to make a choice between wearing a tie or trimming his Santa Claus-gray beard. The beard always won. Wondering about his shirts, I respectfully asked him whether he ever received a salary from his ARI.

"Good gracious. I could never pay myself a salary from ARI funds and donations. You must remember that I am on a full Navy pension so it would be wrong to double dip."

After the meeting, as we traveled back along the I-405 to San Diego, I broached the subject of Dr. Aginski's offer of a $2.6 million donation for the Autism Research Institute. Bernie looked out the window for a few moments and fiddled with his beard. I could see he was calculating in his head. He turned to me and said, "We have so much money in the ARI at this time, donations and such, that I think that amount of money could be used elsewhere. Find another recipient."

Dr. Bernard Aginsky, a widower, passed away in January 2000. I have no idea where his donation ended up. I do know whether Bernie Rimland ever had a second thought about not taking that money. He never mentioned our conversation again.

DAN! changing to parallel other autism research.

Research costs money. Bernie used his resources wisely and was not interested in empire-building. He just wanted to find the cause and the answers. Bernie cured kids.

On the anniversary of his death, I went to his Kensington ARI center. I had two bottles of good wine, a bunch of wine glasses, and a whole lot of chocolates. I walked in and was astonished. The whole tenor and tone of the place had changed. The clutter was gone. Bookshelves were neat and organized. The smell of scholarly interest in documents and old books had evaporated. It was as if the ghost of Dr. Bernard Rimland seemed to have moved to another place completely. The staff were delighted to see me, and happily munched on the yummy chocolates that I had brought for them. I commented on the neatness and the vast changes that I observed. One of the staff shrugged her shoulders, grimaced, and said,

"You have no idea just what changes have taken place, and what is about to happen."

An example of the transformation in attitude is exemplified by an offer for inflatable, aka soft-sided, chambers for DAN! while Bernie was still alive. One day, he called me up and explained to me that a group was coming to do a presentation on these soft chambers, and suggested that I plant one of my staff at the ARI to listen to the blurb from the manufacturer, Oxyheal. My secretary, Crystal was waiting amongst Bernie's staff to greet the technicians, doctors, and such that accompanied the owner of the company. They arrived at the ARI, set up the inflatable chamber, and gave their sales pitch, extolling the virtues of hyperbarics at low pressure and at a low cost.

Crystal reported back to me that Bernie looked dour during the presentation and asked, "What would happen to this with a razor blade?" Bernie and I discussed the concept of inflatable chambers the next time he was at my center, after he had finished his treatment in a chamber. He was not convinced about the soft-sided chambers.

"I worried that the scientific data that they quoted was all from hospital quality chambers. I think you are correct Bob, the physics do not hold up. I could not recommend this device to parents for their children."

The "discovery" (observation) of God's gunpowder + Bernie Rimland and Kerri Rivera.

Throughout history, air was taken for granted. You just breathed in and out and there it was; bugs and birds flew in it, mostly useful to keep your floors and ceilings apart. Even in this day and age, many folks think of it in the same way.

Let´s revisit what is now called the Age of Enlightenment, the 17th and 18th Centuries. About 1774, the kindly and soft spoken clergyman/scientist Joseph Priestly and his close friend Benjamin Franklin. They spent time drinking coffee together once a week in a London coffee house along with other scientists. Together they realized that air was actually a mixture of gases, but mostly nitrogen and oxygen. Priestly and Franklin could kill a mouse in a glass jar in less than five minutes by depriving it of one of those gasses. Put the poor little mouse in a glass jar with a lit candle (which consumed the oxygen) and the flame of life in the mouse departed by about the time the candle went out.

Using precise scales, Joseph Priestly and the French chemist Antoine Lavoisier, gave oxygen its name. It could be weighed on a scale just like you would weigh out a cup of rice. Each unseen gas has a weight. Baros is the Greek word for weight. Words that we are familiar with come from this: barometer, barometric pressure, and hyperbaric (as in hyperbaric oxygen therapy, hyper meaning more than and baric meaning weight of the gas).

Weigh oxygen?

The weight of air (mixed oxygen and nitrogen) is 14.7 pounds per square inch at sea level. Most folks like me would prefer to use the word pressure, however, the math is easier if we use the doctors measure (the same as that used in measuring blood pressure – millimeters of mercury or mmHg). An average blood pressure measure is typically 120/80 mmHg. Let's look at it this way; if air at sea level is 760 mmHg, then 20% of that air (oxygen) is 20% of that amount. So multiply 760 by 0.20 and you will realize that vital, life-giving oxygen going into your lungs is about 150 mmHg.

Oxygen - You cannot see it, or smell it but you have to "eat" a kilogram of it each day to stay alive.

Make no mistake. If you take a substance into your body, ALL of your 60 to 90 trillion cells will be affected. Snort it, chew it and swallow it, breathe it, or inject that substance and it will have a positive or negative effect on your whole body. Cells "consume" the substance. Another word for consume is "eat." We will discuss this process, known as oxidative metabolism shortly and, especially how to produce stem-progenitor cells.

Eat oxygen?

Oxygen is a cellular food. The adult human consumes approximately 0.6 kg of oxygen each day (about 1.2 pounds). We can live about three weeks without the food that we chew and swallow, survive three days without water, but we can only live approximately three minutes without oxygen. Body cells start to die—the brain is the most vulnerable. Even a minute or so without oxygen can cause permanent damage.

Don't worry about the earth running out of oxygen. Back in the 1700s Ben Franklin and Joe Priestly also discovered the fact that sunlight on green vegetation produces oxygen—a process called photosynthesis. They showed this with the mouse and candle in the glass jar. As the candle flame seemed to flicker, about to go out and the mouse lay, apparently dead, if there was a sprig of a green plant, both the candle and mouse came back to life. All of the oxygen that you are going to eat in the next 24-hours is replaced by just one square meter of grass producing oxygen through photosynthesis during that same length of time. In populated areas, where there is not much greenery, life-sustaining winds carry oxygen over the oceans and hills to all humans and animals.

Captain Cook, Joseph Priestly, Bernie Rimland, and Kerri Rivera—Explorers

Before we stop talking about Joseph Priestly, he made another observation about gas and this applies to our subject of autism, Bernie, and Kerri.

Living next door to a brewery, Priestly was intrigued about the gas given off by the fermentation of beer in the barrels. He put a dish of water under the vent-pipe coming out of the barrel. When he tasted the water it was full of refreshing bubbles we now call fizz. In 1767, Priestly discovered how to carbonate a liquid. He taught the Navigator, Captain Cook, how to carbonate water and, thinking that drinking that bubbly water would prevent scurvy, Cook set sail with it in 1772. It did not prevent scurvy, but, just like Bernie and Kerri, everything is worth investigating.

We now know that any gas becomes soluble if it is concentrated or made thick. In this instance, the gas was an extremely light gas known as carbon dioxide (yes, the stuff we breath out and, unlike the 21% oxygen, there is only about .033% of carbon dioxide in the air we breathe). However, if you concentrate it to 100% some of it melts into the water and becomes carbonic acid, as is the case with soft drinks. Pop the lid and the acid turns back into carbon dioxides gas, forming little bubbles in the liquid. Joseph Priestly should have patented his observation. Ten years or so later, Joseph Schweppes patented the process in Germany and most folks think of him, not Priestly, when they have a gin and tonic.

Thereby hangs another Newtonian rule about gas that cannot be changed. "Gas under pressure becomes soluble in a liquid according to its density (or thickness)." – Henry's Law.

And this is how oxygen works in a hyperbaric chamber – Newtonian Gas Laws

Stay with the soda can thought and the thicker gas melting into the sugary drink. When a human climbs into a hyperbaric oxygen chamber, we substitute oxygen for carbon dioxide. Believe it or not, you do not feel squashed by the pressure other than you have to "pop" or equalize your ears. Humans are mostly water and other fluids that cannot be compressed like a gas. What is happening in the chamber is that the oxygen (it should be 100% oxygen) is being made thicker or concentrated. And, just like the soda, Henry's Law kicks in. The oxygen melts and the body supersaturates with oxygen.

Another curious thing about a well-oxygenated body is that it becomes slightly alkaline. Your powers of hydrogen (pH) read about the same as seawater, which is alkaline because of the dissolved oxygen in it. Yes, even fish need their daily meal of oxygen!

The word "saturate" comes from the Latin word meaning "to completely fill." Since only our red blood cells (RBC) carry oxygen, they are almost always full of oxygen in a healthy human. The little pulse-ox device that clips on your finger when you are in hospital almost always reads 99% unless you are anemic.

It takes between one and three minutes for each RBC to leave your heart, make its complete circuit, and be back in your lungs for its next load of oxygen. Remember that Henry's Law also applies here, therefore, oxygen is a gas in your lungs but turns into molecular oxygen when it enters your body's fluids. This is so complex that there is no chemical symbol for it, but rest assured, your body's cells feed on it with a great appetite. (More on oxidative cellular metabolism shortly.)

Supersaturate?

When you fill a glass of water to the brim, it is full or saturated. Right? Yes. Holding it under the faucet and running more water into the glass will only mean that the water slops over the edges. The glass is still full. However, this is not the case with any gas, particularly oxygen breathed in by a human. Sure, just like a glass of water, oxygen can be measured by volume, but there is plenty of room to over-fill our bodies with oxygen—supersaturated.

To illustrate a complex process, let's paint a simple picture—An underground subway system.

Think of your lungs as a subway station. Passengers get off the carriages and others get on. In this instance, remember that air is made up of (for easy math calculations) 80% nitrogen and 20% oxygen. Visualize each gas molecule of either type as a gas-person. The body is already full of nitrogen at sea level and since it does nothing at all (it is inert), the nitrogen-people just come in and out your lungs. However the oxygen-people are dynamic and bustle to climb on board the little red-blood-cell carriage (which has a special oxygen-people magnet—an iron molecule), and away the red blood cell rushes with the oxygen-people ready to jump off to the hungriest of the body's cells.

Since Henry's Law allows a gas to melt into clear fluids (and our body has lots of clear fluids), there is a whole lot of room to add more oxygen-people. For example, if we barred entry to our lungs of the nitrogen-people (simple to do—just put on a mask and breath oxygen out of a 100% oxygen tank), then our lung-subway station would have five times more oxygen-people and that would mean that we increased the oxygen-people with each breath from 160 mmHg to 760 mmHg. Remember that they are dynamic, and that each red-blood-cell carriage has an oxygen magnet in it. The thick crowd oxygen-people all bustle to get onto that carriage, through the wet soapy surfactant in the wall of your lungs, even though it was already full.

Essentially, the oxygen-people fill the red-blood-cell carriage, and into the plasma where they are quickly swept along in that clear plasma fluid. Then, when even more oxygen-people continue to crowd on back at the subway station (i.e. the lungs), the plasma, which normally does not carry oxygen-people (molecular oxygen), then needs to put the overload of oxygen somewhere. From here the oxygen-people go out through the rail tunnels (i.e. the circulatory system) and into the clear fluid (i.e. interstitial fluid) that bathes our body cells. As this fluid fills with oxygen, it dumps it off into the body's largest water compartment—the body's cells (the intra-cellular compartment). These cells now have a veritable feast of oxygen available.

About 90 minutes after you start breathing 100% oxygen, you are supersaturated with five times the normal amount of molecular oxygen. No, you do not swell up since we are talking about molecules in existing body fluid, not added fluid. Curiously, if you put the little pulse-ox back on your finger, it would still only read 99% since it is just measuring the oxygen in your red blood cells. However, using high-tech oxygen measuring equipment (transcutaneous oxiometry), you can even measure molecular oxygen in your urine, saliva, and tears—something once thought impossible.

Now comes the hyperbaric chamber part. You climb in, the door is shut, and 100% oxygen floods in. The technician can look at the physician's prescription and increase the thickness of the gas in that chamber. Double the thickness (i.e. weight or pressure) to 1520 mmHg; ninety minutes later you will climb out of that chamber with ten times the number of oxygen-people (molecular oxygen) in your body. Or, put another way, since your body's cells are going to consume (eat) that additional oxygen, this is the only way you can increase the weight of oxygen-food available in a 24-hour period. One hundred percent pure oxygen at sea level and you will "eat" between just under half a kilogram to just over one kilogram of oxygen.

The deeper/thicker the oxygen is in the chamber the more you get. In fact, following Dalton's Universal Gas Laws, by doubling the pressure, you can actually get your daily oxygen meal at almost two kilograms.

Now the nifty thing about oxygen supersaturation.

Unlike many pharmaceuticals that are weight dependent, (too much of a certain drug will sicken or kill a smaller patient, not enough of the same drug and there will be no therapeutic benefit to the patient) with hyperbaric oxygen no individual can suffer from an "overdose" of oxygen, regardless of whether the patient is a mouse, rabbit, horse, or human. All climb out of the chamber, (depending on the pressure/thickness of oxygen they were treated at) with the same amount of molecular oxygen in their body. Not one person has suffered from an "overdose" of oxygen.

Our oxygen dispensary centers have treated, according to their physician's prescription, tiny babies, the elderly, and everyone in between; we have never seen a negative side effect. Instead, we have observed clinical positive effects for all.

What happens when we actually give people an extra "oxygen feast" by putting them in the chamber? Again, an extremely complicated process has to be simplified for understanding. However, before making things simpler we must first look at the science. Chatelier's principle predicts the effect of a change in conditions on a chemical equilibrium. The principle is named after Henry Louis Le Chatelier, who observed that if a chemical system at equilibrium has a change in concentration, temperature, volume, or partial pressure then the equilibrium shifts to counteract the imposed change and a new equilibrium is established. Any change in the status quo prompts an opposing reaction in the responding system.

Time to change just a couple of words for better understanding. Let us start with the word equilibrium and now call it "the way it was." We can also use that term for status quo and counteract can be changed to "pushing back." So what is really being said here is, if we change something in any chemical environment it will push back hard to be the way it was. Now it is time to make things even easier.

We are all chemical systems.

We have already mentioned cola in a can and advised against giving it to anybody, your child or yourself, because of the acidity of the liquid in the soda. But there is an even more compelling reason—the sugar. There are 39 grams of sugar, about ten teaspoons of sugar, in one can of soda. Would you feed your child that much dry sugar?

"Come on," you might think to yourself, "No way. It does not taste that sweet." It is true. The manufacturers of sodas use a lot of phosphoric acid to disguise the sickly sweetness of the drink. If you still doubt this, take an ordinary penny, or an egg and put it in a glass full of cola overnight. Within a few days, you will find all tarnish removed and instead a bright, shiny penny; the eggshell will be soft and pliable, all its protein dissolved.

Visualize what happens when you allow your small child a glass of cola (or any soda drink). Your little kid becomes supercharged, bouncing off the wall, and for some time you cannot get the child to sit still. In other words, your child has become hyperglycemic. Too much sugar, of any sort, whether it be corn fructose, beet or cane sugar, the results are the same according to Chatelier's principle. Remember, we are all chemical systems and by adding all of the sugar to a small child's body, all of the cells in that body will push back to return to the way they were before the additional sugar. The most efficient way to return to this state is to increase physical activity, causing cells to consume all of the additional added sugar.

Run, baby, run!

Another way, of course, is to rely on the body to use its own chemicals to burn off the sugar. This is predominantly the job of the hormone insulin. If an adult drinks a lot of soda each day (or even has one gin and tonic, which has about half as much sugar as a soda) and does not increase physical activity, diabetes eventually sets in as the body become insulin exhausted, unable to produce more. Then the risk of blindness in old age, amputations, and other terrible consequences may become a reality.

The process of cells using the nutrients we consume is called cellular metabolism. Overloading cells with nutrients that we do not need such as excessive raw sugars (or even food that is easily converted by the body into glucose) and fats, results in obesity; your brain will become sluggish. Now, add extra oxygen and your body will certainly consume it. This is called oxidative metabolism. The added oxygen will push all cells into overdrive; repair cells use the added oxygen to work harder in an effort to restore their state prior to entering the hyperbaric chamber. Repair cells help get rid of the toxins, acids and, excess/unneeded sugars.

After people have been in a hyperbaric chamber, healthy adults comment on the fact that their brain is working more efficiently. Memory becomes vivid and problems are easier to solve. This state is commonly known as the "cappuccino" effect or "brain brightening."

As for small children with autism, almost all of them have a neuronal oxygen transport problem. So the additional feast of oxygen actually makes the good cells, the repair cells, work harder for just a little while after the treatment. This increase in oxidative metabolism dissipates after a couple of hours, but that little bit of improvement lasts: brain cells wire up into complex circuits, blood vessels within the brain become robust, and stem cells are produced. (More on that shortly.)

This is why all oxygen treatments need to take place over consecutive days. There is no point in attending one hyperbaric treatment and then not following it up for another week. Sort of like a seed sprouting from the earth. With each treatment, the positive changes begin to accumulate, and positive results are visible with the passing days.

Can oxygen therapy alone cure autism?

The short answer is no; it cannot. I make this statement based on the treatment of scores of challenged children that have come to my centers across America, and in other parts of the world. Something more is needed—an interdisciplinary approach.

How many treatments in the chamber does a challenged child need to be part of that recovery program?

As noted earlier, we treated our first challenged child, Emily, in one of my centers in the United States. Just one treatment per day at 2 ATA, the pediatrician's decision, made a vast difference to little Emily. Then along came a physician, Dr. Paul Harch, a very bright health scientist. He came to the conclusion 15 years ago that two 60-minute treatments each day at 1.75 ATA for 20 days could cure children with autism. He was so sure of himself that he even took out a patent on that protocol.

I was nonplussed and puzzled. I did not think that you could patent a natural phenomenon such as the effects of hyperbaric oxygen therapy or gravity. Of interest is the fact that the Supreme Court came to the same conclusion in 2012 with what is now known as the "Prometheus" ruling. In essence, the courts had taken all of the enforceable teeth out of Dr. Harch's protocol. This is not to say that there isn't some merit in the treatment pressure, nor is it to imply that Dr. Harch was ignorant of the science of hyperbaric rights in the therapy. So my centers took notice of the fact that he is a physician, and for a little while at least, we did use the Harch protocol on children.

While our little patients saw useful and positive results, there was never a normal recovery by any of the children in that 20-day double ride. This left a lot of the parents disappointed, some angry at what they felt were false claims about hyperbaric oxygen therapy, and rightfully so.

It is significant to note that Dr. Harch, and other clinicians, no longer use the two treatments a day protocol for challenged children, and he no longer claims that recovery is possible in just 20 days.

Now, onto our wonderful Jennifer; the ballet dancer and champion ice-skater. Her mom, Vickie, a bright spirit and highly intelligent woman (actually that describes the whole family), independently arrived at the conclusion that diet was a most important part of the normalization program. All together, over a 12-year period, Jennifer had 135 rides in the hyperbaric chamber. She ice skated at 2am (when the rink was clear), and focused on diet. In a nutshell, while the extra oxygen was feeding one side of cellular metabolism in spurts of 20 treatments at a time, Jennifer's cells were getting the correct diet of nutrients on the other. All of Jen's cells were giving off the right amount of heat and energy, particularly her repair cells.

Bernie and Kerri proved scientifically that the addition of proper nutrients, combined with the removal of deleterious/toxic foods is probably more important than hyperbaric oxygen therapy for children and young adults on the spectrum. Yes, the oxygen boost helps propel the patient to "normal," but the other nutritional changes are really the rocket fuel. It is a long journey, not all that expensive, and certainly worthwhile.

When a hyperbaric chamber is not a hyperbaric chamber.

One final comment about treating neuronal disorders at 1.75 ATA pressure is of utmost importance; this is that 100% oxygen is essential to the protocol. Since Dr. Harch arrived at this treatment depth, there have been thousands of inflatable chambers, so-called mild hyperbaric chambers, sold in the United States and around the world. These are not the same as hospital grade, hard-sided chambers. These bag-chambers do not deliver the needed 100% oxygen. In my opinion, at the very best, if you modify them (against FDA rules) you will only get 34% oxygen.

What have we learned thus far? Time for a review and then THE BIG SECRET REVEALED!

- Oxygen cannot be seen, but we can weigh it.
- Our bodies "eat" oxygen every day because it is a food for our cells.
- The only way we can get additional oxygen is in a hyperbaric chamber.
- This is because any gas becomes soluble and melts into a fluid (i.e. Henry's law); the same reason we can carbonate soda drinks.
- In a single treatment in a hyperbaric-oxygen-therapy chamber, we cannot overdose (and I have never witnessed any negative side effects).
- With the extra oxygen feeding the cells, our bodies get a boost of energy, particularly the repair cells.
- For oxygen in the chamber to be effective, it must be 100% oxygen. Inflatable chambers do not deliver 100% oxygen.
- Hyperbaric oxygen therapy alone will not cure autism, but it does make a big difference.
- There is no such thing as a "one-size fits all" treatment protocol in a hyperbaric chamber that works for all patients. For example, twice a day in the chamber for 20 days will make some difference but not necessarily "normalize" a challenged child.

Did you miss the big secret?

It was already mentioned about one page back—the discoveries of Bernie and Kerri. Let us repeat the secret for you and then push the edges of their really stunning discovery that is backed up by the latest science.

Bernie and Kerri proved scientifically that the addition of the proper nutrients, in the absence of offending foods, in addition to eliminating pathogens and parasites, are most likely more important than hyperbaric oxygen therapy for children and young adults. Yes, the oxygen boost helps propel the patient to "normal" but the other dietary interventions are really the rocket fuel. Not to mention freeing the body of offending pathogens/parasites which wreak havoc on the body. It is a long journey, not all that expensive and, certainly worthwhile.

Nutritional "padding." Hyperbaric oxygen therapy and the production of progenitor and stem cells.

When a baby is growing inside its mother, it has progenitor cells and stem cells. The function of these cells is considered to be, as yet, undecided. Although studies continue to elucidate exactly which mechanisms are involved in determining the fate of these cells, it is generally accepted that their surrounding cells will dictate their development. For example, the big arteries that crisscross the chest area make a decision sooner or later to turn into a heart with all of its compartments. Then, as development moves on different parts of the baby appear. These are called progenitor or stem cells.

There are various estimates on how many different types of cells the developed human has in total; however, it is predicted there are somewhere between 210 and 300. Mind you, when the baby takes its first breath of air, all but about four of these different cell groups stop reproducing. For example, the brain, with all of its neuronal pruning and circuitry needs about 20 year's worth of stimulation to properly wire all of the connections. Surprisingly, a lot of the neurons will be shed or "pruned" since they will not be put to use in the adult. However, neuroplasticity allows new skills to be added or repairs to be made to and by the brain in a lifetime.

However, medical scientists have now realized the great need for progenitor or stem cells (cells that can make decisions to replace worn or damaged cells within the body), and the search is on for these decision-making cells. Many scientists are looking for something they can patent and as a result are missing the point that it is already here. Or they are ignoring it, because but they cannot patent it.

It is called hyperbaric oxygen therapy.

Penn Study Finds Hyperbaric Oxygen Treatments Mobilize Stem Cells

Science Daily — According to a study to be published in the American Journal of Physiology-Heart and Circulation Physiology, a typical course of hyperbaric oxygen treatments increases by eight-fold the number of stem cells circulating in a patient's body. Stem cells, also called progenitor cells are crucial to injury repair. The study currently appears online and is scheduled for publication in the April 2006, edition of the American Journal.

Stem cells exist in the bone marrow of human beings and animals and are capable of changing their nature to become part of many different organs and tissues. In response to injury, these cells move from the bone marrow to the injured sites, where they differentiate into cells that assist in the healing process. The movement, or mobilization, of stem cells can be triggered by a variety of stimuli including pharmaceutical agents and hyperbaric oxygen treatments. Where as drugs are associated with a host of side effects, hyperbaric oxygen treatments carry a significantly lower risk of such effects.

"This is the safest way clinically to increase stem cell circulation, far safer than any of the pharmaceutical options," said Stephen Thom, MD, PhD, professor of emergency medicine at the University of Pennsylvania School of Medicine and lead author of the study." This study provides information on the fundamental mechanisms for hyperbaric oxygen and offers a new theoretical therapeutic option for mobilizing stem cells."

"We reproduced the observations from humans in animals in order to identify the mechanism for the hyperbaric oxygen effect," added Thom. "We found that hyperbaric oxygen mobilizes stem/progenitor cells because it increases synthesis of a molecule called nitric oxide in the bone marrow. This synthesis is thought to trigger enzymes that mediate stem/progenitor cell release."[1]

Nutritional padding: It has long been known that when hyperbaric oxygen therapy is applied, existing cells, the good ones, the repair cells, turn the body into its own pharmaceutical company, providing the right sort of chemicals at the right time. Above all, there is a dramatic increase in the production of the molecule called nitric oxide from the bone marrow. Probably the best way of describing the addition of hyperbaric oxygen therapy, as an adjunct to the correct nutritionals, is simply by putting fuel onto an already existing smoldering fire. Out of the glow of embers and smoke you will see a vigorous combustion as your fireplace heats up and the flames appear.

Now imagine other ingredients that have yet to be discovered as beneficial. For example, stem cells that repair the damaged brain of a person with autism. It could be that adding external stem cells to the recipe of recovery and normalization, with simple nutritional low-cost padding, and putting the little patient in the chamber would be a faster way of achieving what all parents want for their children—to eventually become fully functional and independent adults.

All of this by just a little bit of nutritional padding and helping the body to rid itself of pathogens/parasites.

Now, it is time to turn back to Kerri so she can tell you what she has seen when hyperbaric oxygen therapy is added to the correct nutritional padding, along with chlorine dioxide to keep pathogens under control. That is the big secret to helping your child through the challenges that living in this century have visited upon you.

As Bob mentioned, I have seen miracles happen when hyperbaric oxygen therapy was applied to a child who is ready. Two girls, in particular, lost their diagnosis completely within weeks of completing treatment in the chamber. As I mentioned before, hyperbaric oxygen therapy gave my own son his speech back. Before his first 40 dives he had several single-syllable sounds, but after, he began stringing words together to request his favorite foods.

Today we are seeing that one dive a day at 1.75 ATA (atmospheres absolute) for 90 minutes at depth is better than two 60-minute sessions were first prescribed for Patrick seven years ago. Every three months after the first treatment of 20 sessions, apply ten sessions of 90 minutes, each at 1.75 ATA, until your child is recovered.

A lot of parents ask when is a good time to do hyperbarics. To this I reply that we must first have diet and chlorine dioxide totally under control, and be at least three months into the Parasite Protocol. At that point it's time to start looking for a chamber.

Make sure to do an ATEC before your child's hyperbaric oxygen therapy sessions, and repeat two months after the sessions are over; the results will be obvious.

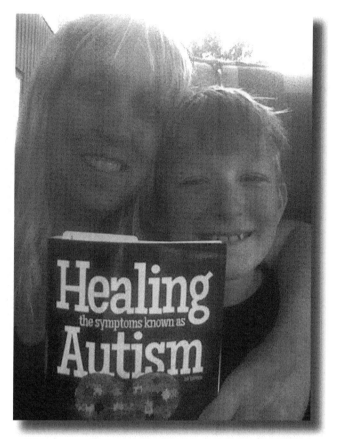

This is my Asperger son Tobias, 10 years old, and
me... when we received the book this summer.

Chapter 12

Step 7 - GcMAF & Autism:
State of the Art & Future
Perspectives for a Natural Cure

by Marco Ruggiero, MD, PhD.
Specialist in Diagnostic Radiology
Full professor of Molecular Biology
Dept. of Experimental & Clinical Biomedical Sciences
University of Firenze, Italy

*"The voyage of discovery is not in seeking
new landscapes but in having new eyes."*

*~ **Marcel Proust***

My family and I have been in biomed for so long, that there aren't too many interventions we haven't already tried. A few years back, Dr. Usman mentioned to me that GcMAF might be something good for Patrick. She explained that GcMAF is a human protein that occurs naturally in a healthy body. It is a special supplement that replaces the missing part of the immune

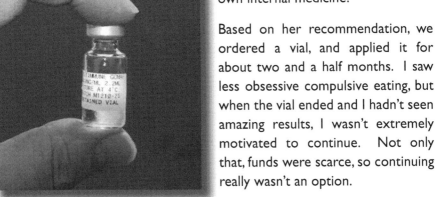

system, and also acts as the body's own internal medicine.

Based on her recommendation, we ordered a vial, and applied it for about two and a half months. I saw less obsessive compulsive eating, but when the vial ended and I hadn't seen amazing results, I wasn't extremely motivated to continue. Not only that, funds were scarce, so continuing really wasn't an option.

Two years went by and I spoke to Dr. Usman again. She said we really should give it four to five months before making a final decision. So, we scraped together the money for a second order. We started again in November of 2012, and reached full dose by December, 26th 2012. Seemingly, as time went on, Patrick started to do new things.

By springtime of 2013, Patrick's BFF's mom was saying how well he was doing, and reminded me that during the prior month Patrick had not been doing the things that he was now doing. As I write this in October of 2013, all of my money now goes to GcMAF. ☺

One of the things that I feel makes GcMAF so exciting is the fact that it helps regrow dendrites in a matter of hours after it is injected. The dendrites are the very things that got fried when mercury entered our children's bodies. With the help of GcMAF, we are now able to restore what was lost. Not to mention, GcMAF boosts the immune system, which we have come to find is often sorely lacking in people with ASD's.

Many people have asked me if GcMAF is now an official part of the protocol. When working towards recovery, I feel that we need to try everything at our disposal that has been proven to heal autism—in the correct order, or course. GcMAF fits that description. According to www.gcmaf.eu, "As of February 2013, on the American National Library of Medicine alone, 142 eminent scientists from 8 nations have published 59 major GcMAF research papers, which can be viewed on the US Government's Pubmed system." There is now enough research to prove that GcMAF has secured its place as a powerful biomedical intervention for healing autism. Therefore, after three months on the Kalcker Parasite Protocol, it is time to start thinking about adding in supplements, HBOT and GcMAF.

We are blessed to have the one and only Dr. Marco Ruggiero, the lead GcMAF researcher, write the remainder of this chapter about this substance, it's benefits and applications in autism and beyond.

The information he presents is extremely important because I feel that GcMAF is the future of medicine—today. What other intervention boasts a cancer recovery rate of 80%? None! Dr. Bradstreet is reporting 85% responders and 15% recovery rate from autism with GcMAF.[1]

Imagine adding GcMAF to the protocol already outlined in this book at the right moment (after working down some of the pathogen load), we should start seeing even higher rates of recovery than 15%. I look forward to seeing what transpires during the upcoming year as more families add GcMAF to their children's protocols. I am excited for more and more people to lose their autism diagnoses.

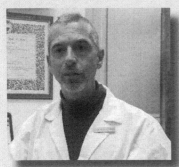

For the past 20 years, Dr. Marco Ruggiero has worked on the vitamin D axis, a metabolic pathway that includes the vitamin D binding protein-derived macrophage activating factor or GcMAF. In the past 3 years he has published studies on the immunotherapeutic effects of GcMAF in cancer, HIV/AIDS, chronic fatigue syndrome and neurological conditions.

Marco Ruggiero holds a PhD in Molecular Biology, is a certified Medical Doctor specializing in Clinical Radiology and is a professor of Molecular Biology at the Department of Experimental and Clinical Biomedical Sciences of the University of Firenze, Italy.

He served in the Army as Medical Lieutenant with specific training in chemical, biological and nuclear warfare. He worked at Burroughs Welcome Co. North Carolina, USA publishing a seminal paper with Nobel Laureate Sir John Vane and, subsequently, at the National Cancer Institute of the NIH in Bethesda, working with Dr. Stuart A. Aaronson and Dr. Peter Duesberg.

Since 1992, he holds the chair of Molecular Biology at the University of Firenze where he leads a research group of about 10 researchers. He has published more than 150 peer-reviewed scientific papers on signal transduction in a variety of experimental and spontaneous pathologic system related with cancer, chronic kidney disease, chronic fatigue syndrome and neurological conditions.

The role of nutrition in the treatment and eradication of the symptoms of autism is well established and other chapters of this book treat this topic in detail. What is far less known is the fact that certain natural components of the diet, certain nutrients, have profound effects on all the systems that are affected in autism and in particular on the brain and the immune system. Their effects are so dramatic that for about 20 years, these natural components have been labelled as "drugs" even though they are essential parts of our bodies, just like hormones or neurotransmitters. I am referring here to the family of molecules that is known as GcMAF, an acronym that stands for Gc-protein-derived Macrophage Activating Factor.

GcMAF has been the object of intense research in the past 20 years for its therapeutic role in cancer, autoimmune diseases, and HIV infection (for review, see: Anticancer Res. 2012 Jan;32(1):45-52). But, only one year ago, in 2012, its dramatic effects on the eradication of the symptoms of autism were published in a prestigious peer-reviewed scientific journal (Autism Insights 2012:4 31–38).

In this chapter I shall provide an overview on GcMAF with particular reference to its therapeutic role in autism and to the future perspectives deriving from the basic and applied research that is revolving around this fascinating molecule.

A Brief History of GcMAF

The first publication on GcMAF in a peer-reviewed journal indexed in the US National Library of Medicine is dated 1994 (J Immunol. 1994 May 15;152(10):5100-7). In this article, a group of researchers from the Department of Biochemistry at the Temple University School of Medicine in Philadelphia, USA, described the effects of a protein, defined as GcMAF, on rat macrophages. Macrophages are key elements of the immune response and the research group led by Dr. Nobuto Yamamoto, the first author of this paper, showed that GcMAF activated these cells. Given the central role of macrophages in the control of all immune responses, GcMAF was considered a powerful regulator of the immune system and the research on GcMAF initially was focused on its immune-stimulant properties. In fact, one year after the initial observation on rats, Dr. Yamamoto, who in the meantime had moved to the Laboratory of Cancer Immunology and Molecular Biology of the Albert Einstein Cancer Center in Philadelphia, authored a paper suggesting that a defect in endogenous GcMAF production contributed to immunodeficiency in AIDS patients (AIDS Res Hum Retroviruses. 1995 Nov;11(11):1373-8.). Consequently, he provided GcMAF to Medical Doctors treating HIV patients and, 14 years later, after 7 years of follow-up, he published a seminal paper describing eradication of HIV infection through GcMAF administration (J Med Virol. 2009 Jan;81(1):16-26).

Immunodeficiency, however, is not unique to HIV/AIDS and, back in 1996, Yamamoto and colleagues, hypothesized that deficient endogenous GcMAF production was responsible for the relative immunodeficiency that is typically observed in cancer patients (Cancer Res. 1996 Jun 15;56(12):2827-31). Quite logically, this observation of 18 years ago, led to the proposal of administering GcMAF to cancer patients with the goal of empowering the immune system that in turn would fight the cancer growth. This approach is known as "immunotherapy" and it is much older than GcMAF since, in modern times, it stems from the observation of Dr. William Coley in 1891. However, it could be argued that the idea of stimulating the immune system to fight diseases is even older since, as it is stated in this recent article, "…cancer regresses when associated with acute infections such as bacterial, viral, fungal, protozoal, etc. Acute infections are known to cure chronic diseases since the time of Hippocrates…" (Indian J Cancer. 2011 Apr-Jun;48(2):246-51).

Whatever the case, administration of GcMAF to patients with metastatic advanced cancer proved efficacious and there are now scores of papers published in the peer-reviewed literature describing the dramatic therapeutic effects of GcMAF in all types of experimental or spontaneous tumors.

Nowadays, the interest for GcMAF in the immunotherapy of cancer is so high that the prestigious scientific journal "OncoImmunology" dedicated the cover of its August 2013 issue to GcMAF. The molecular rendering of GcMAF is on the left of the cover with a caption linking it to an article by Thyer and colleagues published in the same issue and describing successful treatment of advanced cancer patients (Figure 1).

Figure 1

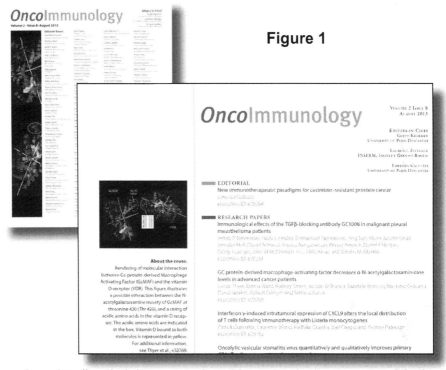

Source: https://www.landesbioscience.com/journals/oncoimmunology/oncoimmunology_2-8.pdf

Consecration of GcMAF in the Olympus of science, however, occurred a few days later, on September 14, 2013, when another article by Thyer and colleagues was published in "Nutrients", an international, peer-reviewed open access advanced forum for studies related to human nutrition (Nutrients. 2013 Jul 8;5(7):2577-89). In fact, this article describing the effects of GcMAF on human breast cancer cells, was ranked in the top 5% of all articles ever tracked by Altmetric. The Altmetric score is a general measure of the attention that an article, book or dataset has received online and reflects the quantity of attention received as well as the quality of that attention. By the time that the GcMAF was ranked in the top 5% of all scientific articles ever tracked, Altmetric had analyzed 1,510,524 articles across all scientific journals. Therefore, we may safely state that in this chapter we are describing one of the hottest topics in today's world science (Figure 2).

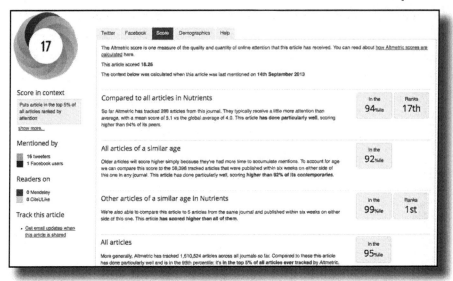

Figure 2

The interest for the therapeutic effects of GcMAF in a variety of conditions derives from the early observation by Yamamoto and colleagues in 1995, who showed elevated level of serum alpha-N-acetylgalactosaminidase (Nagalase) in the serum of AIDS patients. Nagalase is an enzyme that deglycosylates (degrades) the precursor of GcMAF that is the circulating Gc-protein, also known as vitamin D-binding protein (AIDS Res Hum Retroviruses. 1995 Nov;11(11):1373-8). This results in the loss of GcMAF precursor activity and consequent dysfunction of the immune system. Increased Nagalase activity, however, is not observed uniquely in AIDS patients. For example it was demonstrated that the increase of Nagalase activity in the serum of cancer patients is due to the fact that cancer cells release Nagalase and, therefore, Nagalase activity reflects tumor burden, aggressiveness and progression of the disease. Consequently, determination of Nagalase activity is currently proposed as a reliable way of evaluation of cancer severity (Cancer Lett. 2009 Oct 8;283(2):222-9).

In short, in cancer, HIV/AIDS, and in many other chronic conditions, elevated serum Nagalase, degrades Gc-protein that is the precursor of GcMAF. Therefore, GcMAF is not produced inside the body to a sufficient extent and this leads to immunodeficiency. Serum Nagalase, however, does not degrade GcMAF, and this justifies the administration of exogenous GcMAF in all those conditions where its endogenous production is insufficient due to elevated Nagalase activity.

Until 2002, it was thought that GcMAF exerted its effects only on macrophages and that its therapeutic efficacy was due to stimulation of macrophages that in turn would attack and destroy cancer cells as well as virus-infected cells. In 2002, however, a novel effect of GcMAF was described. Kanda and colleagues, working at the Department of Molecular Microbiology and Immunology, Division of Endothelial Cell Biology, Nagasaki University Graduate School of Medicine, Nagasaki, Japan, published a paper, co-authored by Yamamoto, describing the inhibitory effects of GcMAF on angiogenesis (J Natl Cancer Inst. 2002 Sep 4;94(17):1311-9.). Angiogenesis is the process of building new blood vessels that provide the tumor mass with the required supply of blood and nutrients that it needs to grow and metastatize. Therefore, since 1971 it was postulated that inhibition of angiogenesis could be a successful strategy to deprive the growing tumor mass of its supply of blood and nutrients (N Engl J Med. 1971 Nov 18;285(21):1182-6). While there are scores of inhibitors of angiogenesis, some of which in use in the therapy of cancer, GcMAF offers the advantage of performing more than one anticancer effects; in fact, not only it inhibits tumor-induced angiogenesis (Cancer Immunol Immunother. 2011 Apr;60(4):479-85), but it also stimulates macrophages that attack and destroy the cancer cells (Nutrients. 2013 Jul 8;5(7):2577-89).

If these combined anticancer effects were not enough, in 2010 Gregory and colleagues, working at the Department of Ophthalmology and Visual Sciences of University of Kentucky in Lexington, Kentucky, USA, demonstrated that GcMAF directly inhibited proliferation and metastatic potential of human prostate cancer cells (PLoS One. 2010 Oct 18;5(10):e13428). Slightly more than one year later, we were able to demonstrate that GcMAF not only inhibited proliferation and metastatic potential of human breast cancer cells, but it also reverted their neoplastic phenotype; in other words, cancer cells treated with GcMAF became normal (Anticancer Res. 2012 Jan;32(1):45-52).

On the basis of the peer-reviewed scientific literature quoted above, we can now state that GcMAF exerts multiple effects that are responsible for its efficacy in anticancer therapy:

1. It stimulates macrophages that attack and destroy cancer cells, as originally postulated by Yamamoto and colleagues.

2. It inhibits tumor-induced angiogenesis thus depriving the growing tumor mass of blood and nutrients.

3. It directly inhibits cancer cell proliferation and metastatic potential and it retro-transforms cancer cells into normal healthy cells.

Given this plethora of effects on cancer, it is no wonder that the majority of GcMAF research has been focused on its anticancer properties. There are, however, a few research articles suggesting that GcMAF might exert also other biological actions with therapeutic implications. In addition to the studies on HIV and AIDS quoted above, GcMAF has received attention for its potential role in the therapy of bone disorders (Blood. 1996 Oct 15;88(8):2898-905), and autoimmune diseases such as Lupus Erythematosus (Clin Immunol Immunopathol. 1997 Mar;82(3):290-8).

Despite these scanty evidences on the possible role of GcMAF in conditions other than cancer and AIDS, it was not until 2012, however, that GcMAF proved dramatically effective in the therapy of autism.

GcMAF & Autism

GcMAF, being derived from Gc-protein, also known as vitamin D binding protein, belongs to the so called "vitamin D axis", a nutritional metabolic pathway described in detail in a recent review (European Nephrology, 2011;5(1):15–9). My research group had been working on the vitamin D axis since 1996 (Epidemiol Prev. 1996 Apr-Sep;20(2-3):140-1), that is since the beginning of GcMAF research. Just like our colleagues in the USA and Japan, we were mainly interested in the role of the vitamin D axis in bone metabolism and cancer (Radiol Med. 1996 Nov;92(5):520-4. Oncol Res. 1998;10(1):43-6). Therefore, it came as a surprise when Dr. Nobuto Yamamoto first mentioned to me the effects of GcMAF on neurodegenerative diseases such as Parkinson's and Alzheimer's diseases.

In the hot summer of 2010 we visited Dr. Yamamoto in his hometown of Philadelphia, and we had the honor and the pleasure to spend two very intense days with this old-style exquisite gentleman. Dr. Yamamoto gave us a detailed history not only of his decade-long research activity, but also of the entire field of immunotherapy, starting with the pioneering work of Dr. William Coley at the end of the nineteen century. During these intense and fruitful talks, Dr. Yamamoto mentioned the dramatic effects that he had personally observed by administering GcMAF to a patient suffering from Parkinson's disease. According to Dr. Yamamoto, the effects had been almost immediate and dramatic up to the point that he himself was amazed. Regrettably, he had been unable to clinically document the case and, therefore, this remained an anecdote. From this anecdote, however, an entire new field of GcMAF research was about to rise; that is the study on the role and implications of GcMAF in treating neurologic and neurodegenerative disorders.

The first solid evidences for a role of GcMAF in treating a neurodegenerative disorder were simultaneously presented by Dr. Paul Cheney and Prof. Kenny de Meirleir at the meeting of the International Association for Chronic Fatigue Syndrome and Myalgic Encephalomyelitis (CFS/ME) held in Ottawa in September 2011. A few days later, in collaboration with Dr. Paul Cheney, we presented in Padova, Italy, a study demonstrating that food-based GcMAF dramatically improved the symptoms of CFS/ME, and this work was published in the official journal of the Italian Society of Anatomy and Histology, one of the oldest and most respected European scientific societies, founded at the beginning of the twentieth century (It. J. Anat. Embryol. Vol. 116, No 1, 2011).

CFS/ME is a complex disorder that shares many features of autism. In fact, it is characterized by immune system dysfunction, widespread inflammation, and multi-systemic neuropathology (J Intern Med. 2011 Oct;270(4):327-38. In Vivo. 2013 Mar-Apr;27(2):177-87). Dysfunction of the immune system involves abnormal functions and distributions of T lymphocytes, B lymphocytes, natural killer cells, and monocyte/macrophages (Nihon Rinsho. 1992 Nov;50(11):2625-9. Brain Behav Immun. 2012 Jan;26(1):24-31). The etiology of CFS/ME, just like the etiology of autism, is still unknown and multiple factors are thought to be responsible for its onset and progression, thus lending credit to the hypothesis that both etiology and pathogenesis are multifactorial (J Intern Med. 2011 Oct;270(4):327-38). Heavy metal exposure and viral infections are among the factors that contribute to CFS/ME etiology and pathogenesis, and a role for human endogenous retroviruses has been recently hypothesized (In Vivo. 2013 Mar-Apr;27(2):177-87). Both chronic heavy metal exposure and viral infections are considered responsible for the immune system dysfunction and neuropathology that are typical of CFS/ME (Med Hypotheses. 2012 Sep;79(3):403-7. In Vivo. 2013 Mar-Apr;27(2):177-87).

In addition to these areas of overlapping, it had been noticed by Doctors treating autism and/or CFS/ME, that in several families the two conditions are often associated with parents of autistic children suffering from CFS/ME. Interestingly, this happens also in families with adopted children with autism, thus lending credit to the hypothesis that environmental or infectious factors may contribute to both conditions.

Whatever the case, it had been observed that CFS/ME patients had elevated levels of serum Nagalase together with a number of immunological alterations, and it was hypothesized that they could benefit from GcMAF treatment. The results presented in Ottawa and in Padova confirmed this assumption and ever since immunotherapy with GcMAF is a stronghold of CFS/ME treatment.

At about the same time, Dr. Bradstreet, a leading authority in the field of autism, began to study the levels of Nagalase in autistic children and their responses to GcMAF treatment. The results obtained in a first cohort of 40 subjects were reported in a seminal paper published in 2012 (Autism Insights 2012:4 31–38). This paper represents a turning point in the understanding of autism pathogenesis and treatment.

The first significant finding is the observation that the average level of Nagalase in autistic subjects was more than two folds higher than the normal level, thus lending credit to the hypothesis that immunodeficiency or immune system dysfunction is a hallmark of autism. The second finding, probably the most important in recent years, is the observation that GcMAF treatment significantly improved the symptoms of autism and this improvement was associated with a decrease of Nagalase levels.

The therapeutic response to GcMAF was statistically significant and showed the typical bell-shaped curve that is expected when a biologically effective treatment is at work. About 15% of subject did not respond; this means that their symptoms were not ameliorated by GcMAF treatment. However, more than 15% of children responded so dramatically that all the symptoms of autism were eradicated in a matter of weeks up to the point that the children could no longer be defined as "autistic." According to the very word of the authors, in the children in this group, "This response was demonstrated at school, during therapies, home and outside the home as substantial improvement to the point that many or most of the criteria of autism were no longer present."

The remaining 70% of children were distributed according to the so-called Gaussian distribution in the groups showing "slight," "moderate," or "considerable" improvement.

This paper demonstrated for the first time that GcMAF treatment was able to eradicate the symptoms of autism in a matter of weeks, thus reinforcing the idea brought forward in many chapters of this book that autism is a curable condition indeed.

Quite obviously, the dramatic results obtained by Dr. Bradstreet did not go unnoticed and, in April 2013, he presented further results at the First GcMAF Immunology Conference held in Frankfurt, Germany. According to Dr. Bradstreet, as the time of follow-up and the number of subjects increased, a shift toward the right (that is the "best") part of the curve could be observed. This means that the percentage of those showing "considerable" to "very considerable" improvement increased.

From the point of view of the general practitioner, the issue could be considered closed: GcMAF cures a significant percentage of autistic children now and that figure is rising.

However, since I am a researcher in addition of being a Medical Doctor, the successes of Dr. Bradstreet in treating autism and the research papers published by Immuno Biotech laboratories are in the middle of an exciting series of observations that are leading to a completely new understanding of how GcMAF works and what autism truly is.

In fact, the undisputable efficacy of GcMAF in treating autism raises a number of questions on the mechanisms involved at the cellular and molecular levels. The most important questions are:

1. The efficacy of GcMAF in curing autism is due only to its immune-stimulating effect?

2. Or, is GcMAF acting directly also on neurons as it does on cancer cells?

3. Does GcMAF revert the neuro-anatomical alterations that are typical of the autistic brain?

4. Why a certain number of autistic subjects do not respond to GcMAF?

5. Can we devise strategies to have these non-responders respond?

6. Can we devise strategies to further improve this already dramatic therapeutic effect?

The Effects of GcMAF on Human Neurons

GcMAF is a protein and, as such, it was thought that it would stimulate cells from the outside. In other words, until 2013, it was conjectured that, on their external surface, cells had a receptor that bound GcMAF and conveyed the signal to the inside of the cell and, ultimately, to the nucleus and the DNA, thereby modifying the cell behavior. However, despite 20 years of research, such a receptor for GcMAF had not been identified. And this might appear truly odd considering that the entire human genome had been sequenced, that is studied in every single detail, more than 10 years ago.

In our first publication with Dr. Yamamoto, presented at the XVIII International AIDS Conference in Vienna in 2010, we had demonstrated that the response to GcMAF in human mononuclear cells (that is macrophages) was dependent on polymorphisms (that are the individual variations among humans) of the vitamin D receptor (VDR) gene. This observation was not surprising considering that vitamin D, its receptor, and GcMAF all belong to the vitamin D axis.

In order to further investigate this relationship between GcMAF and the VDR we began studying the molecular assembly of GcMAF that is the "shape" that the molecule assumes in its physiological conformation. Having done this, we looked for complementary areas in the GcMAF and VDR molecules and... voilà! The two molecules complemented each other as two elements of a puzzle.

We published this observation in the "Nutrients" paper that is now in the top 5% of all articles ever tracked, and the picture of the two molecules interacting with each other is in the front cover of the OncoImmunology August 2013 issue. The molecular mechanisms through which GcMAF and VDR interact and the consequent complex web of intracellular signaling are topics for specialists and rather difficult to divulge; the basic point, however, is that we had demonstrated how is it possible that GcMAF exerted so many different effects that can be exploited to treat a number of diseases so different from each other.

From this observation we deducted that all cells having the VDR would have responded to GcMAF and, given our interest for the effects of GcMAF in neurological conditions such as autism and CFS/ME, we began our study on human neurons. In fact, human neurons express (i.e. "have") the VDR and therefore, they are candidate to be stimulated by GcMAF.

We cultured human neurons in Petri dishes and we challenged them with ultra-pure GcMAF; in this type of experiments there were no other variables. That is, there were only neurons and GcMAF; the cells of the immune system or other molecules were not involved. By doing so, we would have been certain that whatever effect we observed, this was due uniquely to GcMAF.

As I have shown at the congress "Curando el Autismo" in San Juan de Puerto Rico in August 2013, GcMAF at extremely low concentration significantly increased neuronal cell viability and metabolic activity. These effects on cell viability were associated with dose-dependent intracellular cAMP production (cAMP is an intracellular second messenger). This means that GcMAF increased the production of energy inside human neurons and made them more active, more viable. Increased viability and metabolic activity following GcMAF stimulation as well as cAMP formation were accompanied by morphological changes, meaning that stimulated neurons changed their shape.

In the absence of GcMAF, human neuronal cells under the microscope appeared as small, relatively undifferentiated cells with large nuclei. After 24h stimulation with GcMAF, neurons showed a significant change in morphology that was consistent with the induction of neuronal differentiation and increased connectivity. The cytoplasm was enlarged and cytoplasmic elongations could be observed. After 72h incubation with GcMAF, these morphological changes were more evident and well differentiated cells could be observed.

After incubation with GcMAF, the cells appeared to establish contacts with each other. Taken together these results indicated that GcMAF increased neuronal cell viability, metabolic activity and differentiation, with the first effects being observed at 24h. It is worth noticing that the assay that we used to determine cell viability, measured mitochondrial activity, and mitochondrial dysfunction is known to be hallmark of ME/CFS (Int J Clin Exp Med. 2012;5(3):208-20), and possibly of autism as well. Therefore, the effects of GcMAF that we observed explain the reason why GcMAF is so effective in CFS/ME and autism; it counteracts the molecular alterations that are the pathogenetic basis of both conditions.

I wish to spend a few words here on the effects of GcMAF on neuronal connectivity. It is well assessed that this is one of the basic alterations in the brain of autistic subjects; neurons do not establish contacts with each other and therefore the neurological signal cannot be transmitted from one area of the brain to another thus causing a "disconnection" (Rev Neurol. 2012

Feb 29;54 Suppl 1:S31-9). GcMAF re-establishes neuronal connectivity by stimulating the formation of what are called "cytoplasmic elongations" that are like small "arms" that protrude from the neurons and establish contact with each other as if neurons were tending arms to "touch" each other and exchange information.

In Figure 3A, human un-stimulated human neurons in culture can be observed; they are small and roundish. After stimulation with GcMAF (Figure 3B), they are much larger because increased energy production leads to increased protein synthesis in their cytoplasm. But, perhaps more important, they have a highly irregular, elongated, triangular, shape with spikes that touch each other. The areas of contact between the two neurons can be clearly observed in the central part where they establish connecting bridges. Please notice that both pictures were taken with the same magnification.

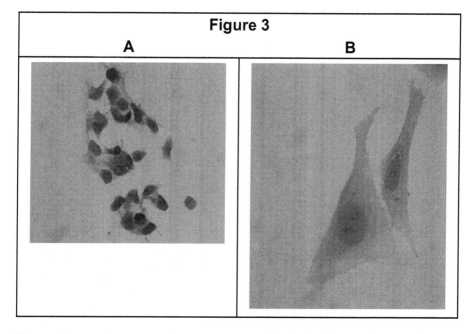

Figure 3

A   B

These observations provide an answer to the first two questions raised by the article published by Dr. Bradstreet: the therapeutic effects of GcMAF in autism can be ascribed to at least two different actions of GcMAF. On one side, it rebalances the immune system that is typically dysfunctional in autistic subjects; on the other side, it directly stimulates human neurons increasing their metabolic activity and their connectivity. But, as it always happens in research, these "answers" led to other "questions": does GcMAF cross the blood brain barrier? That is, does it arrive to the neurons of the central nervous system? Before challenging this question further, however, let's proceed with order and let's try to provide an answer to the other questions that were raised by the Bradstreet's paper.

GcMAF and the Neuro-Anatomical Alterations of the Autistic Brain

If the etiology of autism is still undefined, the pathogenesis and the brain alterations associated with autism are better understood. Several studies using sophisticated imaging techniques demonstrated that there is atypical structural brain connectivity within cortical white and grey matter and it is postulated that such an alteration of brain connectivity may represent one of the principal neural substrates underlying autistic symptoms (PLoS One. 2013 Jun 18;8(6):e67329. Proc Natl Acad Sci U S A. 2013 Jul 22.).

The observed atypical brain connectivity is localized to particular areas of the brain and the alterations in the fronto-temporal regions are associated with the severity of social and repetitive symptoms of autism (Proc Natl Acad Sci U S A. 2013 Jul 22.). Atypical brain connectivity in autism is also associated with reduction of grey matter volume in different areas of the brain (Cerebellum. 2013 Apr 10.). In the bilateral superior temporal gyrus significantly decreased functional connectivity was accompanied by the strongest trend of grey matter volume decrease (PLoS One. 2013 Jun 18;8(6):e67329), thus reinforcing the hypothesis that study of grey matter volume may provide indication of functional connectivity.

However, the studies on brain connectivity and grey matter reduction quoted above were conducted with sophisticated Magnetic Resonance Imaging (MRI) equipments using complex softwares. Because of their cost and complexity, these techniques are not suitable for routine examination and this appears to be in contrast with the need to provide the general practitioners with the instruments to study autism. In fact, given the current epidemiological trend, it is highly probable that even primary care providers will see with increased frequency a patient with autism spectrum disorder in their clinic (Curr Probl Pediatr Adolesc Health Care. 2013 Jan;43(1):2-11). This consideration prompted us for the search of accessible methods to study brain alterations in autism and to study the response to different treatment including GcMAF.

To this end, we developed an easily accessible method to study the brain cortex using transcranial ultrasonography. This technique was first applied to the diagnosis and treatment CFS/ME a syndrome that, as we know, share neuropathological similarities with autism (Toxicology. 2008 May 2;247(1):61-72). In particular, we proposed to use ultrasounds to study the grey matter in the temporal lobe, and to evaluate signs of neuronal layer disorganization and brain inflammation (Med Hypotheses. 2012 Sep;79(3):403-7). It is worth noticing that these same neurological alterations, i.e. minicolumn structural changes and inflammation are frequently observed in autism (Front Immunol. 2013 Jun 10;4:140. doi: 10.3389/fimmu.2013.00140. Print 2013). Therefore, we hypothesize that ultrasounds could be used in autism in order to study the brain alterations that have been described using more sophisticated and less accessible techniques.

First of all, we assessed the safety of the technique; to this end we used sub-thermal ultrasounds. These are considered inherently safe and have been used for fetal imaging in utero, and virtually every part of the body, including brains of newborn babies through fontanelles. Their inherent safety and any lack of correlation with the onset of autism have been confirmed by meta-analysis of thousands of cases. A recent randomized controlled trial on over 1.400 cases demonstrated beyond any reasonable doubt that there is no link between the prenatal ultrasound scans and the autism phenotype (J Autism Dev Disord. 2012 Dec;42(12):2693-701).

Then, in a collaborative work with Dr. Bradstreet, we decided to focus our attention on the temporal cortex in order to compare our results with those already published by Hameroff and colleagues and by ourselves using this technique (Med Hypotheses. 2012 Sep;79(3):403-7. Brain Stimul. 2013 May;6(3):409-15). In addition, having to choose a particular area of the brain for this initial study, the temporal lobe was particularly interesting because of its accessibility to ultrasounds and its involvement in the pathogenesis of autism (PLoS One. 2013 Jun 18;8(6):e67329. Print 2013).

In the typical adults subject, meninges appeared as a well-organized array of layers of about 2.6 mm thickness. The meninges were separated from the cortex by a structure that shows echogenic and morphological feature consistent with the sub-arachnoid space. The cortex of the temporal lobe appeared as a well-organized array of alternate, hyper-echogenic/hypo-echogenic, layers. The thickness of the cortex was 5.0 mm. This value of thickness and the anatomical positioning of the probe led us to hypothesize that we were observing the temporal areas designated by von Economo as TG and TE, i.e. those areas involved in the control of eye movements and balance in standing position (area TE), social behavior, mood and decision making (area TG) (von Economo C. Temporal lobe. In: Triarhou LC, editor. Cellular structure of the human cerebral cortex. Basel; 2009. p. 114-132). It is worth noticing that the layers within the column-like structure of the healthy subject appeared well-organized and parallel to each other.

However, the images obtained in a representative autistic subject showed that the thickness of the cortex of the temporal lobe was significantly reduced, as it had been observed with MRI (PLoS One. 2013 Jun 18;8(6):e67329. Print 2013). Other images showed a concomitant increase in the spinal fluid in the sub-arachnoid space that was twice as much as in the healthy subject. These findings are consistent with the very recent observation that infants who developed autism spectrum disorder had significantly greater extra-axial fluid characterized by excessive cerebrospinal fluid in the sub-arachnoid space (Brain. 2013 Jul 9.).

Taken together, the results obtained in autistic subjects demonstrate that our technique was able to visualize the excess extra-axial fluid in a manner comparable to MRI; however, at variance with MRI, the observation with ultrasounds was immediate and intuitive and could be easily performed with no discomfort during a routine examination.

Another finding that we observed was a relative disorganization of the neuronal layer arrangement in the temporal cortex of autistic subjects. It was possible to observe that the neuronal layers had a different orientation and that there were black areas of about 0.4 mm that could represent areas of poor connectivity.

Since this technique has been applied only recently to the study of autism, there is no statistical analysis indicating whether GcMAF or any other effective treatment can reverse the anatomical alterations that we have observed in the brain of autistic subjects. Therefore, there is no sound scientific answer to this question; there are only some anecdotic evidences suggesting that this might indeed be the case. Autistic subjects treated with GcMAF and showing considerable clinical improvement showed a normal brain anatomy. Future observation will tell whether these anecdotic evidences have a statistical meaning.

Ultrasounds, however, in addition to their role in early diagnosis and follow-up, might also have a role in the therapy of autism and in particular in improving the response of those subjects who do not appear to benefit from GcMAF treatment.

GcMAF Non-Responders

As odd as it may appear to non-researchers, the presence of non-responders is often the best assurance that we are dealing with a real biological phenomenon and not with placebo effects or worse. In fact the bell-shaped curve presented in the article by Bradstreet and colleagues it typical of any effective treatment and it confirms the validity of the results. This having said, however, there is the need to provide an answer to those who do not respond. And, in the effort of providing an answer to non-responders, improvements in the overall efficacy of the treatment for everyone will eventually follow.

At the moment, there are two hypotheses that could help explaining why certain subjects do not respond to GcMAF in terms of improvement of symptoms of autism.

The first hypothesis is related with the VDR gene polymorphisms. As we proposed at the AIDS conference in Vienna in 2010, and later published in 2012 (J Nephrol. 2012 Jul-Aug;25(4):577-81), the individual responsiveness to GcMAF depends on the individual variations (polymorphisms) in the VDR gene. In other words, there are subjects harbouring variants that are associated with little or no response. However, this lack of response is relative and not absolute. In fact, it has been observed with vitamin D that these individuals respond to higher doses of the vitamin, thus indicating that the VDR is "less" responsive, but still functioning. This would mean that the so-called non-responders might need a higher dose or a longer time of GcMAF treatment to obtain the desired therapeutic effects. Prolonged observation of a higher number of cases will tell whether this hypothesis is correct.

The second hypothesis is closely associated with the first one as well as with the question briefly outlined in a preceding section: "does GcMAF cross the blood brain barrier?" In a recently submitted paper, we proposed that the interconnection between GcMAF and VDR signaling is responsible for the transport of GcMAF through the blood brain barrier. In fact, transport of macromolecules across the blood brain barrier requires both specific and nonspecific interactions between macromolecules and proteins/receptors expressed on the luminal and/or the abluminal surfaces of the brain capillary endothelial cells (Int J Cell Biol. 2013;2013:703545. doi: 10.1155/2013/703545). Since VDR signaling appears to enhance brain to blood transport at the blood brain barrier through both genomic and non-genomic actions, it can be hypothesized that the interaction between GcMAF and VDR (Nutrients. 2013 Jul 8;5(7):2577-89. doi: 10.3390/nu5072577) may favor GcMAF transport into the brain. This means that subjects with a less responsive VDR because of unfavorable genetic variants, would also have a less efficient transport of GcMAF to the brain.

This latter consideration, however, opens the way to a possible solution that might also help increasing the effectiveness of GcMAF in those who already respond to it.

In fact, now that we know the physiological molecular assembly of GcMAF, we can design specific GcMAF molecules that are more efficient in crossing the blood brain barrier and, therefore, are more effective in treating neurological conditions such as CFS/ME and autism. These molecules exploit the fatty acid binding site in the GcMAF molecule, and use one of the most beneficial fatty acids, oleic acid, the basic component of olive oil, to target brain cells.

Most interestingly, GcMAF/oleic acid molecules do not only stimulate human neurons with a much higher efficiency than GcMAF, but they also regulate glial cell metabolism. Glial cells are the connective tissue of the brain and glial cell dysfunction is involved in the pathogenesis of autism. In particular, glial cell dysfunction seems to be responsible for the neuronal underconnectivity typical of the autistic brain (Neuron Glia Biol. 2011 May;7(2-4):205-13). In short, we can postulate that the development of these novel GcMAF/oleic acid molecules will prove beneficial not only for the GcMAF non-responders, but also for improving the therapeutic efficacy of GcMAF in all neurological conditions where GcMAF treatment is indicated.

In addition to these novel, more physiological, brain-targeted, molecules, there are other strategies that can improve GcMAF transport into the brain with consequent increased therapeutic efficacy. Just a few days ago, in a journal dedicated to advanced radiological research, it was published a report demonstrating that ultrasounds, just like those described in the preceding section, transiently open the blood brain barrier. This phenomenon is exploited to favor transport of chemotherapeutic drugs into the brain of individual with brain tumors and it proved safe and efficacious after extensive testing.

On the basis of this observation, one could devise a simple treatment protocol using the same ultrasound system that is currently used for transcranial ultrasonography. In analogy with what is performed to deliver chemotherapeutic drugs to brain tumors, ultrasounds could be used to facilitate the transport of GcMAF through the blood brain barrier and to focus its delivery into those areas of the brain that are known to be altered in autism.

In this manner, during a regular examination, the health professional could exploit our technique to assess the neuro-anatomical alterations in the autistic brain and to deliver GcMAF to those areas. The use of more physiological, brain-targeted GcMAF molecules that can be administered sublingually, would greatly improve the efficacy of the treatment and it will most likely reduce the percentage of the so called non-responders to GcMAF.

As noted above, however, the use of ultrasounds to treat neurological conditions is not completely new. In fact, we and others have demonstrated that non-thermal ultrasounds have significant effects on mental states (Brain Stimul. 2013 May;6(3):409-15), modulate neurotransmission (Neuropsychobiology. 2012;65(3):153-60), cardiac frequency and blood pressure and improve skeletal muscle strength (The Journal of IiME, vol. 6 (1), p 23-28, 2012). These effects can be observed with ultrasounds alone, that is in the absence of other treatments.

In a protocol for the treatment of autism and CFS/ME, we propose to use our ultrasonographic technique together with timely administration of sublingual GcMAF/oleic acid molecules. In this manner, we are able to exploit the direct effects of ultrasounds on the neuronal microtubules (Brain Stimul. 2013 May;6(3):409-15), together with the ability of ultrasounds to favor the transport of GcMAF/oleic acid into the brain and, more precisely into those areas where the neuroanatomical alterations are observed.

What is GcMAF?
A drug, a hormone, a natural component, a nutrient?

How to define a molecule that is formed every time a wound is licked? This is the most evolutionary conserved protective behavior in animals, humans included. The enzymes in the saliva convert the Gc-protein in the blood that is on the wound into active GcMAF that prevents infection of the wound and promotes repair (PLoS One. 2013 Jul 18;8(7):e69059).

For many years researchers considered GcMAF only a key regulator of the immune system because of its activity on macrophages and its denomination reflects this early conjecture. However, as it often happens in science, the original denomination of a molecule proves incorrect with the passing of time and the accumulation of scientific evidences. Vitamin D is a notable example; it is not an vitamin and it does not contain any amine group (even though the suffix "vita" applies, in that it is indispensable for life). Now it is rightly considered a hormone produced by the body and, to be more precise, a secosteroid hormone that has a mechanism of action similar to that of classical steroidal hormones. GcMAF, being a part of the vitamin D axis might soon become another example of scientific mislabeling. In fact, we now know that it exerts its actions in many other cell types in addition to macrophages and that its role go well beyond activation of macrophages.

And even though there are no doubts that it is a powerful stimulant of the immune system, it would not be surprising to realize that this might not be its most relevant physiological role. In this respect, GcMAF shares the destiny of its precursor, the Gc-protein. Gc-protein is a serum alpha 2 glycoprotein composed of a single polypeptide chain, structurally related to serum albumin, that performs a variety of actions in several cell types. It is synthesized in the liver and has been detected on the surface of several cell types, yolk sac endodermal cells, and some T lymphocytes. In B cells, it participates in the linkage of surface immunoglobulins. In addition to vitamin D, it binds actin and acts as an actin scavenger. These characteristics are of paramount importance in human pathology since actin is the most abundant protein in eukaryotic cells and it is a major cellular protein released during cell necrosis that may cause fatal formation of actin-containing thrombi in the circulation if the actin scavenging capacity of Gc-protein is exceeded. Not surprisingly, therefore, several studies suggest an association between Gc-protein and resistance or susceptibility to chronic obstructive pulmonary disease, thyroid diseases, diabetes, multiple sclerosis, and sarcoidosis (for a review on Gc-protein and the vitamin D axis, see: European Nephrology, 2011;5(1):15–9).

From these considerations it derives that the potential indications for GcMAF treatment might be far too numerous than those currently envisaged. And also this parallels the fate of vitamin D, once thought only to prevent rickets and now involved in almost all aspects of human physiology and pathology up to the point that a (serious) scientific article on this subject was entitled: "Does vitamin D make the world go 'round'?" (Breastfeed Med 2008; 3: 2392–50.).

Apart from issues of biomedical terminology, it is now emerging the concept that GcMAF is an essential component of that nutritional pathway that is the vitamin D axis. It is not a case or a coincidence that the article on GcMAF that has received the greatest attention was published in a scientific journal named "Nutrients". With the proceeding of research it is becoming apparent that GcMAF participates in such a variety of physiological events that each proposed definition is limited.

But, if we accept the concept that GcMAF is a natural nutrient, indispensable for brain and immune system development and function (and possibly for many more essential physiological events), two questions spontaneously arise: "Where do I find it in nature?" and "How can I consume it?"

The second question already has an answer: now that the physiological molecular assembly of GcMAF is known, there are on the market several GcMAF products that can be used sublingually or simply eaten. Modern biotechnology has reproduced the physiological conformation of GcMAF so that it can be absorbed in a natural way without recurring to intravenous or intramuscular injections. GcMAF injections are reserved for those cases where a strong and rapid stimulation is required.

The other question is more intriguing and leads to the final section of this chapter.

My Own Personal Experience with GcMAF

As it happens in many people of my age exposed to the radiations from the Chernobyl incident, I have several thyroid nodules. Being a radiologist, it was easy for me to perform ultrasonography on my thyroid and what I saw on the screen was not nice. In addition to small lesions in my right lobe, in my left lobe I observed a massive mixed (solid and cystic) protruding nodule substituting for most of the lobe. The anterior-posterior diameter was about 3 cm, whereas the longitudinal diameter was greater than the length of the probe (4 cm). The structure was grossly inhomogeneous with cystic areas and hypo-reflecting areas alternated with iso- or hyper-reflecting areas. The margins bordering the residual normal thyroid tissue appeared well defined with an area of edema (inflammation) surrounding the nodule. The blood vessels were located around and inside the nodule and few or no blood vessels could be observed in the large hypo-reflecting areas suggesting the presence of metabolically inactive tumor tissue. Consistent with these findings, laboratory tests showed signs of immunodeficiency and anemia. And, it has been reported that anemia is among the predictive elements of malignancy in thyroid nodules (Tunis Med. 2002 Sep;80(9):536-41).

It was immediately clear to me that I needed a powerful stimulant of the immune system as wells as an anticancer agent, and GcMAF was my first thought. However, at that time, GcMAF was synthesized only in academic research laboratories and it was not available on the market as the pure, highly active, quality controlled product that we know today. Therefore, we decided to look for natural sources of GcMAF.

We already knew that GcMAF is naturally formed when a wound is licked because saliva contains the enzymes that convert blood Gc-protein into active GcMAF. Licking my thyroid, however, quite obviously, was not an option.

Because of these hindrances, we hypothesized that GcMAF could be obtained through a natural food fermentation process that exploits the characteristic of certain microbial strains to produce the enzymes that convert food Gc-protein into GcMAF (Hollis and Draper, 1979). According to our hypothesis, fermented food-derived GcMAF would activate the macrophages widely diffused in the walls of the entire gastrointestinal tract and, in particular, in the Waldeyer's-Pirogov tonsillar ring (or pharyngeal lymphoid ring). Our first goal was to assess the feasibility of obtaining natural GcMAF through home-made food processing procedures. To this end, we devised a strategy to prepare a fermented food product using those microbes, known to mankind for their healthy properties for millennia, that express the enzymes involved in GcMAF synthesis (Hollis and Draper, 1979).

After having prepared this fermented food at home, I began consuming it on a daily basis.

Since at that time we too considered GcMAF mainly for its immune-stimulating properties, the first objective was to assess the efficacy of this procedure on certain markers of immunodeficiency, the so called CD4 lymphocytes. The general public became familiar with CD4 lymphocytes because of their involvement in HIV infection and AIDS, and CD4 cell number is considered a reliable marker of immune system function. The role of CD4 cells in the immune system has been widely popularized up to the point that the webpage of the AIDS Authority of the Government of the United States of America states; "CD4 cells or T-cells are the "generals" of the human immune system. These are the cells that send signals to activate your body's immune response when they detect "intruders," like viruses or bacteria. Because of the important role these cells play in how your body fights off infections, it's important to keep their numbers up in the normal ranges..."

In our observation, the reference laboratory considered normal value for CD4 cell count 500 - 1500 cells/μL. Before consumption, my CD4 count was low, close to the threshold of AIDS definition (372 cells/μL). CD4 count rose from the abnormal value of 372 to the normal value of 609 cells/μL after three weeks of consumption of the fermented food that I had prepared. Such an increase continued up to eight weeks with CD4 cell count reaching 853 cells/μL. After many years, they are still in the normal range.

The trend toward normalization of blood parameters was observed also in other abnormal haematological values. My values (low or abnormal) changed as follows:

	Before Consumption	After 3 Weeks	Normal Values
Red Blood Cells			
(x106/uL)	4.55	4.85	4.6 - 6.2
Haematocrit, %	42.9	45.9	40 - 52
Haemoglobin, g/dL	14.8	15.6	13 - 18
Platelets/uL	165,000	206,000	140,000 - 440,000

The neutrophil cell count decreased from 77% to 55% in about 12 weeks, indicating a normalization of parameters suggestive of a pro-inflammatory state. Overall, the observed changes in haematological parameters were consistent with those positive modification of immune responses in humans that might represent the potential mechanism by which food fermented by probiotic bacteria confer health benefits.

Being a researcher, I am very well aware that this report is a mere anecdote that, in the era of evidence-based medicine, has low value or is not even considered to be medical evidence. However, a very recent study on the evaluation of clinical practice challenges the deprecation of stories like that reported above. Thus, it is well known that some studies present large and impressive statistics obtained from many observations while others report a small number of noteworthy events, as we did in this study. However, according to this authoritative epistemological approach, "all of these stories become evidence of what works in medicine" (J Eval Clin Pract. 2011 Oct;17(5):920-6).

Conclusions

In August 2013, a paper published in the very prestigious American Journal of Immunology reported a series of clinical cases successfully treated with GcMAF (Am.J.Immunol., 9:78-84.2013). Among these, there were pathologies already known to be responsive to GcMAF treatment, such as cancer, autism, and CFS/ME. Other neurodegenerative diseases such as multiple sclerosis and amyotrophic lateral sclerosis, however, had not been treated with GcMAF before, and this is the first report on such a successful treatment. This paper, together with all the other recognitions reported above, places GcMAF as one of the most effective tool to fight diseases that were considered incurable until very recently.

In other chapters of this book it is clearly stated that autism IS curable, and the successes of GcMAF in curing autism further strengthen this concept. What is emerging and what I hope to have been able to convey, is that GcMAF is not an exogenous drug that "fixes" some problem, but rather a very natural component of our body that is essential for, at least, brain and immune system development and function. In many conditions, including autism, GcMAF is not produced to a sufficient extent and therefore it has to be administered from the outside. With the advent of a courageous little biotech company that has perfected the synthesis of natural, fully physiological, GcMAF molecules that can be eaten, GcMAF treatment will become all the more and flexible to fit the individual needs. Eventually, GcMAF will become part of an integrated nutritional plan as it was intended by nature during evolution.

Consistent with this concept, I wish to conclude with an example from the realm of nature.

According to the Genetic Science Learning Center of the University of Utah, "Some mother rats spend a lot of time licking, grooming and nursing their pups. Others seem to ignore their pups. Highly nurtured rat pups tend to grow up to be calm adults, while rat pups who receive little nurturing tend to grow up to be anxious. It turns out that the difference between a calm and an anxious rat is not genetic—it's epigenetic. The nurturing behavior of a mother rat during the first week of life shapes her pups' epigenomes. And, the epigenetic pattern that mom establishes tends to stay put, even after the pups become adults."

It seems that licking their pups while breastfeeding in the first week of life is the decisive factor; in the saliva there are the enzymes that convert milk Gc-protein into GcMAF. What is more natural than this?

Subcutaneous GcMAF has been available through FIRSTiMMUNE for several years. Their website is:

www.gcmaf.eu

They now also produce a sublingual version of GcMAF called GOleic. They also have Bravo probiotics, and more. Please visit their website for more information.

"If you're not stubborn, you'll give up on experiments too soon. And if you're not flexible, you'll pound your head against the wall and you won't see a different solution to a problem you're trying to solve."

~ Jeff Bezos
Founder of Amazon

Chapter 13

Beyond Recovery:
<u>The Maintenance Plan</u>

*"Success is not final, failure is not fatal:
it is the courage to continue that counts."*
~ Winston Churchill

We see these questions on our boards from time to time:

Will my son have to take CD for the rest of his life?

or

Will we be sorting through poop forever?

The answer is No!

Once your child has recovered, you can move to the maintenance phase. Since we live in a toxic world, it is important to continually detox the system, and keep the body free of parasites. While this can look different for every child and every family, the following are some general guidelines designed to keep our kids healthy once they are recovered.

Diet

While some families go back to giving their children foods that aren't permitted here, many do not. Wheat, dairy, and soy aren't "healthy" foods for any of us to be consuming. After reading Olive Kaiser's section on gluten, you may have a tough time giving your child any bread products ever again. That said, once the gut is healed, it should be able to tolerate many of these foods again, to the extent that a "healthy" person would.

CD

Even into the recovered stage of autism, many of the families keep using CD (oral, baths, enemas) to reach an ATEC of zero... or until there are no behaviors left from the autism. Once that is accomplished, then a maintenance plan of one oral dose on Monday and one oral dose on Thursday is enough. Typically, such a dose is 3 drops for children and 6 drops for adults—all in one dose on each of those 2 days. However, each family does this a little differently depending on weight and what the optimum dose was while on the full protocol.

The more I learn about how toxic our planet is (i.e. GMOs, toxins in the air, drinking water, parasites in the environment, etc.), the more I realize how critical it is to be on a at least a limited long-term detoxing program. This is especially true for someone who was, or may still be immunocompromised. I do believe that once a child recovers from autism, their immune system can do the job that it was designed to do. However, healing takes time, and every case is different. Some people ask me if recovered children still take CD once recovered—and to be honest—many do not.

Parasite Protocol

It is impossible to avoid parasites in our world. As Andreas and Miriam explained to us, their larvae are nearly indestructible in nature and can live for years. A strong immune system, as well as sufficient stomach acid, may prevent a parasitic infection from taking hold in the body. To make sure, it is best to do a "mini protocol" every 3 months. You can do the full 18 days every 3rd month or a 1-week mini version—whichever you prefer.

Other Supplements

While ocean water is necessary when detoxing with CD, it is extremely beneficial to all of us as our soils are almost completely devoid of nutrients and are contaminated with heavy metals and toxins. Also, it has been theorized that many GMO crops are lacking in nutrition as well. The 90 bioavailable nutrients in OW can certainly go a long way in keeping our bodies healthy. I especially love that it helps with conductivity in the brain. And, it is conducive to speech and cognitive function as well.

Depending on each individual's needs it may behoove a family to keep giving MCT oil or Vegan 3,6,9 omegas. Certain supplements may still be required if there is a history of seizures.

Chelation

Gentle chelators like Bio-Chelate™ can continue to be used into the recovery phase as heavy metals are present in our air and water.

Hyperbarics

Nothing brings down inflammation quite like a hard hyperbaric chamber. However, 10 to 20 sessions can be very cost prohibitive for some families, making it a very personal decision as to whether or not to continue with HBOT after recovery.

GcMAF

I never felt better than when I did a course of GcMAF injections on myself. Energy went up and so did my ability to concentrate. Again, GcMAF is a fairly expensive intervention and that will factor into each family's decision as to whether to keep using it. or not

In a nutshell, I would at least continue with CD two times a week, and a mini parasite protocol every 3 months, just as a preventative. Staying healthy is as important as getting healthy.

Um, YEAH so just took an ATEC. We have officially been on the protocol for 12 months now and finishing up our 11th PP. ATEC of THREE!!!!!!!!!! 57 to 3 in 12 months. Henry's speech is what is keeping us from 0. He has great conversation with people that are patient and don't interrupt him so we are so close to a BIG ZERO!!! 57 to 3 in 12 months!!!! Far cry from the severe autism diagnosis he got at 2.5 years old. Here is to the doctor that told me my son should be medicated, would never speak, and will probably need to be institutionalized. I hope YOU never say those things to another person!!!!! All you need is hope, determination, and LOVE.

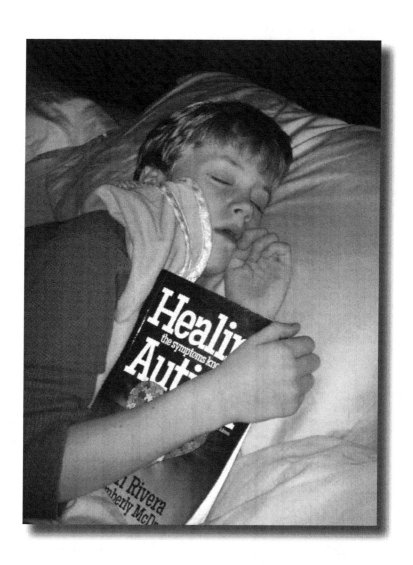

Chapter 14

Miscellaneous Information
<u>You Should Know</u>

*"Always bear in mind that your own resolution to succeed
is more important than any one thing."*
~ *Abraham Lincoln*

Seizures

An estimated 40% of children with autism suffer from some form of seizures. Seizures can be absolutely terrifying for both child and family and deleterious to the health of a child who is already suffering from various issues. I have talked to many different professionals about seizures and in turn have heard just as many different opinions on why this happens. Many doctors are unsure, while some simply don't express their opinions. Some say it is a virus in the brain or heavy metals, inflammation, or pathogens/parasites. In a presentation by Dr. Andreas Kalcker, he stated that high levels of ammonia in the body can cause seizures and the high levels of ammonia in the body come from parasites. Since we know that CD kills pathogens/parasites, neutralizes heavy metals, and helps to reduce inflammation, it is not surprising that we have noticed reduced, or even eliminated seizure activity in children with seizure disorders that use CD in combination with the Parasite Protocol.

MCT (medium chain triglyceride) oils, which come from the Ketogenic Diet out of UCLA, are also a very important piece to healing the body and eliminating seizure disorders. There is plenty of information on the Internet that discusses the results of people (on the spectrum and otherwise) using MCT oils for seizure disorders.

The following is a list of things that parents on The Protocol have used successfully to reduce/eliminate seizures in their children.

- CD
- Parasite Protocol
- MCT oil

- GABA
- Hyperbarics at 1.75 ATA
- Ketogenic diet
- SCD diet (grain free)
- L-Carnitine
- P5P with magnesium
- L-Carnosine
- Taurine
- DMG
- Pycnogenol®

The first four in this list have proven to be the most important and have shown consistent results. If you have a child suffering from seizures, you would be wise to review and consider these interventions immediately. The others have also proven very helpful and can be added in one-by-one, (always leaving three days between each new supplement) while you watch for a decrease in seizures.

When we introduce GABA, we increase the dose daily in search of the appropriate dose for the individual. While establishing the correct dose for one intervention it is not appropriate to add in other supplements. Watch out for sleepiness or undesired behavior with GABA. In these cases, I would personally discontinue its use, as with everything there is not one formula that is right for every child. Similarly, if you see hyperactivity or undesired behavior with DMG discontinue its use.

All of the above supplements/interventions have proven very important for eliminating seizures, in different combinations, for different families. Whether the seizures are grand mal (tonic clonic) or petit mal (absence), they start to fade away as a result of the Protocol.

Sometimes, when a family starts corresponding with me, their child may already be taking some of these supplements, and they continue to do that. They may have already taken some of these and seen no improvement. Some other families live in parts of the world where these supplements are unavailable, and in that case we focus on CD and killing parasites.

As I mentioned, a critical piece for some of the children with seizures has been the implementation of the Parasite Protocol. This has also led to a reduction or cessation of seizure activity in many children with seizures.

Interestingly, once some moms were made aware of the parasite/seizure connection it was easy to time seizure activity/anxiety/aggression to full and/ or new moons. As Dr. Andreas Kalcker talked about in the parasite section, the full moon period is when parasites are mating, many in the gastrointestinal tract, and therefore "wormy behaviors" (anxiety, SIBs, depression, tantrums, aggression, and teeth grinding to name a few) will generally be higher around that period. New moons can also cause an increase in these behaviors.

Children who have a seizure disorder or are self-injurious need to avoid food coloring, eggs, tomatoes, pork, and chocolate. When adding in the supplements for the seizures that we listed above, follow the same rules as before, never adding more than one supplement every three days, and always carefully observing and keeping track of any and all changes in your notebook so we know what causes what.

After starting anti-parasitics with the help of her daughter's doctor, one veteran mom introduced the CD protocol; a combination that has been extremely beneficial for her daughter, who suffered from frequent grand mal (tonic clonic) seizures.

Her Advice:

Most of my understanding of how parasitic infections can lead to seizures involves my own tracking of seizure activity patterns in my daughter, which coincided with new moon and full moon periods. Then, since MOST doctors want references to what they feel are 'reliable sources,' I started by Googling "NIH parasites seizures," which brought me to:

ncbi.nlm.nih.gov/pubmed/18754958
Helminthic parasites and seizures. [Epilepsy. 2008][1] - PubMed - NCBI

I would strongly suggest that you document patterns of seizure activity against the Farmer's Almanac of Full Moons (you can even look up past Full Moons) and marry that information with info from sites like the one above. Also, I would highly recommend you hunt down a pediatric infectious disease specialist in your local area (start by researching pediatric staff at local hospitals) and bring with you all information/insight to your first appointment.

Her Testimonial:

From her very first drop of activated CD in early July 2012 (actually her very first one-eighth drop to be exact), I witnessed an improvement in my daughter. Within about two hours of drinking her first ounce of the activated CD water solution (one activated drop of CD mixed into eight ounces of water), I witnessed her sitting still in our kitchen and observing me in such a way unlike she had ever done before. She was calmly observing me instead of running around the kitchen. She was taking my actions in. She was studying me. Her eyes were focused on me, rather than constantly scanning everything else in the room. Both her facial expression and her body language were calmer than I had ever witnessed before. She was more focused, more centered. She appeared content.

This change that I witnessed in her was so noticeable and so sudden, that I couldn't help but think to myself, "So this must be why the first word in MMS is Miracle." It was that amazing of a change in those moments.

Shortly after those incredible moments, my daughter went on to eating contently and then jumping on the neighbor's netted trampoline. She has enjoyed the neighbor's trampoline for years; yet on that particular day, only a few hours after her first drink of a tiny amount of CD, I noticed something quite different in her behavior. As I observed her from the windows of our house, I could see that she was jumping less than usual and instead looking around a lot more. She was calmly looking around at the neighbors' houses, down at some birds in the grass, up at the trees, the clouds, etc. It was all as though she was perhaps truly noticing them for the first time. She had glanced at these things before that day, sure, but she never before appeared to be studying them in the manner she was in those moments on the trampoline that July afternoon. She did engage a bit in some of her tic-like spitting movements with her mouth while on the trampoline, but to nowhere near the intensity, nor duration that would more typically have consumed her prior to that day.

When she came back into the house after using the trampoline and observing her world, I asked her, "why were you spitting out there?" To my surprise, she then very calmly replied, "because it's sensory." Wow! She truly was more connected somehow to her world than ever before. Something good was happening to my girl—only hours after drinking one-eighth of a drop of activated CD with one ounce of water. From those moments on I felt encouraged in my heart and soul that CD could possibly be a very important catalyst toward improving my daughter's health and well-being.

With the help of a caring local doctor, we had already begun some trials of anti-parasitic medications on our daughter in early May 2012, prior to starting CD, in response to behavioral struggles that had been consistently intensifying around full moons every month. (Later, we noticed new moon behavioral intensities as well). We had seen some improvement with anti-parasitic medication, yet CD seemed to somehow boost our daughter toward further improvements that much quicker. In fact, our daughter's ATEC score before starting CD measured 79 on July 8th, 2012 (the day before starting CD), but as of September 30th had dropped down to 55 (only two and a half months later).

Now, in early December 2012, our daughter still appears to be on an overall upward trend of improving health and stability, attributable to the synergy of CD and anti-parasitic medications. Natalie's interpersonal skills have improved, her growth rate has improved, her focus has improved, and her frequency of seizures has lessened.

In fact, at this writing she is 53 days seizure free, which is quite an improvement considering before she was on a terrifying pace of grand mal (tonic clonic) seizures occurring every 2-3 weeks. These are very dangerous, life-threatening events. Her seizures were rapid onset, heading toward grand mal within seconds. They could happen anywhere, i.e. while in her car seat coming back home from a Dr.'s appointment, while driving away from Costco, while running in the backyard playing with the dog, or swinging high on the swing set in the backyard with a neighbor girl. Yet another occurred while wading in the lake (with life vest on), another hit while in our neighbor's four-foot swimming pool with me and her brother. She was right next to me, walking around and then suddenly, she was in the throes of a rapid-onset grand mal seizure that required me to lift her out of pool into her NT (neurotypical) brother's arms. May these be the last my daughter ever knows of seizures.

It is our hope that, in time, CD will be able to take on the lead role as the primary health-support for our daughter, if not, perhaps even someday the sole healthcare support to her. We're looking forward to the days when we may be able to remove or reduce many, or perhaps even almost all, of her current supportive medications (i.e. antibiotic, antiviral, anti-seizure, etc.). With the caring support of parents of The Thinking Moms' Revolution, as well as some excellent local doctors, we suspect that our daughter's life will continue to improve. In the almost 14 years of caring for our daughter in her various states of medical fragility, we have never ever had this much Hope. We feel fortunate to have been swept up into this Revolution and embraced warmly by so many Thinking Moms who are also in the process of working toward more healing for their children. Working to heal illness is so much nobler than working to mask illness, wouldn't you agree? God Bless Jim Humble, Andreas Kalcker, Kerri McDaniel de Rivera and all the TMR families!

UPDATE: January 30th, 2013

I too am so thankful for Kerri and her whole 'crew'. Thanks to Kerri for bringing CD to all of our kids on the spectrum worldwide. My Natalie is now OFF of her former roller-coaster ride of prescription anti-fungals, OFF of her former roller-coaster ride of prescription antibiotics, OFF of prescription antiviral, OFF of prescription low-dose naltrexone, etc. Her belly distention has disappeared, she's gained weight, she's gained height and she's now almost 103 days seizure free (as of 6:16pm tonight). She still has a ways to go toward more improvements, but she's happily climbing up from bottom of the trenches; she's climbing up from what seemed like the very bottom of the abyss that vaccine injury/injuries had placed her in. Thank you Kerri, Andreas Kalcker, Jim Humble and all of the moderators on the supportive websites!!!

UPDATE: February 1st, 2013

My Natalie's long run of 105 seizure-free days has ended. After being off of Albenza® less than 24 hours, BOOM! a grand mal (tonic clonic) seizure occurred yesterday evening. This same thing happened the last time we stopped Albenza®, sooooo we're not sure if it's withdrawal related or parasitic activity related. We're going to closely watch her behaviors this week for signs of parasitic burden. We put her on Alinia® now, just to give her some sort of parasitic coverage while we wait to likely restart Albenza®, soon. She did fine on Alinia® 200mg BID in the past. I'll keep you all posted, but for now we unfortunately need to restart the clock on my Natalie's 'seizure-free days' tracking. I'm bummed, but thought I should keep you in the loop on this; as I've been soooooo excited over the past three months about her freedom from seizures, which I believe was due to the synergy of CD and Albenza®. I'll touch back if/when we learn more.

UPDATE February 2nd, 2013

O.K. so, I just wanted to kind of round out this long thread a bit with my thoughts, for whatever they're worth: I really truly suspect that perhaps too sharp of a drop off (lack of weaning) from the systemic med, Albenza® lead to the seizure. Natalie is stable right now on a low-dose interim of Alinia® 200mg BID for now until all insurance approvals are in for the delivery of more Albenza®. This leads me to believe that the several courses of Albenza® over the past months likely HAS lowered her overall parasitic load/burden fairly well thus far (it's a pretty broad-spectrum anti-parasitic, from what I understand). However, I don't think for a minute that Natalie's broad spectrum anti-parasitic medicine needs are finished. For this reason, we'll resume Albenza® as soon as we're able.

Although further discussion/negotiation between myself and Natalie's pediatric infectious disease doctor is required, my thought is that she may need an entire year on Albenza. However, certainly in the future, whenever we stop Albenza®, I'm going to plan for a slow weaning off period so as not to disrupt Nat's delicate nervous system. Also, I'm kind of thinking that perhaps if our kids 'wig out' when CD is eventually dropped that maybe we've not lowered the overall parasitic burden enough, as yet to allow their immune system to 'kick in gear' and properly function??? I don't know, obviously, just theorizing with the brain matter God has given me.

SUMMARY & UPDATE FOR SECOND EDITION: December 1st, 2013

From birth to age 7 years, my daughter Natalie unfortunately had her share of health and developmental struggles. Her diagnoses began with 'Failure to Thrive' shortly after birth, followed thereafter by a Mitochondrial Encephalopathy Partial Complex III Deficiency diagnosis by age 7 months, then Hypothyroidism as well as global developmental and cognitive delays obvious from there. Despite significant medical and developmental challenges, Natalie entered a Kindergarten designed for the 'mild cognitively impaired' (formerly referred to as educatably mentally impaired 'EMI') with daily opportunities for mainstreaming with the typical Kindergarten classroom next door. After a fall 2005 Flu shot early in that same Kindergarten year, however, all bets were off. She regressed very rapidly in every way: medically, developmentally, and behaviorally. Within months of that shot, a laundry list of additional diagnoses began to form: Sensory Integration Disorder, Autism, Epilepsy, P.A.N.D.A.S., P.A.N.S., and Combined Immune Deficiency, to name a few. After much study by a large team of educational specialists, Natalie was reclassified by school professionals by the following April of 2006 to the 'SXI'' category of disabilities (Severely Multiply Impaired), having deteriorated terribly from her former classifications of POHI (Physically or Otherwise Health Impaired) and 'CI' (Cognitively Impaired) within only months of that Flu shot. Her significant healthcare needs and behavioral challenges since have necessitated assignment of a one-on-one Para-educator to her case, even while she's been schooled within high adult-to-student ratio basic education special- needs classrooms over the past several years.

In 2011, between the ages of 12 and 13, I began to notice patterns of apparent P.A.N.S. flares in Natalie, which seemed to coincide with the New Moon and Full Moon weeks. When I began to study this phenomenon a bit more closely, I also recognized a pattern of seizure activity that tracked these timeframes as well. In reading about potential parasite activity that is thought to link to the New Moon and Full Moon timeframes, I requested anti-parasitic medications for Natalie. Thankfully, a local Pediatric Infectious Disease doctor kindly accommodated my request. Each time that the doctor prescribed various anti-parasitic medications for Natalie, she would improve. The improvements were noticeable both at school and at home. It was incredible to witness. However, each and every time that she was off of such medications, she would regress back to her former state of illness (displayed primarily by significant behavioral regressions). So, we found that we needed to try to keep her on various anti-parasitic medications more often than off of them, in order for her to enjoy overall improved health and neuropsychiatric stability. Even so, there was still some sort of physiological strain that she was very definitely experiencing, but we were unable to decipher what it could be. This was frustrating, of course; to witness her continued rollercoaster of ups and downs in health and her various psychiatric disturbances each month.

It wasn't until a friend suggested we get Natalie started on CD, that the health and behavioral 'rollercoaster ride' began to show signs of smoothing out. In July 2012,

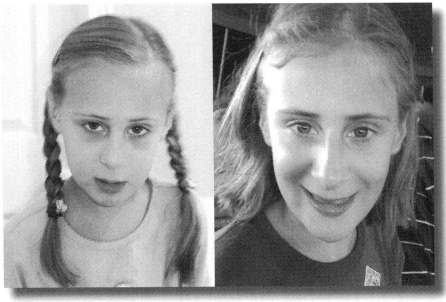

Natalie in 2006 (left) and in 2013 (right)

after her first drink of CD (only one-eighth of a drop), Natalie began to show initial signs of relief from whatever it was that was still ailing her. Her connectedness and overall psychological state of being changed within hours of that first one-eighth drop of CD. After that first day, we of course then continued with a very slow and conservative ramp-up of CD (orally, then baths, then enemas) alongside various anti-parasitic medications and all of the components of the Kalcker PP (with frequent swap out of Mebendazole with Albendazole, predominantly). With each passing month over the past sixteen months, we've been able to witness improvements in Natalie; perhaps a bit more slowly than some of the younger and/or potentially less health-compromised kids that Kerri's protocol has healed, but improvements nonetheless. Before CD, Natalie's ATEC score was a 79. As of this writing, her ATEC score is a 39. Even more astounding to us than that improved ATEC score have been the changes witnessed thus far in her overall health status and health regimen. Here is a list of some of the improvements that I can very easily recall as I write this (there are likely many more that I could comment upon, if I had more time):

1. Daily prescription anti-fungal medications no longer needed.
2. Daily prescription antibiotic medications no longer needed.
3. Daily prescription antiviral medication no longer needed.
4. Daily prescription LDN (low dose naltrexone) immune modulator removed.

5. *Daily prescription Leucovorin removed without ill effects noticed, as well as several other daily supplements that might have been ultimately not helpful.*

6. *Prescribed Immune Globulin (weekly subcutaneous, formerly monthly intravenous for years) removed.*

7. *Distended belly gone & improved posture (no longer hunched over).*

8. *Formerly very frequent tongue sores/lesions lessening more & more.*

9. *Seizures formerly as high as every 17-21 days in her worst times; now she's enjoyed seizure-free stretches as high as 105 days (3.5 months) followed shortly thereafter by a seizure-free stretch of 168 days (5.5 months). Prescription anti-seizure medication reductions have also been enjoyed as well as fewer headaches resultant of those reductions.*

10. *P.A.N.S. flares controlled with the combination of CD and anti-parasitic meds. Neuropsychiatric symptoms of flares very dramatically declined.*

11. *Overall appearance of improved health, improved language and interpersonal skills, improved attentiveness (per Neurology's opinion at recent appointment).*

12. *Improved stamina and strength (core, legs, etc.) noticed at Special Needs Performance Cheerleading practices, physical therapies, etc. Her ability to peddle adaptive bike has also improved.*

13. *No more nose bleeds, no more ear infections, no more apparent seasonal allergies, fewer headaches (as noted above).*

14. *Incredibly improved sleep and need for naps only once in a while now (as opposed to formerly daily).*

15. *Improved growth rate and normalized appetite.*

16. *Improved language (more descriptive words, more sentences).*

17. *Healthier-looking skin overall; softer, less dry, improved color & ability to tan.*

18. *Improving oral muscular abilities, able to swallow pills/capsules.*

19. *Capable of successful dentist appointments and now even Orthodontist appointments, with calm and ease.*

20. *Increased success rate during therapies (Speech Therapy, Occupational Therapy, Physical Therapy, etc.).*

21. *Less rigidity overall, fewer transition issues, cooperates more often than she ever used to.*

With all of the well-documented improvements noticed in Natalie at home, at school and in doctors' offices, I don't have the same level of fear as other parents might surrounding our open use of CD, as Natalie's doctors are all well informed and quite supportive. We've also formally notified her social worker (both verbally at a home meeting and in writing) of our use of Kerri's CD Protocol (including Kalcker's Parasite Protocol and of course a GFCFSF/low sugar diet) while under Natalie's local medical team's support and medical monitor. We're 'out of the closet', so to speak, when it comes to our use of CD for improving Natalie's health. It's been quite obvious to Natalie's doctors; actually, that Kerri's protocol has been extremely complementary to their medical efforts for improving Natalie's health and overall quality of life.

There's of course no way to predict with certainty how far my sweet Natalie will be able to ultimately improve via this protocol, but based upon what we've witnessed thus far, I do feel that her current best hope for continued improvement lies within the pages of this book; as these healing strategies of Kerri Rivera's have brought Natalie toward more health (physical, neuropsychiatric, emotional and even some initial cognitive improvements) than any other medical effort attempted since her 2005 Flu shot injury. All other medical efforts for Natalie over the years, I feel, perhaps only temporarily patched her severe illness. Kerri's methods actually work to attack disease, kill it and remove it. Yes, that's right. Eight years after Natalie's tragic rapid spiral downward, it's now finally a time of healing for Natalie. Thank you, Kerri Rivera, for all of your help given to our girl and to so many children around the world.

Self-Injurious Behaviors (SIBs)

Self-injurious behaviors (SIBs) can be absolutely devastating for families with children on the autism spectrum. Common self-injurious behavior includes: headbanging, hand biting, pinching, slapping head/ears, eye poking, hair pulling, scratching/rubbing, throwing one's body on the floor, etc. The horror of watching your own sick child further inflict pain onto himself, and the helplessness of not knowing what to do to help him is heartbreaking. I have met with families through the clinic who have had terrifying episodes of SIBs in front of me as well as at home, and many of these families as well as others are now using the Protocol to help their children with very good results.

There are many theories as to why some children have SIBs. The article "Self-Injurious Behavior" by Stephen Edelson on ARI's website discusses several different theories and supporting research.[2] The theory that most fits what I see on the ground is that of pain alleviation. Many of our kids are in chronic pain and cannot tell us. Sadly, we haven't always had answers to help them.

If we follow this thinking, and assume that many of these children suffer from severe gastrointestinal pain, or headaches (supported by head banging, gut clutching, etc.) we can hypothesize that much of this pain can come from pathogenic overload, parasites wreaking havoc on the body and the resulting inflammation.

Families applying CD in combination with the Kalcker Parasite Protocol are reporting a dramatic reduction in SIBs in their children. I believe there is an important connection to be made here, as we eliminate pathogens and parasites SIBs decreases. More research is needed, but for families facing the horrors of self-injurious behavior, this combination could be of great value. (More testimonies on decreased SIB's can be found in Chapter 2, and the Miracles and Testimonials section at the end of the book starting on page 357.)

Prior to starting CD, we had tried almost every autism biomedical protocol. We saw several DAN and GI specialists and numerous other practitioners. We spent tens of thousands of dollars on consults, supplements, diets, medicine and medical procedures not covered by insurance. My daughter either had no response or negative ones and she continued to get worse. She developed extreme self-injurious behaviors that progressed to the point of her needing to be restrained several times a day in an attempt to prevent her from pinching or biting herself until she drew blood. Her body was covered with bruises and cuts. She would also pull out big clumps of her hair. She would be up for hours screaming in the night with these behaviors. She was severely malnourished despite the fact that two registered dieticians had deemed her daily caloric intake adequate. She was 14 years old and weighed a little over 70 pounds. I honestly did not think that CD would be any different than anything else we had ever tried but figured things could not get much worse.

Since starting CD her self-injurious behaviors are almost entirely gone. She went from having to be restrained almost daily to once in the last 5 months. Her former multiple daily 45 minute self-injurious tantrums are now a few minutes of crying or protest and happen once a week if at all. We have noticed gains in language and cognition (20 point drop in her ATEC score). After years of fluctuating between loose stools and constipation, she is now regular and has gained almost 10 pounds. She sleeps through the night and we are able to take her places that we would have never dared to before. If my daughter can make gains this drastic in 5 months at age 14, I can't wait to see what the future holds.

Julie, Colorado, USA

PANS, PANDAS and PITAND

PANS stands for *Pediatric Acute-onset Neuropsychiatric Syndrome*. It encompasses PANDAS (Pediatric Autoimmune Neuropsychiatric Disorder Associated with Streptococcal Infections) and PITAND (Pediatric Infection Triggered Autoimmune Neuropsychiatric Disorders), where PANDAS is a subset of PITAND. Dr. Susan Swedo, Chief of Pediatrics & Developmental Neuroscience Branch at the National Institute of Mental Health (NIMH), and her research team identified a subtype of OCD in children during the 1990s that is triggered by infection. Streptococcal infection has been most studied; however, any infection can trigger this condition.[3]

I have run across these diagnoses a lot since I have started helping families in first world nations. There seems to be an overlap in some autism and PANS/PANDAS/PITAND cases. I have heard that around 25% of children with ASD's also suffer from PANS/PANDAS, and/or PITAND. Some practitioners would put that figure even higher. However, since further research is needed, and this field is still developing it is impossible to say for certain at the moment.

According to the International OCD (Obsessive Compulsive Disorder) Foundation some of the symptoms of PANDAS/PANS may include:

- Acute sudden onset of OCD.
- Challenges with eating, and at the extreme end, anorexia.
- Sensory issues such as sensitivity to clothes, sound, and light.
- Handwriting noticeably deteriorates.
- Urinary frequency or bedwetting.
- Small motor skills deteriorate - a craft project from yesterday is now impossible to complete.
- Tics
- Inattentive, distractible, unable to focus and has difficulties with memory.
- Overnight onset of anxiety or panic attacks over things that were no big deal a few days ago, such as thunderstorms or bugs.
- Suddenly unable to separate from their caregiver or to sleep alone.
- Screaming for hours on end.
- Fear of germs and other more traditional-looking OCD symptoms.

I know several moms who have been able to reduce/control/eliminate their children's symptoms with CD. In fact, families began to eliminate the antibiotics that they were using as they reached full dose of CD. I am by no means suggesting anyone reduce or remove a prescription medication without a doctor's supervision. I am simply reporting on what I have witnessed.

We know that CD kills bacteria, so we could hypothesize that CD could have a similar effect on the PANS/PANDAS/PITAND symptoms that an antibiotic would. What has worked in these cases is upping the number of doses of CD given a day so as to kill pathogens around the clock. For PANDAS/PANS/PITAND use two baby bottles a day. If your max dose is eight drops in an eight ounce bottle, and a PANDAS flare presents, prepare two baby bottles with eight drops in each and give one dose every hour over the course of 16 hours. Some families are doing 16 doses a day even if there is no flair and the child is doing excellent.

As noted previously, in the absence of research, we cannot recommend doing nothing for these children. Their suffering is intense and the risk of long-term damage cannot be ignored. We also do not know if some of these children remit spontaneously later in adolescence. We do not know if some of them grow into adults with the most treatment resistant OCD due to permanent basal ganglia damage. While we research those questions, offering treatment options at the local level, especially in the first few months after onset, could be critical to the long term success for these kids.[4]

We parents are pioneers in the research surrounding PANS/PANDAS/PITAND, so it is critically important that we document what we are doing with our children and what is working for them. In fact, A MOM was the first to discover the connection between strep and OCD/tics. Her child was the first documented PANDAS child. Dr. Susan Swedo reinforces that physicians should listen to what the mothers have to say![5] Speak up to your doctor, share your findings, join our forum to learn, and share what is working for you. Parents are driving the biomed movement (and always have) for ASDs as well as PANS/PANDAS/PITAND. In fact Dr. Bernard Rimland was a parent and the first to suggest biomedical interventions for people on the spectrum. We as parents can help countless other families by sharing our experiences.

You will find more info on PANS/PANDAS/PITAND at:

www.pandasnetwork.org

and

ocfoundation.org/PANDAS

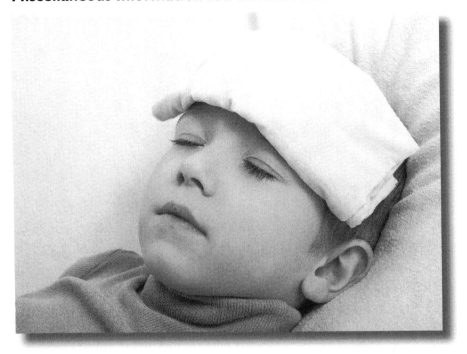

Fever Therapy

Dr. Kenneth Bock and Nellie Sabin, in their groundbreaking book *The Road to Immunity: How to Survive and Thrive in a Toxic World*, explain how to use fever therapy and how it is an incredible tool for healing.[6] When a mom emails me to tell me her child has a fever, it tells me that the immune system is reacting to an invader, and we have an excellent opportunity to kill pathogens in the body. Having a fever is part of an effective immune response. This is also true in infants as well as small children. Using over-the-counter (OTC) fever reducers interferes with the body's own ability to fight infection.

This section was excerpted from the aforementioned book.

> Fever has long been recognized as an important tool in the process of healing. The process of heating the body is called "hyperthermia." Hyperthermia, or ordinary fever, can be very effective against cancer cells, various pathogens, or invading organisms that cannot "tolerate the heat." Hyperthermia may not kill all pathogens in the body, but may reduce the number of invaders in the body to a manageable level for the immune system. Hyperthermia may also be responsible for stimulating the immune system to produce cytokines i.e. antibody production, and release of toxins from fat cells.

What Temperature Constitutes a Fever?

According to Dr. Robert Sears, the following are normal temperatures in children over 3 months:[7]

Normal temperature: 97° to 99° F (36° to 37.2° C)
Low-grade fever: 99° to 100.9° F (37.3° to 38.3° C)
Common fever: 101° to 103.5° F (38.4° to 39.7° C)
High fever: 103.6° F (39.8° C)

Fever Therapy in Practice

If your child develops a fever, it is not a failure of the body that needs to be corrected, but a mechanism that brings the body closer to healing. Rather than administer an OTC remedy to reduce fever, apply a cool, damp washcloth to the forehead and neck, replace them as they warm, and let the body do its job. Some parents put damp socks on their child's feet.

During a fever you can dose orally, as well as do one CD bath and one CD enema in one day. Keep dosing CD every hour (16 to 24 doses a day), unless the person stops eating. Even if you must reduce the number of drops, even if you are only giving one drop, keep dosing every hour. CD baths, as well as baths in general, are also your friend if your child has a fever. Some parents have given several baths throughout the day while a fever is present with great results. Bath the child if the fever spikes. Always be vigilant that the temperature does not rise too high or too fast so as to cause febrile seizures, we have to use common sense and trust our instincts. Bath and keep a cool damp wash cloth going 24/7 until the fever passes.

According to the National Institute of Neurological Disorders and Stroke febrile seizures are convulsions brought on by a fever in infants and small children. The majority of children with febrile seizures have rectal temperatures greater than 102° F. Approximately 1 in 25 children (4%) will have one febrile seizure. Although febrile seizures can be frightening to parents, the vast majority of febrile seizures are fast and harmless. There is no evidence that short febrile seizures cause brain damage. Large studies have found that children with febrile seizures have normal school achievement and perform as well on intellectual tests as their siblings who don't have seizures.[8]

If your child has a febrile seizure, experts recommend that you try to stay calm, keep the environment around your child safe (place them on the floor if they are not, and clear objects out of the way), and allow the seizure to resolve spontaneously without restraint. Try to look at your watch so you will know how long the seizure lasted. Do not put anything in your child's mouth as it may break, obstructing their airway.

Skin Issues

I have been hearing about skin issues right and left: rashes, hives, redness, acne, eczema, psoriasis, pustules, etc. It is very easy to assume that since skin is on the outside of our bodies that these reactions are caused by exterior factors (i.e. irritation from a detergent, mold, etc.). However, the skin is our largest detox organ, and many pathogens seek exit through the skin causing many of the above conditions.

The scenario that I keep hearing is the following: We just started the Kalcker Parasite Protocol. Little Johnny has a rash with white heads on his legs. What do I do? When the families keep up with the parasite protocol, and continue dosing daily with CD these eruptions disappear, and this is generally accompanied by improvements in behavior, or hyperactivity/anxiety.

We need to think about skin issues as outward manifestations of inner toxicity, and use our protocols accordingly. Skin issues can be a good indicator that something is being flushed from the system, or something needs to be flushed from the system. The Kalcker Parasite Protocol combined with CD tends to eliminate skin issues at the root.

The following paragraphs were excerpted from leakygut.co.uk, written by Dr. Gloria Gilbere ND DA hom PhD[9]:

> Experts agree that most chronic skin disorders, specifically psoriasis, is the external manifestation of the body's attempt to eliminate internal toxins that have accumulated within the lymphatics and blood stream by "seeping" through intestinal walls in a condition known as leaky gut syndrome.

> In working with clients around the world, the protocols that have been most effective are those that include repairing the intestinal walls by first beginning a protocol to eliminate candida yeast and parasites.

> The most effective cleansing protocol is obtained by clearing out these "uninvited" health-depleting microorganisms in order to release the accumulated pressure on the liver and the intestines—allowing free passage and thus reduction of overall toxic load.

The following paragraphs, authored by Dr. Edward F. Group III, DC, ND, DACBN, DABFM, were excerpted from parasite-cleanse.com/intestinal-parasite-symptoms.html[10]:

Symptoms of Intestinal Parasites Related to Skin

The presence of intestinal parasites, at times, manifest as allergies, tumors, and various other skin conditions.

Intestinal parasites cause the human body to release hormones and immune system defenders, which in turn irritate the skin and cause various skin conditions such as acne, hives, rashes, itching, weeping eczema, ulcers, swelling, sores, lesions, blisters on lips, and dermatitis. It also deprives the skin of its usual glow.

Intestinal parasites cause irritation and inflammation in the stomach making it difficult to digest certain types of foods. The presence of undigested food particles in the stomach causes the body to produce increased levels of eosinophil, an immune system defender. These eosinophils inflame the body's tissue and cause skin rashes.

Intestinal parasites trigger the body's immune system to develop a tumor-like mass known as granuloma to encase parasitic larvae or eggs. Granulomas usually develop in the colon, rectal wall, lungs, liver, peritoneum, and the uterus.

> Btw, you were bang on re his allergies and PP (parasite protocol). He had this horrible red lip thing because of food allergies. He would make it worse by rubbing it. It would get really bad. After first PP (Parasite Protocol) - NO MORE RED LIP ISSUES!

Families often tend to panic when dealing with sudden "unexplained" skin issues. If you are seeing chronic or acute skin issues I think there is enough evidence to look towards parasites as the main or at least a contributing culprit. Therefore, if we work towards removing the parasites causing the symptoms, rather than treating the symptoms topically we can expect an alleviation of the symptoms.

If you are seeing acute or chronic skin issues and you have not started a Parasite Protocol, I would suggest you revisit the parasite chapter and go over the recommendations with your healthcare provider. Keep dosing CD, in some cases upping the dose has helped resolve the issue faster, and in the case of severe irritation using a CD spray topically can provide relief (10 activated drops per ounce of water in a spray bottle) and a CD bath can also help. I have seen most, if not all skin issues resolved with CD and/or the Kalcker Parasite Protocol.

Healing Adults with Autism

Common thinking in the biomed community and the autism community at large is that autism is only "curable" or "recoverable" up to a certain age. I have heard that two to nine years old is the "golden window" for autism, and that after nine years of age improvement would be possible, but not recovery. The neural pathways would be set, the damage done, and the child would retain the autism diagnosis for life.

Not anymore. This year a 15-year-old recovered from autism, as well as two 17-year-olds. In addition, I am helping an amazing mother of a 31-year-old with autism that began the Protocol and for the first time in 28 years was seeing real progress with her son. In fact that young man's ATEC score dropped from a 65 to somewhere in the 20s in his first three months on The Protocol. I want to prove that autism recovery is possible at any age. It may take longer, and the road may prove more challenging, but it's already happening. Families that have been using biomedical interventions for more than ten years are finding the Protocol and sharing their gains.

Older children and adults on the spectrum start the same way as the little kids—clean up the diet first, and then on Day one of CD, give one drop in eight ounces of water over eight doses throughout the day. It is so important to start low and slow even with adults because they have often been chronically ill much longer than young children and have deep rooted pathogenic and parasitic infections. This means that when we start giving CD they might experience a detox reaction considering the amount of pathogens that will be dying.

Working with Neurotypical Adults

Can CD benefit parents and other adults not on the spectrum? Absolutely. You can literally find thousands of testimonials on the Internet (Jim Humble's website, www.jimhumble.org or www.curezone.com, etc.) on people who successfully detoxed, or healed a myriad of illnesses using CD.

Many parents who have seen improvements in their children have decided to use CD, or the Kalcker Parasite Protocol for themselves. I have done CD oral, baths, and enemas on myself, especially when I feel "something coming on" and with great results.

It's important to keep in mind that just because we weigh more than our children doesn't necessarily mean we should jump in and go to full dose from one day to the next. The best way to start an adult who may have 40 or 50+ years of accumulated toxins/pathogens/parasites is low and slow. Use the baby bottle method and start day one with one drop spread out over eight doses and go up from there. Chart your progress, see how you feel, go low and slow. When we as adults use the protocol it can be great for us, but also a window into how our children are feeling.

I love to see a mom or dad begin CD with their child. Both begin at one drop on day one in eight ounces of water, 1/8 or a drop per dose, for eight doses throughout the day. Starting with our children gives us a much better understanding as to how our child is feeling, and when we up the dose how that feels as well. This includes enemas. Once parents see how good they can feel after an enema, it helps garner confidence, if we had doubts about using them for our children. Applying our own enemas can help to remind us just what a powerful tool they are for healing.

Many of the parents doing the protocol for themselves write me to tell me about their remission from fibromyalgia, chronic fatigue syndrome, Lyme disease, life-long constipation, etc.

We all do the parasite protocol in my house so as not to re-infect my son, as parasites can be highly contagious. Last year I did a round of parasite medications prescribed to me by a doctor. During the course of treatment I felt a tremendous amount of anxiety and some depression (feelings I had never felt before) right before I passed worms, I can assure you it felt awful. That experience motivated me to encourage parents to get these invaders out of their children's bodies.

As soon as I started passing worms and detoxing more with CD, I started to feel good again. The cough that I had had on-and-off for years miraculously disappeared. Seriously, go low and slow, a toxic body can only process so much at a time. Too much too fast can cause headaches and diarrhea. The way I see it, there is no need for that, listen to your body and go at whatever pace you need. Don't just "push through," low and slow wins the race. Always remember to drink water when doing any sort of detox!

Tax on a Marriage

During the first five years after an autism diagnosis married couples face an estimated 80% divorce rate, and a 90% chance of divorce beyond the tenth year of marriage. My family was almost a statistic. Even before we had a diagnosis, our family was suffering. Due to Patrick's constant screaming and tantrums, he wasn't sleeping at night, and that meant that no one else was sleeping either. He had also stopped being the affectionate baby that he was for the first two years of his life, which was emotionally challenging for all of us. We were all over stressed and sleep deprived, not to mention having symptoms of post traumatic stress disorder (PTSD).

If I could give any advice to families dealing with a new diagnosis it would be to start The Protocol and CD immediately. The sooner the affected family member starts to heal, so will the rest of the family, similar to the sun coming out after a storm—this too shall pass.

Financial Stress

Not only is an autism diagnosis emotionally stressful on a marriage, but it can be extremely financially stressful as well. The Protocols outlined here can be extremely cost effective, even if including ocean water. Recently, one of the moms using The Protocol did some calculations comparing what she spent previously (see table on page 342) using another biomedical intervention with many supplements, etc., to what she spends now (see table below).

The Protocol - Estimated Cost				
Product	**Size**	**Price**	**Reorder Schedule**	**Current Cost per Month**
CD	1 bottle	$22	1/mo	$22.00
Diatomaceous Earth	2.5 lb	$15	1/3mo	$5.00
Rompepiedras	50 ml	$24	1/2mo	$12.00
Vortex Ocean Water	1 L	$40	1/mo	$40.00
THERALAC®	30 caps	$36	1/mo	$36.00
Natures Way® Neem	100 caps	$4.09	1/5mo	$0.75
Pyrantal Pamoate (Combatrin®)	32 oz	$35	1/6mo	$5.00
NOW® Castor Oil	16 oz	$8.23	1/6mo	$1.38
Mebendazole	90 tabs	$28	1/5mo	$5.60
TOTAL				**$127.73**

Defeat Autism Now! based Protocol - Estimated Cost				
Product	**Size**	**Price**	**Reorder Schedule**	**Current Cost per Month**
Actifolate	60	$15.00	1/2mo	$7.00
Calm PRT	120	$89.00	1/5weeks	$78.00
Caprilex™	90	$16.00	1/6weeks	$10.60
Cytoflora™	4 oz	$79.00	1/mo	$79.00
Designs for Health Lithium Synergy	120 caps	$22.00	1/mo	$6.00
DMG	90	$16.00	1/5mo	$10.60
Douglas B-Complex	60	$21.00	1/6mo	$21.00
Douglas CoQ10	60	$49.81	1/6mo	$12.50
Enhansa™	150 caps	$58.00	1 / 75 days	$29.00
Enzymedica Virastop™	120 caps	$32.11	1 / 4 months	$8.00
Garden of Life Probiotics	81g	$32.17	1/mon	$32.17
GI Revive	225g	$52.00	1/mon	$52.00
Homocycsteine Supreme	60 caps	$20.00	1/4months	$5.00
Kirkman Digestive Enzyme	200 caps	$60.00	1/3months	$20.00
Kirland Vit E	500	$13.65	1/16months	$0.84
Klaire Multivitamin	180	$28.00	1/3months	$9.00
Liver Life	4 oz	$50.00	1/2months	$25.00
Magnesium	240	$13.25	1/6months	$7.00
Metagenics Adreset®	60	$33.00	1/4months	$8.00
Milk Thistle	100	$25.00	1/3months	$8.00
NDF+	1 oz	$80.00	1/6months	$15.00
NeuroProtek®	4 bottles	$140.00	4/4months	$35.00
NeuroScience Avipaxin	60	$58.00	1/2months	$28.00
NeuroScience EndoTrax	1 bottle	$27.00	2/month	$54.00
NeuroScience Kavinace	120	$65.00	4/4months	$32.50
New Beginnings Copper	50 ml	$20.00	1/year	$1.75
NOW MCT	32 oz	$17.00	1/6months	$2.80
Nutribiotic GSE	4 oz	$16.99	1/6months	$3.00
OSR	30	$60.00	1/2months	$30.00
Oxycell Glutathione Cream	1 jar	$33.00	1/2months	$16.50
Pharmax Cod Liver Oil	8 oz	$13.33	1/mon	$13.33
Source Naturals B6 (p5p)	240	$15.00	1/6months	$2.60
Source Naturals Evening Primrose Oil	90	$7.45	1/6weeks	$4.97
Source Naturals Gaba	100g	$18.00	1/4months	$4.50
Source Naturals Lysine	200	$10.00	1/mon	$10.00
Source Naturals Quercitin	200	$25.80	1/3months	$8.25
Speak EFA	60	$42.00	1.5/month	$63.00
TheaNAQ	90	$54.00	1/month	$54.00
Therabiotic	120	$69.00	1/2months	$35.00
TravaCor Jr.	120 caps	$24.00	1/4months	$7.00
Vit B12 shots	1 refill	$45.00	1/3months	$15.00
Wobenzyime®	120	$60.00	1/2months	$30.00
TOTAL				**$894.91**

Tips for a Non-Toxic Home

Many of our children on the spectrum have chemical sensitivities, and even if they don't, it's wise to limit their exposure to toxins during the healing process as much as possible. Toxins are not good for anyone at any point in their life. The benchmark investigation "Bodyburden: The Pollution in Newborns" by the Environmental Working Group[11] (see Appendix 13, page 499) explains why this is so important for children with developing brains and immune systems. The following is a list of products to use instead of toxin filled, name brand cleaning products.

Floor cleaner: Add one cup of white vinegar and baking soda to a bucket of water (add a squirt of liquid soap if you like).

Air Freshener: To remove odors from carpets spread on baking soda and then vacuum the carpet. Simmer cloves and cinnamon as air freshener.

Removing Toilet odors: Borax

Trashcans: Spread baking soda in the bottom, then spray to disinfect with a solution of borax and water.

Dish soap: I use liquid dishwashing soap and white vinegar to cut grease. If you buy dish soap make sure it's biodegradable.

Disinfectants: Borax with water is an excellent disinfectant, or spray CD.

Laundry detergent: Soak the clothes for an hour in borax soap before putting into the washer.

Oven Cleaner: Dissolve two teaspoons of liquid soap (not detergent) and two teaspoons of borax with enough warm water to fill a spray bottle.

Windows and Mirrors: Club soda in a spray bottle

Toilets and Tubs: Baking soda with apple cider vinegar

96% Alcohol: Kills parasites on enema catheters, etc., and is great for cleaning bathrooms.

Videos

I have had many parents ask me if I think it is a good idea that their child watch "Genius Baby" or other videos that are supposed to help with their development. I do not believe these videos to be appropriate for a developing brain. Studies were done in Cuba that found that excessive TV watching before three years of age can cause the symptoms of autism. When the TV was removed from the children that presented symptoms of autism, the symptoms disappeared. They also reported that TV watching could cause neurological discharges in the brain.

I can also tell you that the only time my son stims or flaps is when he is allowed to watch TV. When he was younger, and deep in the throes of autism, the only thing he wanted to do was watch TV, while running back and forth and squealing. Any other activity was met with screaming and tantrums. He is much more interested in other activities now, and easily transitions from one to the next, including school. However, he still requests to watch YouTube in the evenings when all of his activities are complete, and that is truly the only time he flaps his hands anymore. To me it is very obvious that TV is a source of over stimulation for him. However, it is hard to deny him a truly preferred activity, especially when he enjoys videos on cooking and foreign language! The least amount of screen time (TV, computer, iPad, etc.) the better, however, we do what we can.

Therapy Options:

ABA is not the only therapy for children with autism.

Many parents worry because ABA/IBI is either not available, or not affordable to them. I firmly believe that something is better than nothing. At the same time, I have seen many children recover without any ABA or IBI. Here are some of the options that have worked for families in conjunction with the protocol:

- ABA - Applied Behavior Analysis
- Occupational Therapy
- DIR® Developmental - Individual Difference, Relationship-based Model
- Floortime Therapy
- TEACCH - Treatment and Education of Autistic and Related Communication Handicapped Children
- Son-Rise®
- PROMPT - Prompts for Restructuring Oral Muscular Phonetic Targets
- Sensory Integration Therapy
- RPM - Rapid Prompting Method
- Supportive Typing

There are many other options not mentioned here. Human interaction is key for our children on the spectrum to find joy with us in our world.

I have known many families to have varying degrees of success with all of the above therapies. Some are better for younger children and some for older children. Depending on the areas most lacking in your child's development, you can investigate any one of these types of therapies. Families in many countries where insurance doesn't cover any type of therapy have had to be trained themselves in how to apply therapy. Sometimes an aunt, sister, cousin, or neighbor steps up to help out. No ONE therapy has been fundamental to all of the recovered children and for that reason I say something is better than nothing when it comes to therapy.

Even household chores can be therapeutic and task oriented. Simply because a person has autism doesn't mean they can't have responsibilities and learn new skills while helping out in the home.

A word on laboratory testing

I can't stand to watch people waste money that they could be using for healing their children through various interventions on laboratory testing. If you have all the money in the world, and want to chart your child's progress through laboratory testing, so be it. However, the rest of us sometimes have to choose between expensive testing and treatment. So many families have come to me after spending thousands of dollars they didn't have on testing to tell me their child has viruses, bacteria, and candida. Am I surprised? Never. I have yet to see a child with regressive autism that does not have pathogens/parasites. No matter which pathogens are present, we use CD.

Testing for parasites is woefully lacking at this time, and in fact, the only practitioners who have consistently diagnosed parasites have been veterinarians and practitioners of alternative medicine (also Metametrix labs have identified parasites in some cases).

Generally speaking, if a child doesn't have viruses, bacteria, yeast, parasites, heavy metals and allergies they don't have autism.

Stay Up-To-Date
Subscribe to our Newsletter!

Just go to www.cdautism.org and enter your name and email address...

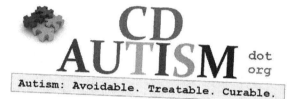

Chapter 15

<u>Final Thoughts</u>

*If you knew how powerful your thoughts were
you would never think a negative thought again.*

~ Peace Pilgrim

What would be your message to families of children with autism who have just read the book, but not started the protocol?

Do not wait! Get started now! Autism is <u>Avoidable, Treatable and Curable!</u> You don't have to spend fortunes on lab testing, imported foods nor supplements. Even if the medical community can't decide if your child has autism, PDD-NOS, ADHD, Asperger's, PANDAS, etc.... don't wait! Start the diet. Even if you cannot do more than that, it will help. Some children have lost their diagnosis with just diet. There are parents all over the world doing biomedical protocols for autism, get together with them, join the forum at...

www.cdautism.org

...or the CDAutism Facebook group. The Internet helps us all to be close and share information. Don't let anyone tell you the diet doesn't work, just keep going and don't stop. There is never an excuse to not do what is right for your child. "Their future depends on our courage."

The final chapter of this book is yet to be written. Until the day we have recovered every victim of regressive autism, there is no success. Just progress. Here I have expressed what I have seen and what the road of autism recovery has brought to me. I have learned a lot and continue to learn. Our children need us to keep learning and searching until we find what unlocks them from their autism. Not everything works for everyone. However, I have seen that this protocol works for most. Especially when it is done exactly as it should be. If you have found this book you have an advantage that I did not have with my son. When I first learned of Patrick's diagnosis I lost precious time and money that I didn't have to lose, trying interventions that didn't yield results. In the nine years that my son has been in recovery I have yet to come across another protocol that has helped as many children to recover from autism in such a short amount of time—less than three years, to be exact! As of the date of this writing in May of 2013, 93 children have lost the diagnosis of autism and every month more and more are recovering.

Please remember that if your journey is autism you will never walk alone. I am here too. Just one click away...

www.cdautism.org

I wish everyone who is ill to have the fastest recovery possible from whatever it is that ails them.

To be continued...

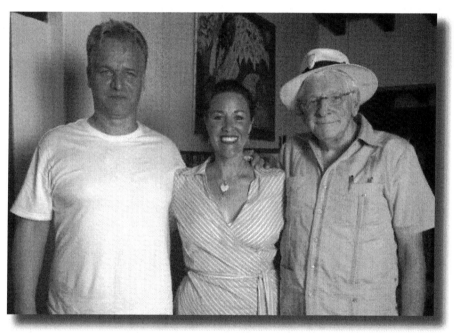

Dr. Andreas Kalcker, Kerri Rivera, Jim Humble,
in Puerto Vallarta, Mexico 2012.

Chapter 16

Healing Beyond Autism...

When TRUTH is found, understood and accepted is when we realize it
was not even close to what we thought it would be...
~ Miriam Delicado

As Jim Humble has been proving for many years, chlorine dioxide is a molecule capable of healing many common ailments. When combined with the other elements of this protocol, in the correct order, it has shown to be even more effective. We have decided to include this bonus chapter because it is time to start sharing this information with everyone, as pathogens and parasites are the root cause of many of the diseases that are causing suffering in our world today.

As parents saw improvements in their children's health from the protocol, some of them decided to use it on themselves as well. Similarly to when the flight attendant tells you to put on your own oxygen mask first before helping others, it is important to take care of yourself if you want to be able to help your children heal, grow, learn and mature.

Over time, parents who followed in their children's footsteps started to have some undeniable gains in their own health. This was an added bonus many didn't expect, and we couldn't resist sharing their stories with you.

After reading the parasite chapter, you may have been surprised to see how many common symptoms can be caused by parasitic infections. Imagine what would happen if we could get this information into the hands of people who have seen many doctors, used various drugs, and applied countless protocols for years while only masking the symptoms of the underlying cause. So, there should be no surprise if going after the real cause was life changing in real ways.

The following testimonials are a small sample of how some of these people's lives have been changed. Serious afflictions such as Lyme disease, fibromyalgia, chronic fatigue syndrome (CFS), depression, cancer, and chronic infections, are just some of the conditions that improved or completely cleared up. By cleaning up toxic pathogens and parasites, as well as removing foods that feed these invaders, it should be no surprise that disease triggering inflammation is reduced so true healing can take place.

I am so excited for you to read these, and I know that some of you will recognize yourselves here. Please know that healing is possible! We have a public Facebook group called *CD Health* where adults using the protocol for themselves can share questions, doubts and success stories. I highly recommend that you check it out if you are looking for support or some guidance getting started.

Testimonials Beyond Autism

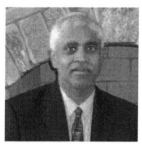

After we saw our son recover from ASD using CD, I tried CD myself and it helped me recover from Lyme and its co-infections. Some of our extended family heard about our success and they have had very good results using CD for treating Hypertension, Diabetes and Liver problems. My younger NT son used to bang his head in sleep since he was born, CD has now resolved the problem. I think anyone who tries CD sincerely, can only benefit in treating so many hard problems. One very beneficial side effect I have seen with CD is the resolution to seasonal allergies and improvement in the immune system to the point where kids do not fall sick or catch colds. In this regard CD is much better than yearly flu shots which have so many toxic elements in them and still do not protect adequately.

—Nilesh

To say I was anxious about the impending birth of Baby #2 is an understatement. I felt like I had failed our first born on so many levels and was a mess believing that I'd do the same for our new daughter.

But alas, she was born a perfect and healthy baby girl. So was Callum, our son, but unlike Lila who had zero interventions, Callum had antibiotics from my labor, the Vitamin K shot, HiB, and DTaP. And it was the DTaP vaccine at 15 months that took the shine from our sweet boy's eyes.

We discovered Kerri's protocol when Lila was 3 months old and more worries cropped up about how to best protect her from the die off that was going on in our house.

At 5-months, she developed an eczema patch underneath her chin, became chronically constipated, and her normally cheerful disposition became irritable.

As soon as she hit the 20-lb mark, I started giving her 20 drop CD baths, low dose oral CD, and 3 drop CD/150 mL water enemas. To my horror and surprise, Lila started passing 1" baby roundworms almost daily.

In a family with both NT and ASD children, the NT child always has some type of quirky behavior. Now we know why! Parasites do not only affect the ASD population, they affect everyone. Having CD in my tool chest gives me the power to prevent so many things that may have been in my daughter's future.

Don't be afraid to treat your babies! Her eczema is gone and she's pooping regularly once more.

I write and share my story in that it might help or save someone else's life. That it may just be the key to help someone see what may be what is happening for them as it was and is happening to me. If it helps just one person onto their path to recovery and health then it will have been worth sitting down at this computer and sharing it.

For the past 10 years or so my world has been collapsing in on me, and getting smaller and smaller, and accelerating the past 5 years. I have felt as if I were under a thick coffee mug on the edge of a table about to fall off. On a scale of 0 to 20 with 0 being death and 20 being fully alive and cognizant, I felt as thought I was at 3 staring at 0. For the past 5 years at least I have done so much research, listened to so many radio interviews, done so many different modalities, bought so many products, paid a lot of money to different therapists, ate weeds, made my own concoctions, etc. My mother would always say to me wow you should be so healthy to which I would reply no mum, actually I am not. I began feeling like a phony. I ate real good took all the right stuff, got plenty of rest foraged for my own food and spring water, got exercise, walked barefoot, etc, but always felt exhausted and looked worse and worse. I was fighting with everyone it seemed and chasing people away including family.

Four months ago my wife decided we should go away on a weekend getaway and relax. We fought the whole drive up there and when we got there she threw me my room key and said you're on your own. I spent the whole weekend in bed and on the trip home we both decided to end our 20 year relationship and marriage. I was good with that and looking forward to being on my own. I was finally chasing the last person who mattered to me away.

A week later an angel came into my life. I have been listening to oneradionetwork.com for the last 5 years and on this day Patrick Timpone had a lady by the name of Kerri Rivera on and she spoke about how she was curing kids with autism and that the kids had parasites. I looked up the symptoms of autism and realized I had quite a few of them. I immediately began the mms enema protocol which she recommends. I could not believe what then came out of me. I kept this up for a week and still there was no let up with the amount of parasites, biofilm, and who knows what coming out of me. After a week of this and seeing no let up on what was coming out of me, and having just done an mms enema I laid on my bedroom floor and the grief just poured out of me. My wife came in and lay down next to me and just held me. I knew then that something had changed, that my life and my marriage were now on a healing path. That the pain, the toxins and parasites were now leaving my body.

It has now been just over 3 months and there has been no let up on what has been coming out of me. If I were to have scooped it all up and put it in a jar I am sure it would fill a one gallon jar with hardly any water in it. I now feel I am at about a 9 with 20 in my sights. I thank God that this info came into my life and I took action on it. It has saved my life and my marriage. I love my wife, and cannot imagine not having her with me. And I love my life and am looking forward to not only getting to the 20 mark but what is beyond the 20. What is possible when one's brain is at full capacity and not being inaundadated with toxins? Much love and appreciation goes out to Patrick Timpone at oneradionetwork.com, Kerri Rivera and her work with autistic kids (adults too Kerri), and to Andreas Kalcker. Thank you all for showing me and pointing to the keys I needed to free myself from what has been a nightmare.

A big part of my healing has been reviewing my life and realizing that this has been going on for most of it and answers so many questions I have had. As a child growing up I had pain in my stomach and what the doctors eventually did was take out my appendix, which most of us know now is needed to keep the healthy flora in our intestines. And they told my parents that it was all in my head. So whenever I complained about stomach aches and pains was told that it was all in my head. School was a nightmare for me, as socially I felt I didn't fit in or belong, and a lot of easy concepts that most others got, I just couldn't get. I always had the feeling like I was missing something. I felt as though I was stupid or something just wasn't right with me. I now know there are many just like me. The words Autism, add, adhd, ocd, etc were not a reality back then. And I know those are just words or diagnosis of toxins and parasites. Get rid of the toxins and parasites and the diagnosis goes away. Easy peasy. Thank you all for listening to this chapter of my story. I look forward to many more chapters in my life story. Please feel free to pass this along to anyone who it may help. Much love.

—Bruce

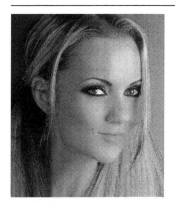

When starting the protocol for my son's Autism, I decided to do it along with him.
I was suffering from Hypothyroidism, Adrenal Fatigue, a Hormonal Imbalance, and Severe Anemia. My cortisol was at a 3. One week into the protocol, my cortisol was at a 14, and my iron levels were normal without supplements. My thyroid medication dosage was decreased twice. My vitamin levels were all normal. My uterine fibroid cysts were completely gone after a few months on the protocol. I continue to see improvement in my health. This protocol has been a Godsend for my family.

—Maggie Kaye

CD has been life changing for my 18 year old son who has autism and Lyme, although his ATEC today is only a 3, down from a 68 at the start of cd, but I never thought it would be so instrumental in my dad's life also.

My dad, William, has a malignant melanoma in his eye and has received radiation for treatment for the last few years. I talk about cd all the time but they never took this treatment seriously, at least for anything besides autism until now. My dad gets terrible ear infections that he sometimes has to go to the hospital for. They tell him each time that he has "swimmers ear" and they give him abx, sometimes it seems to work, sometimes not, and he goes back to the drs or hospital for more abx....over and over. Recently he was leaving here for his 7-hour trip home, and he was very worried that he would not make it home with the painful infection that had begun, and he would have to stop on the way and visit a strange hospital. So I mixed up some cd, and told him to drop a few drops of the cd mixture in his ear periodically on his way home. To his surprise, the infection cleared up by the time he got home and there was no need to even call a doctor.

Of course, my secret plan is to get him on the cd protocol to finally deal with the tumor in his eye and that's the plan we have started. Whether he uses it and shrinks the tumor and saves his life with cd or not, he's a true believer now that cd cures infection.

I have been taking CD and the parasite protocol for 5 mo., and here are my observations. I have had long-term chronic sinus issues which has caused sever sleep problems. Also, a few months ago, I had a severe toothache in the upper left area. The dentist examined and found no fault with the tooth, even though there was severe swelling in the area. The infection originated from my sinus, and by taking my CD regularly hourly, was quickly solved. (My hourly CD doses were compromised by travel) I have also noticed improvement in my sinus condition, resulting in better sleep, although I have not fully recovered yet. Right now my sleep is somewhat interrupted by peetox. I will continue CD and PP for the 18 mo. Previously; I had used several naturopaths, with either negative results or limited results that disappeared when the medications were discontinued. So far I am happy with CD and would recommend it to people to try.

—Ed Canada.

A friend started eardrops with her 13-year-old pug 3 weeks ago. The pug Lucy was almost deaf from ear infection after ear infection, on constant drops, had seizures. After 3 weeks on CD eardrops, went to the vet, no ear infection, hearing is improving!! Winning!!

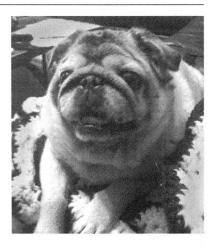

Since I was a child, I had been anemic and reading the book "Healing the symptoms known as autism" on the Parasite chapter, I saw that anemia is a sign of parasite infection. Since my son is taking CD I also took CD to know how my son feels and maybe cure my anemia. I had no problem going up to 24 drops in less than 2 weeks. I stopped taking my iron pill after 1 month of taking CD. I also did parasite protocol as I do not want to reinfection my son. Since, I stopped taking my iron pill I never had any dizzy spells and I feel great.

I used to wake up at night too to use the bathroom, now with CD no more night waking. In 2009, I was informed by my Doctor that I need to go and see a specialist as there was some suspicious stuff in my Pap Test and if not removed it can lead to cervical cancer. I was booked in the hospital for the procedure. After taking CD reaching full dose, I had been discharging this horrible smell, like rotten egg, whenever I urinate. It took about a month before it stopped. Whatever that was, CD cleansed me and I think that discharge is related to my diagnosis on the pap test result. I am very grateful for CD for giving me my health back. I am still continuing taking CD as I want to be healthy and I will also try to complete the Parasite protocol for 12 months, I just finished my 5th PP and have been seeing lots of parasites mainly pinworm and ascaris. Now, I know the root cause of my anemia especially. I would encourage people to try the Protocol and see where the healing leads you. Thanks to Kerri Rivera, Jim Humble, Andreas Kalcker and people who used the CD before me as you gave me courage to use the CD.

—G.M, Canada.

Two days before our first set of cd bottles arrived (we bought it to start Kerri's protocol with our autistic daughter), our son (6) got sick with scarlet fever. We didn't give him antibiotics because we just finished our research on cd and were excited to use it instead. My sons face was swollen and red, he had a moderate fever and rash all over his body. After the first dose of 1 activated drop of cd within one hour his swollen red face subsided completely and in the evening the fever was gone. His rash got dry and after 3-4 days it was not visible anymore. Our physician told us that scarlet fever without antibiotics lasts up to three weeks. We were done within 4 days, without damaging his gut flora, as it would have using antibiotics. CD has taken care of many infections in our family since then and most important - brought our daughters ATEC down from 100 to 46 in nine months. I'm beyond grateful for its discovery.

For the past six years, my life has been plagued with anxiety/fear, depression, pressure in my chest, making it difficult to lay flat and sleep, bloating which caused me to look 7 months pregnant and which made my abdomen very tight and uncomfortable. Headaches, weight gain, sore joints, no energy, fibromyalgia pain, and dizziness causing me to feel drugged and off balance.

The anxiety and fear were debilitating literally making it impossible for me to sleep. I would go night after night not sleeping, just dead on my feet suffering with so much anxiety and very frightened wondering what in the world was wrong with me.

When Kerri's book, Healing The Symptoms Known As Autism came into our lives, I read it wanting to help or autistic son. I soon realized I had so many of the symptoms that I needed to do the protocol.

I started on the cd taking a very small amount, 2 drops every hour, about 12 doses per day, and worked up to between 60 and 90 drops a day, I also took cd baths and did enemas. I increased the cd every day by just a drop or two. Very soon I started to calm down significantly. I started sleeping! I started losing weight! For about 5 weeks I thought I had died and gone to heaven. In two months I lost 20 lbs.

But when my anxiety started coming back I set up a consultation with Kerri. I learned I needed to begin the parasite protocol to kill the parasites. The cd just killed the little ones.

With Kerri's help in several consultations I was able to tweak the protocol in her book and apply it to me for my personal needs. I started on low doses and increased it for what I needed to sleep.

As of today I have only been taking Mebendazole, the medication that kills parasites, for 3 and a half weeks. I sleep at night. Some nights are a little choppy but I get 4-5 hours of sleep. I am not depressed. My emotions are not all over the place. I am coping. I'm functioning without sever headaches, only mild ones. I still have bloating but not as severe. I feel like I will live and that I am not dying anymore. I hardly ever feel depressed.

To date I take 200mg Mebendazole at breakfast, lunch, dinner and bedtime, plus a 200mg implant right before I get into bed. The implant has been the turning point in my healing. (Consult with Kerri for directions regarding the implant.) I also take 2 neem tea capsules with each meal. Also, one dose of Combantrin everyday at lunch. I take castor oil as needed each day 1-2 Tablespoons to keep things moving, plus a cd bath at bedtime, 150 drops soaking for 20 minutes.

Trying to differentiate what is die-off and what are actual symptoms from the parasites is challenging. Pay close attention to how you feel after you do or take something. After an hour note how you feel. Worse, better? You have to listen to your body. Consult with Kerri often and keep her informed by email. You may have to tweak the protocol every few days so write everything down, day, time, how much, how you feel etc.

All of my symptoms are not gone 100% but they have greatly improved. The anxiety, which was the worst and most debilitating symptom, is the greatest improvement I have had. I know I will be able to heal completely and get my life back. I have just begun!! I have had so much progress in just a few short weeks that I still cannot believe it!! And...I have lost 2 more pounds!!

Thank you Kerri for all of your love, support and guidance!! I could not have attempted this without your knowledge and help!! You are an angel!!!! I AM HEALING!!!!!!

Your devoted friend, Marcie

My mother 84 yrs of age- who has dementia was very, very serious last week. Her lungs were filled with mucous and she could not spit it out. We thought this was the end and my sister invited the priest to bless her. The doctors suggested that I place her in a hospice, but I refused! They also offered antibiotics, but I bought some CDS and gave it to her every hour. I placed a humidifier with 40 drops of activated CD by her bedside day and night. And massaged different parts of her body with CD and DMSO. soaked her feet just once in CD as it is difficult. She cant sit straight. To everyone's surprise she made it through. Just a little bit more to clear up! Thank you everyone for sharing wonderful tips on loving and caring for our loved ones! This is a wonderful extended family! love the CD!!!!!!!!!!

I want to thank all of those who were kind enough to share their personal stories with us. There are many more, but you get the idea. I am so excited for you to read them, and I know that some of you will recognize yourselves here. It just goes to show that healing challenging illnesses is possible. We have a public Facebook group called *CD Health* where adults using the protocol for themselves can share questions, doubts and success stories. I highly recommend that you check it out if you are looking for support or some guidance getting started.

Appendix 1

<u>More Miracles & Testimonials...</u>

The only limits you have are the limits you believe.
*~ **Wayne Dyer***

To date, 115 children have lost their diagnosis of autism by using CD and some or all of this Protocol. Autism IS curable!

This section is comprised of testimonials, miracles, and short blurbs on gains made by children using The Protocol. In many cases, these are candid emails from parents to Kerri sharing their joy at their child healing. These were gathered over the past 3 years, and have come from families all over the world. Some were translated by the parents of the child to English, and some were translated by my sister or I. We have done our best to honor these exactly how they came to us, unless a correction was needed for clarification, these were not edited. Many are anonymous for the protection of the families and their children. Names were used when permission was given. These families were generous enough to share their experiences with all of us to spread hope and joy, as well as to prove that children all over the world of all ages are healing from the symptoms know as autism. Please enjoy and share.

Please note that many of these testimonials were collected some time ago and therefore some contributors use the term MMS instead of CD. Due to time constraints it was impossible to request permission to change the acronym of MMS to CD in their testimonials. As we mentioned previously, MMS and CD are the same substance. Where the acronym MMS is used in the following testimonials please know that chlorine dioxide is the substance responsible for the healing.

We have added many new testimonials since the first edition came out. Those new testimonials are located at the end of chapter 2 and continue on the next page, followed by those appearing in the first edition.

(continued from Chapter 2, page 40)

45. *Things I wish I'd known before starting this protocol:*
* *My son would drop juice and pick up a water regimen immediately.*
* *My son would sleep through the night every night.*
* *My son would not be constipated again.*
* *My sons ATEC score would be halved in 7 weeks.*
* *My son's speech would be at age level.*
* *My son wouldn't need his daily rx med again.*
* *My son would be excited about and participate in his birthday celebration.*
* *My son would come into the bathroom and say, "I'm ready to wash my butt" unprompted.*
* *My son would drink ocean water.*
* *My son would get acclimated to school and would initiate conversation with his peers.*
* *My son's dark circles under his eyes would disappear. He would start to look and act like a healthy boy, and others would take notice.*
* *My son would be affectionate, tell me he loves me, crack jokes, and be connected to me like never before.*
* *The people who opposed our diet and protocol choices would be unable to deny that this works and we're on the right track.*
* *My marriage would be saved by rolling our sleeves up and tackling this together.*
* *I would find a way to heal my own ailments.*

The future is bright

46. *My son with autism is 31 years old. Although he is fully verbal, he had a lot of issues: SIB, Aggression, he was not able to sleep. We have been trying different kinds of protocols since he was 3 years old. Unsuccessfully. I heard about Kerri Rivera and the CD Protocol last September. We started right away. We were continuously in touch with Kerri who kept giving us the faith, that even at that old age it is possible to heal and even recover. In September, when we stared CD he had an ATEC of 87, 4 months later we measured 63, and now, after 8 mounts, he has an ATEC of 28. There are some SIB's and aggression left, but it happens only rarely. If we could get rid of it, my son would be recovered. He became an interested young man, his memory improved. He keeps giving proper answers to my questions, something he never did before. I can see his real personality now: he became a nice, lovable, open-minded young man from a very sick raging, roaring, screaming, suffering boy. There are no words to say thank you to Kerri to show us the end of the tunnel. I think I'm on the best way to recover my 31-year-old son!*

Mark, 31, Hungary

47. *Dear Kerri, I am very grateful to you for your benevolent service of helping to recover kids with Autism like myself. You have really improved the quality of lives of many hopeless kids. I really feel the difference now that my ATEC score is a*

I and I am still making inroads in executive functioning and social skills. Without someone like you, we would have not known about CD and it would have taken several years to cure me solely with chelation. By that time, I would have been out of high school and probably in a community college taking rudimentary general education courses and would have had a bleak future ahead of me. But now, I am doing well in school and am taking college level courses. And I am not the only one in my family that has had benefitted from using CD. My brother used to have mild seizures in the form of head banging and most of that has now stopped. My father has used it because he contracted Lyme's disease twice. And my grandparents have used it to treat Alzheimer's, Diabetes, Blood pressure and Hepatitis C. So again, I cannot thank you enough for everything you have done that has not only changed my life forever but has made a profound difference in the lives of others afflicted with Autism.

48. My seventeen-year-old son was a healthy happy baby until he received vaccinations at age three. The day after the vaccinations he began having horrible anxiety problems. Day by day he lost skills and regressed. He developed problems with fine and gross motor skills, and social skills, memory and sensory integration. He also had multiple learning disorders and struggled in school. He spent all of his time in his room by himself and he did not make eye contact.

We tried many interventions to try and help him. Biomedical interventions, antibiotics, therapies homeopathy and Biofeedback all had limited benefits for my son. The only thing that helped him some was a gluten free, casein free, sugar free diet. While reading Healing the Symptoms Known as Autism we learned that most of the interventions we tried did not work because we were feeding the parasites that were causing my son's autism with vitamins and supplements.

While I was watching videos about Chlorine Dioxide I came across a video of Kerri Rivera talking about the protocol she uses with autistic children. As I watched the video everything began to make sense and I knew the protocol would help my son.

We bought Kerri's book Healing the Symptoms Known as Autism, gathered the supplies and my whole family started the protocol. To our amazement we saw improvements in my son overnight. We had taken the ATEC test for my son right before we started the protocol and it was a 43. In just one month of Kerri's protocol my son's ATEC dropped to a 5! We will continue with the protocol for the recommended time and we expect to see my son's ATEC drop to zero before we finish.

His social skills, motor skills, thinking, behavior, attention span and stimming have all improved immensely. His sleep patterns, digestion, physical appearance and weight have also improved tremendously.

Kerri Rivera's book gave us the tools we needed to reach in and pull my son away from the grip that autism had on him. We will forever be grateful to Kerri. She devotes her life to helping children with autism and always has an open line of communication for anyone who needs help. She is the voice for so many children that don't have a voice. Thank you from the bottom of my heart!

49. FUA!!!! BIG moment... crazy morning, ughhh we miss the Bus I was so mad because my other daughter had preschool at 9:30 so my morning was a mess, I had to leave in Pj's and make them eat breakfast in the car....but then in our way to school my son saw a School Bus passing by our side and said "school Bus is gone, L is sad" OMG OMG OMG......did he just said this 30 words sentence?????

(actually 7 words but seems like 30 to me!!!) Ok...WAIT then I get to school not mad anymore, I walked with him still in shock, I couldn't believe what I just heard....and when he saw the line of kids by the wall he point at them and said "my friends" OMG OMG OMG....ok WAIT....then we get there and he takes the teacher hands, gives me a kiss and said "bye mommy" OMG OMG OMG .... WAIT then the teacher ask him L, remember back pack by the wall, so he goes to the wall with his back pack in his back and does exactly what he was ask to do!!!! O M G

FUA...THAT'S RIGHT.... 223 days in this Protocol, searching poop, dosing, enemas, writing in his food diary every little thing he eats, therapies ABA, speech, occupational, hours hours of work, hard work...all just to witness this miracle of healing...to see him think, react, analyze a situation, be happy, spontaneous and smart by himself (no prompt or reinforcer necessary).... THANK YOU Kerri Rivera since the first day I found you in YouTube I have never stopped believing....I LOVE YOU WITH ALL MY HEART!!!! YES COMADREEEEE!!!!! I can feel it...we are close...it's happening.... so happy I missed the Bus this morning... this is the best day in my son's way to recovery so far!!!!!

HOPE FOR ALL!!!!

---

50. My son is 23 and we have tried many, many approaches to heal him over the years. Typically we would see some initial progress, but then the rate would slow down and he would plateau again, slipping further and further behind. Lyme disease and co-infections, as well as various viral, fungal and metabolic issues complicated everything. We had to resort to psych meds, even, for his depression, anxiety and mood disregulation.

We started Kerri's protocol in the summer of 2012, and had to cut the number of drops again and again to something he could tolerate, since he has MTHFR genetic issues with detoxing, until he was at 1/64th of a drop per dose. By October 2012, he was at full dose and after two weeks, began to talk about learning to drive, to offer to do a chore at home, to draw again. So it has been about a year for us, and the improvements are continuing, his ATEC score went from 77 pre-meds to 11 now, and our lives are all much better thanks to this book and Kerri's dedication to the cause of healing the children. Please, if you are reading this, don't be afraid to try one more thing!

---

51. My son started Kerri's protocol 10 months ago. At the time we started the protocol he was doing a home based therapy program for 60 hours a week. We did not send him to school because he was not able to handle all of the outside stimulus, unable to follow directions, and unable to communicate effectively. He stimmed most of his day and only spoke in 2-3 word sentences to get needs met only. When he started the protocol his ATEC was 57. It quickly dropped and the improvements were mind blowing. In 5 months time his ATEC was a 9. Today at 10 months after starting the protocol his ATEC is a FIVE!!!! He now attends school with out any kind of extra support and exceptions made for him. He is truly just one of the other children. I have been volunteering in his school and I have had 5 different office people tell me that he stops and greets them on his way to different specials (p.e, library, art, gardening). They told me he initiates the greetings and says: hello, good morning, buenas noches, and all with a big smile on his face. I have even been told by 2 of them that he greets them by name. Did I mention that he leaves the classroom on his own to go to specials??? Yep, my one time *severely autistic* child finds his name and places it in that specials category

basket, leaves the classroom and goes to specials on his own???? When he is done with specials he goes back to his classroom and does his work. Holy CRaP!!!! A dream come true.

Thank You Kerri!!

---

52.   My 6 year old son's ATEC went from 45 to 22!!! Wow I knew he was doing better but more then half!!

Thanks Kerri Rivera!!

---

53.   I don't know what to chalk it up to--we just finished our 3rd PP and did our 2nd shot of GcMAF on Saturday--but my 9 y/o son has started taking pictures with my iPhone. They are not just random shots; he is finding objects or angles and taking pictures. They are FASCINATING! He has also figured out how to use the reverse feature, and has taken a series of self-portraits, which he flips through and says to himself "Who's that?"

---

54.   My 16-year-old son is doing great on your CD protocol. ATEC down from 89 to 37. Best thing that ever happened after doing 8 years biomed with him.

---

55.   We started CD with my precious 5 year old 'O-ster' in June 2013. Some of the completely new developments we have seen since we started....... He is aware of how to burp and toot, and thinks it is funny. He is apologizing for things he does wrong. Even a day later, he will remember and apologize. He goes to the bathroom on his own. He is completely pottytrained, even at night. He does household chores happily. He sent people on my contact list emails that said 'I love my mommy.' He has better problem-solving, more motivation to draw pictures. If he gets messy, he just goes to the bathroom and washes his hands and wipes off his shirt by himself without saying anything. He dresses himself. He does somersaults (just a few months ago, it was impossible for him to even get in somersault position), can open baby gates, can get in crab walk position, can jump off of furniture with both feet. He greets us when we come home and is excited to see us. He MISSES us when we are gone and talks about it during the day. He's making up 4 line rhymes. He cares what he wears and picks out his clothes! He is not running back and forth as much. We have normal trips to restaurants. I can leave our front door open now, and not worry that he will run away. He tries to help put our dog in his crate and fetches with him. He wants to come with me if I leave the house to go somewhere. He will now eat almost anything I put on his plate. He used to vomit at the mere thought of things like GF pasta or rice, and he wouldn't allow any food on his plate to touch another type of food on his plate. He will now eat bowls full of tomato sauce, onions, burger, rice, garlic and peppers all mixed together. Our family can eat dinner together now. I no longer have to make separate meals. He even eats raw peppers! He yells 'watch me!' and does things like diving onto the bed or jumping off of something. He looks at cloud formations to see what pictures he sees in them. Last week he heard a toddler crying in Target. He wondered why the child was crying and wanted to go find her. He misses his little sister when she is not at home. He wants her to play with us when we are playing. He is completely aware of what is going on now. He is much more aware of danger. He notices the weather. There is a sense of calmness about him that he did not have before. His tantrums are much less severe and much less frequent. I was supposed to be his aide this year in preschool, but I have been able to just drop him off at school. There are many more new things that he is saying and thinking and doing.

Our quick biomed history- He regressed after vaccines at 12 months. Starting at 18 months of age, he was gfcfsf for 1 year, then scd for almost 3 years. It feels like we have tried everything with supplements over the last 4 years. Some things helped a little, but nothing really tackled his pathogen load, even though he was on an awesome diet. His ATEC was 66 in Dec 2010. Low dose chelation brought it down to 33 in 3 months. The ATEC stayed at 33 for 2.5 years. We did 112 rounds/weekends of low dose chelation during that time. ATEC June 2013 was 34 (before starting CD), July 2013 was 30, October 2013 was 20! We are on our way down. This is the first time that I have physical proof that we are getting rid of the pathogens that have controlled and poisoned his body and brain for most of his life. It feels so good to finally help him. I am hoping to write our complete recovery story in Kerri's next book. I thank God that we saw Kerri at AutismOne.

---

56. *Nick texted me yesterday for the first time, on his own. "Hi from Nick" - that's a 2013 FUA fo sho. – Alison*

    (this text was accompanied by an ATEC drop from 69 at 6 years old to 14 at 8.5 years)

---

57. *Yesterday my son told me I worried too much, I said you worry too much Too Noah! He responded, my hair is red, yours is gray, so who is the worrier, hahaaa! The windshield wipers keep wiping away the autism, what's staying around it seems, is completely lucid speech and unbelievable comebacks! He never could say things like that before, not at all, he really was in there somewhere.*

---

58. *Something really beautiful is going on in our household right now...Caleb is totally blossoming socially on every level. There is a calmness in his body. He is alert, responding to his name, sharing his toys with other kids, wanting to give affection without prompting, soothing Lilia when she is crying rather than batting at her. We even have gotten a few spontaneous silly phrases!!!! Oh baby, oh baby, oh baby!!! We are on our way!!!!!*

---

59. *We started the diet on the 1th of March, CD on the following week. Adam started to ask questions in April. Since then he keeps asking continuously...His ATEC dropped down from 49 to 38.*

    Tunde, Hungary

---

60. *OMG OMG OMG!!!!! My son is singing!!! He was ZERO verbal... I mean ZERO!! His shadow teacher told me a week ago that he started to mimic, I said to myself "yeah he was babbling and she thought he is mimicking!..." Yesterday she told me he started to sing and I said to myself, "Yeah right, she is absolutely illusionist or exaggerating!!!" She knew I will not believe her because he is just humming at home! So she sent me a video which was a shock for us. He is singing the song "A is for apple, a a apple... B is for ball, b b ball... C is for cat, c c cat... D is for dog, d d dog..." I don't have enough words to thank you and thank Kerri Rivera and this incredible protocol!!! Thank you for saving my child. xoxo*

---

61. *...My son is doing his first CD PP. We picked him up from preschool he was extremely happy. Hugs & kisses. Then...runs up to a classmate and touches his shoulder and says, "bye Johnny", runs to another classmate and says, "bye Kevin." Then he skips to the car. These improvements in his socialization is new. We are so pleased and I wanted to pass along these social gains with you all. His atec at start is 58.*

62. My little sweetpea is almost 4...and completely NON VERBAL...upon picking her up from therapy today, her teacher said she was having a great last few days... and both therapists said her eye-contact has been different...like in a really good way!!! I've also noticed her looking at me...straight into my eyes for what seems like forever...almost as if she has never seen me before?! They also said that she has been looking at them and has been opening her mouth trying to make sounds...as if she wants to say something very badly...but can't...but with a lot of prompting...she did say "Hi!"...all I know is that somewhere in there is this amazing person waiting to be let out! I often worry if we are ever gonna make it...finances and healing your family can be very overwhelming...especially on one income. But for the love of my daughter we just cannot give up...feeling very hopeful and blessed today...and very grateful that something is finally working.

63. Hi Kerri,

   I wanted to write and thank you for discovering and sharing your protocol. This protocol has saved my almost 5-year-old son.

   My son suddenly started having absence seizures that would freeze his breath. From the day he had his first noticeable seizure, he was hospitalized every seven weeks for uncontrollable status epilepticas, a life threatening condition. They would pump him with seizure meds, Ativan, and Valium for hours before the seizures would finally stop.

   Since starting CD five months ago my son has not been hospitalized once. He went ten weeks seizure free. He had a few mild seizures that he brought himself out of without any extra medications. He currently broke this record and has made it another thirteen and a half weeks seizure free. I true miracle.

   Everything we searched for to treat his Lyme disease in the past would either cause seizures or not help to prevent them and I now know why. As you predicted after starting your protocols we discovered that he not only has Lyme, he is also incredibly loaded with parasites. So much so, that it scares me to think of what may have happened to him if we didn't find you.

   I'm so amazed to watch him subtly emerge. Since we started, he went from saying about 20 words to saying 69 words, along with two and three word combinations, and over the past month he has begun to answer simple questions. His vestibular system has gotten much better; he'll actually swing. He just started jumping off curbs. His eye contact is perfect. He's gained two pounds in the past three months, something he hasn't' done since being diagnosed with failure to thrive at a year old. He is playing with his three year old sister; it's so adorable to watch them chase each other around the house, hug, chase each other, hug, get in the dog crate together, hug, take turns pushing each other in their wagon, and kick the ball back and forth. Last night the three of us played catch together for over 10 minutes. I'm so happy for her to have her brother to play with.

   This protocol changed his life, my life, and our family's life.

   There are no words to thank you enough for all your help along the way – he's on his way…

   Love, Love, Love

   Update: as of December 3rd, 2013 this little guy is 18 weeks seizure free!

64. My name is Dawn. Below is a shortened version of what we've been through
     prior to and since Kerri Rivera coming into our lives and changing our family
     forever.

     I am Noah and Eli's mom, caregiver, advocate etc., that's been my job for 17
     years. Prior to having children with special needs I had a career that I loved and
     my plan was to continue my career, how deluded I was, my life has been forever
     changed by my children and their symptoms as my entire existence over these
     years has been to save my son.

     My son Noah born August 19, 1996 has struggled and suffered with what is now
     known as the symptoms of autism. His symptoms began at 8 months of age with
     a rare blood disorder known as neutropenia, he had a low white blood count. As
     he continues to improve, I too, along with our entire family seem to be healing
     as we bore witness to his daily struggles of self injurious behaviors, aggressions
     and rages, learning disabilities, speech and auditory delays, 2 steps forward and 4
     steps back.

     Healing the symptoms know as autism with the Chlorine Dioxide and Kalcker
     Protocol have been a cathartic exercise for me as well, no amount of therapy
     would have soothed my soul like witnessing my son's return from the daily brink
     of death.

     My hopes and dreams for my son dashed with vaccines before he was old
     enough to speak. I'm 50 this year, however I'm older then those years, and my
     views and outlook on life have changed forever. Imagine fighting for my son's life
     against those trusted factions of our society supposedly put in place to protect
     us, i.e., government agencies, churches, schools, teachers, principles, school
     boards, doctors, hospitals. I'm changed forever by the daily battles, but somehow
     they are small now in comparison to the beast of the symptoms that ravaged
     my boy with red hair, often referred to by me as my favorite Martian. As he
     continues on his healing path, so do those of us who have loved him so dearly,
     despite his outwardly awkwardness, he is the innocent victim left to suffer for
     what is often referred to as the "greater good", he's responsible for so much
     more in my life then just the symptoms known as autism.

     It was a Saturday morning in May of 2003. Noah, at the time 6 yrs. old, had slept
     with us because of seizures on and off through the night. Like so many times
     before, I was very concerned he would go 'status epileptus', a state of continuous
     seizures. He ate cantaloupe for breakfast that day. I remember it vividly even
     11 years later. His seizures would come about every 20-25 days. First he would
     complain of a stomach ache, and I could hear the gurgle of his stomach. They
     usually lasted a few minutes and then went away. This day, the Saturday before
     Mother's Day, he didn't come out of the seizure. We administered his anti-
     seizure medication but it didn't work. We called 911, the fourth such call in
     Noah's brief life. When EMS arrived, Eli, then 3 years old, ran to his bedroom
     upstairs. I remember the technicians working on stabilizing Noah. They ripped
     the shirt from his body as they worked on him and carried him out to the
     ambulance. As I followed them to the ambulance I happened to look back to
     see Eli watching from his upstairs window as they placed his brother in the
     ambulance. He stood motionless. Darryn scooped him up and followed us as we
     drove swiftly through traffic to Texas Children's emergency room, about 25 miles
     away. I remembered thinking, why don't people heed the right of way? I looked
     back as they worked on Noah. His seizures continued until we arrived at the
     hospital. Once we arrived he was taken straight to the ER, ICU room, where

four doctors began to work on him. Darryn and Eli arrived as I stood next to the bed while the doctors worked to save his life. I took Eli out of the room and we sat in a chair looking in at what was happening. His eyes were as big as I have ever seen them and he sat perfectly silent in my lap, we colored. I overheard the doctors explain to my husband that they were having problems stopping the seizure. They wanted permission to use a drug that could stop his heart. Darryn asked if there were any other options. The doctor shook his head. He asked what they would do if the heart stopped. The paddles. So he was given the drug. No heart stoppage. His breathing became shallow and the seizures finally stopped after 6-7 straight hours. A couple of hours later Noah woke up in his hospital bed, connected to monitors and the like, in a drugged stupor. By this time my parents had arrived (like so many times before) and had taken Eli home. Darryn stood next to Noah's bed rubbing his chin nervously. Noah asked if he could use the restroom. Darryn said yes, and in the next second Noah leapt from the bed, almost a perfect swan dive, toward the floor. Luckily, Darryn was there to catch him. Noah's life was saved twice in the same day. After the drugs wore off, he was released from the hospital. Noah missed a week of school while he learned to walk again.

I never knew the impact this had on Eli until Father's Day that same year. About a month after the seizure we planned to attend with some friends one of those workshops at Home Depot where the kids make a gift for Dad. He was excited to do the workshop. As we approached the store we noticed the local fire station had an area of the parking lot roped off for tours of ambulances and fire trucks. Eli became frightened and started crying, and began backing up, finally screaming and contorting. This from a child that hadn't given us a peep of trouble before. I had to leave our friends standing in the parking lot as my second son became inconsolable. At the time it hadn't occurred to me that he remembered the incident with his brother just a month prior. He too suffered, and sadly he was 3 years old at the time, unbeknownst to me, Eli has probably remembered more then I realize even today.

Noah had his first seizure in March 1998 at 18 months of age, shortly after a round of vaccines. (His doctors continually assured us that vaccines had nothing to do with Noah's problems, but I know otherwise.) Seizures were not Noah's only problem, however. He was diagnosed with neutropenia (the lack of neutrophils or a type of white blood cells) in 1997. He has suffered from acid reflux for as long as we can remember. He was hospitalized for 4 days at 4 years old for a roto-virus infection, something most children get through at home in a couple days. He had a cyst removed from his thyroid. His tonsils were removed due to frequent infections. In 2005, he was diagnosed with Lyme disease. In 2008 his pediatrician discovered his blood was missing carnitine, a key component for the body's metabolism. We took him to a specialist who diagnosed him with mitochondrial disease. His seizures stopped after we started giving him medication for the carnitine deficiency. But his behavioral symptoms continued and even worsened which always indicated a deeper underlying illness plaguing Noah. But what?

Early in 2013 Noah began to show some psychiatric symptoms that frightened us to the point we had to consider putting him in a home. He had frequent panic attacks (all day, minute to minute), tics, and sudden bursts of outrage over insignificant things. He often didn't make sense while speaking, and secluded himself in his bedroom. He fantasized uncontrollably about his videos, and spoke over and over about what we were going to do about the characters (not what we would do if we were in the stories). He had repeated events of unrealistic fears. We took him to see an energy medicine specialist. The energy medicine protocol involved various supplements and dietary changes, as well as electrical pulses to adjust his body voltage (an approach similar to acupuncture). During one of our visits we learned of MMS, which this doctor indicated could be used in small doses to treat colds. Symptoms improved, but very little. But then they worsened again dramatically. We took him to his pediatrician who diagnosed PANDAS, and prescribed antibiotics. This helped but only temporarily. His psychiatrist prescribed anti-anxiety medications, with only marginal results. He was unable to attend school through all of this, and needed someone by his side constantly. His pediatrician prescribed Albenza thinking parasites may be involved (despite a negative stool test). This improved his behaviors some but only marginally. There was also the side effect of hair loss. Noah became completely bald, like a cancer patient.

To see your son regress into psychotic behavior is something no human can ever imagine. Facing people everyday as they watched Noah regress and comment, it was a slow slip and then suddenly he was in a dive toward insanity. I felt he was slipping away. I scoured the Internet for answers. I had heard of Kerri Rivera but thought antibiotics were the only treatment for my son, like the vaccines, I had been told by doctors that the only treatment for Lyme was antibiotics. I emailed her and she answered immediately to "start the protocol." We began the CD protocol in June 2013. The protocol takes complete dedication, it requires steadfast commitment, and it's the best gift I have ever given Noah. I have learned so much about illness and it's roots through treating my son with the protocol.

Noah's behavioral symptoms started to improve immediately. He had fewer and fewer tics and outbursts. He was noticeably calmer. He now answers the phone, takes messages, and helps me scan food items at the grocery store. He even got behind the wheel of our car for a practice drive in the school parking lot. He asks a lot of questions. So much has improved in such a brief time. Prior to the CD protocol I scored Noah as a 38 on the ATEC test. Since then, he has improved to an 8. Darryn (Noah's Dad) scored Noah a 55 before we started, and two months after beginning it was a 22. It's amazing that a few brief months ago we were considering having him put him into an institution. Although we try not to think too far in advance, now we can hope our son can someday lead the normal life he was meant to.

I can't help one final story about Noah. Yesterday he asked me what autism was. We've never explained to him that he has it, because he would not have been able to understand it even if we tried. While I searched for an answer, he said "you know, Mom, Sponge Bob couldn't get his boating license because of his autism." I belted out a loud laugh and said "Ok. Noah, you know you have a little bit of autism too." And he said "Yes Mom, I know that," and smiled.

While he still has much to make up, years of life to regain, experiences to live, we're so pleased and grateful to Kerri and the others responsible for these protocols for these improvements, his life is being restored. I would encourage anyone to follow the protocols as closely as possible and do not delay. It is so fitting that the only opportunity I've ever been given to tell a little of what my family has been through would be afforded to me by the very person that actually saved my son…she gains nothing from what she has done for us, except the knowledge that she saved a boy's life that she has yet to meet, by saving my son, she has saved my family.

65. *Shay is doing so well it's surreal. In the past week the balance has shifted so that he is now recovered more of the time than not. He is having a 2-4 hour block every day or two where he is back in his old state (weeping, raging, zero-to-flipout, shrieking, obstinate, defiant, OCD, mean, potty-mouthed, etc.). The rest of the time he is lucid, has perfect mental clarity, is as funny as can be, does his math quickly, has perfect handwriting, gets along with his sister, is generous, expresses himself clearly, plays well, understands how others feel, etc. It is a mind blower Kerri.*

Although Shay doesn't have the awareness to know when he is in the autistic state, he is now clearly aware when he is in the recovered state. He comes up to me and says quietly, "Mom, it's gone again. Do you think it will come back?" I tell him yes, that it will be like this for a while, coming and going, until one day it will be gone and it won't come back. Shay and I have been discussing which "number" he is going to be in the line of children that recover. :) He is also planning a big "Goodbye Autism" party for himself.

Bella is getting over her meltdowns much more quickly. Sometimes I say "no" to something and then flinch, waiting for the screaming, but it's small, or sometimes she cries and gets over it within minutes. This is a big improvement for her. In her own words, she has noticed that she feels less anxious.

66. *We started the protocol 9 months ago. My son had 2, 3 horrible days every month. He wouldn't stop crying all day long, and he could not get any sleep at night. After talking to Kerri, we realized that these terrible days were always the days of the full moon. We saw improvement straight after the first PP. After 6 months, all of the bad behaviors were gone. I realized that the PP helped my child to improve month by month.*

And to prove that it is not only me who can see the changes, my son's therapist from school told me the other day: "Well, when is full moon again? So that you would start the Mebendazol? I love when he gets it, he is doing so well with it".

Staring atec in February was 50, now his atec is 34. Thank you so much, Kerri!

Betti, Hungary

67. *We are celebrating 3 months on CD and 2 PP's done! Our little angel has (or I should say had) extreme ADHD...we are not seeing much of that anymore. Our life altering issue is her lungs. This child has undergone over 35 surgeries in 8 years. 17 of those to surgically remove mucous from her lungs. She is hospitalized every 6 weeks with pneumonia. We have O2 in our home. She even had a port placed for IV meds at home. Our life has revolved around illness. In 8 years the docs have done every test in the book to figure out the cause. We've turned up nothing. In July, we flew to NYC to see a medical mystery doctor. He told us it's all nutritional and had us do some parasite testing. The testing turned up zilch, but thanks to Jean Marie, we ended up here. Long story short, we are making huge strides. We are not there yet, but to give you an idea, normally her pneumonias take 4 months to clear, this time it was only one month! She's only needed one antibiotic in 3 months, normally it's 8 antibiotics in 3 months. She's doing better in school too, which is just a bonus. Today she came home and told me she was able to run in gym, something she hasn't done for years! Thank you Kerri Rivera and Jean Marie and all the mods for welcoming us to this group and for helping us to take back this child's life. Bless it! Bless all of you!*

68. *30 days of gratitude, Day 4...I am thankful for an evening alone with my son. It's rare that we have time together alone. He jumped on the bed and danced around while I packed for my trip in the morning, talking and singing the whole time. The dinner table was lonely by ourselves so we decided to eat in front of the fire. I said, "This is fun, isn't it?" and he said, "I love this and I love you, Mom" Moments like this were non-existent before our journey brought us to Kerri Rivera who is an angel on earth. She gave us the direction we needed to heal our son.*

69. *I observed my kiddos at school today. Get this........my once severely autistic 6 year old choose and received a Spanish lesson that lasted 27.5 minutes (I timed it). The whole lesson he was sitting on his bottom, following instructions, answer questions correctly (in Spanish), smiling, great eye contact, and really enjoying his time with the Spanish teacher. FUA to the max! This time last year Henry was speaking in 1-2 word sentences to get needs met. Now he is talking in complete sentences in English and Spanish!!!!!!!*

70. *In the past, if I gave Nate a hug and told him I loved him, he would sort of hug me back, awkwardly jutting his backside out (to reduce physical contact) and patting me on the back and saying, "I love you, too." He would then escape as soon as possible.*

    After a few days of being on 7 drops (last week) Nate approached me with full eye contact, threw his arms around me, gave me a prolonged bear hug and spontaneously said, "I love you, Mom". I hugged him back and we stood there, just enjoying the moment, while I quietly balled my eyes out.

    Thirteen years. I had waited 13 years for that moment.

    And now he has been doing it almost every day since that first hug.

    This alone is the world.

71. *There's a lot of people jumping on the "Thankfulness Train" this time of year. Here's my contribution. There's only one major thing I can think of this year that I am thankful for. Of course, there's so much to be thankful for, but one thing that really stands out. That would be this protocol. God led us to see Kerri Rivera at Autism One this year. I only went because it was basically the one thing I didn't know much about. The day before Kerri presented, I saw my friend Laura at Karaoke Night (so fun by the way!). She told me she was doing CD and I'm pretty sure I looked at her like she was crazy! Saw Kerri the next day and I was hooked. We started the protocol June 3rd. Laura got me in this group. Thank you Laura, for your patience with me and for letting me know about this group! Thank you, Debbie who has talked to me many times about the protocol, about my son's aggression, reassuring me that things will get better and they have! Much, much better. We still have further to go, but there is light at the end of the tunnel. My four kids and myself are doing the protocol. We all have Lyme. We are all feeling so much better. We are no longer spending thousands of dollars a month on empty treatments. We are getting our lives back; our finances under control, and my son with autism went from an ATEC of 47 to 20 in four months. Thank you and love you all. And to Kerri Rivera, there are no words. Thanks and love isn't enough. You can be assured of my prayers for you, Patrick and your family for life. That's the least I can do for all you have done for all of us.*

72. *Small progress this week! My son had his ABA therapy yesterday and at the end the therapist gives him a "high five" before he leaves. The therapist asked my 3-year-old normally non-verbal son for a "high five". My son looked at him, gave him a high five and said "HIGH FIVE!" plain as day. My husband almost fell over sideways in shock! He also put his toys away without being asked to, and that too is a big change. CD is the best!"*

---

73. We have been on the protocol since Aug 30th of this year. We've done one PP. My DS is 8 with severe apraxia and autistic.

ATEC: 4/2013: 62 starting some biomed

ATEC: 8/15/2013: 51 before CD

ATEC: 10/6/13: 24

Some WOW moments for us so far:

  * Playing soccer with other kids at school three weeks after the start of the protocol. *Really "on" in conversations...adding information when we didn't think he was listening because he was playing on his iPad.

  * Talking about other things in his day besides Minecraft or Plants Vs Zombies.

  * Going from a battle with homework that would last over three hours to picking him up at daycare with his homework already finished. And correct. That he did on his own.

  * His ST saying he is able to follow three step directions better and was able to talk/ask Who and What questions for nearly the entire hour...I actually had to tell the ST what we are doing because it was obvious to her it was more than just diet.

He's just happier. We're all just happier.

---

74. We came back from our Intensive in December of last year on a high. After a week with the Son-Rise® team, Jordan was saying 20 different words; he was more confident, and more mature. He had such an amazing time learning and growing. Every morning he would take his facilitator by the hand and walk him/her into the playroom. He really grew up that week. I loved watching him grow through love and laughter. What an amazing, wonderful thing to witness.

We, also, learned at our IAHP appointment that Jordan was reading at about a third grade level. What a trip! The evaluator held up a paragraph for Jordan to read. It was so fast I didn't even have time to read it. Then, she held up a question for him to read, then, a sheet with the answers. She, then, asked him to point to the answer and he did. He was three for three. My son taught himself to read. What?! We were, also, very surprised to find out that between running our Son-Rise® program and incorporating exercises from IAHP, Jordan improved 433% from September to December. WOW!

Between the two experiences on the east coast, I felt like I didn't know my own son. I always believed he can accomplish anything and yet I had tremendously underestimated his ability. I was so excited to get home and start his program. I knew that if we focused and put everything into his therapy for two years, he would be ready to go to mainstream kindergarten.

I was so excited; I was beyond hopeful; I believed he was on his road to healing.

On Christmas Eve, Jordan was crouching down and just froze there. I called his name, no response. I ran over to him and noticed his lips were turning blue. Immediately, I tipped him over, hit him on the back and did a swipe in his mouth to get out what he was choking on. There was nothing there, but he gasped for air and began breathing again. Did he just have a seizure?

January 15 has become a day I will never forget. We woke up to Jordan throwing up and he didn't want to get out of bed. He just wanted to sleep; he must have caught the flu and needed to sleep it off? Finally, around 10am he got up and ran around the house like nothing was wrong so we began therapy. While I was in the playroom with him we were jumping on the trampoline and he suddenly stopped and looked at me with a panicked look on his face and reached out for me. Clearly, jumping was too active for his upset stomach so I brought him to the family room with Kaiyan and my helper.

Suddenly, he looked off and froze again. He then threw up again and passed out. Oh shit, he just had a seizure, and another one, and another one, and another one. All the while staying unconscious. I brought him to the ER where he slept and had another mild seizure. While he was passed out they gave him a CT head scan to make sure there wasn't a bleed or something in his brain. Everything was fine.

Shortly after, he woke up. He was playing, running around the ER as if nothing had happened. He went through what little water I had brought and was asking for food and water. A good sign, I thought. The ER wouldn't allow him to eat or drink anything "just in case". Anyone who knows anything about seizures knows that no food and drink could very well cause a seizure...and it did.

This time the ER Doctor went into full-blown panic mode, probably because she saw what happened. They began trying to get blood out of him. On a good day this is almost impossible. Now, they are trying on a kid that didn't have any fluids in his system to help expand the veins.

And so it went, needle poke, dig around in the arm searching for a vein, Jordan would hold his breath from the pain and have a seizure. Seizures are typically the brains way of trying to get oxygen; the pinpricking was inadvertently inducing seizures because of the breath holding. This went on for two hours: needle poke, dig, hold his breath, seizure. They poked him 27 times: in his neck, head, ankles, thigh, anywhere they could think of.

This of course wasn't enough. They insisted on doing a spinal tap to check for meningitis, which we had been declining all day. Now they are telling us that the way he had been seizing for the past two hours is classic for meningitis and not doing it could be fatal. They crunched him in the tightest ball they possibly could and held him so tight he couldn't move...or breath. After the fifth poke, I began to get faint and had to sit down. They didn't know what they were doing. When I sat down I could really see how they were holding him and asked if he was breathing. The nurse looked down and said, "he's blue, get the oxygen" and they put oxygen near his face.

I immediately thought, "they're killing him. They don't know what they're doing." That's when I reached out to every FB group I'm on and asked for prayers. That was the only thing that was going to save him.

When they, finally, let him go he had the worst seizure he's had to date. He was actually convulsing. As they went for blood the 28th time, I told the nurse that's enough. This has gone on far too long. She agreed, ran and got the Dr., they wheeled him into to the CPR room, and called for a crash cart. I think I said, "what the fuck?" She said it's "just in case".

They proceeded to get a drill and drill a hole through his shin and into his shinbone so they could put in an IO (IV into the bone). They pumped him full of all kinds of drugs and, at long last, drew blood.

He looked up at me with a longing in his eyes and reached out for me. I went over and put my hand on his chest and he passed out. He was transferred by ambulance to our local children's hospital; we were allowed to follow the ambulance, but couldn't ride with him. He remained unconscious until he arrived into his private room at the hospital.

The first thing he did when he woke up was reach out for my hand and give me a kiss. My little boy!

The blood they had finally taken revealed low electrolytes and bicarbonate at a life-threatening low level. Screaming and crying can drop bicarbonate, which he did for two hours in the ER; lack of food and drink can drop bicarbonate levels, which he wasn't allowed to have in the ER. Low bicarbonate levels can cause seizures. What a recipe for disaster!

The hospital ran every test they could think of and no reason was found for the low bicarbonate or the seizures. We came home after five days, followed by several follow up appointments over the next two weeks. Everything seemed to check out fine until I brought his labs to his DAN (Defeat Autism Now) Dr., she looked at the blood test, pointed to something and said, "Lyme, every time I see this in one of my kids, it's Lyme."

We had the (one of many) $800 test at the best lab in hopes we wouldn't get a false negative, which is very common with Lyme. Jordan came back positive! Now we had something to go on. I was excited to finally have an answer to what was going on with my little boy. Lyme is known for seizures and abnormal electrolyte levels.

We scheduled an appointment with a Lyme Literate Medical Doctor (LLMD) and were ready to start healing our guy. Two days before the appointment, we woke up to Jordan vomiting. He didn't want to get out of bed. He finally did and ran around like nothing was wrong and then he had another seizure. We were told to take him for blood tests immediately the next time he had a seizure. We took him to his DAN Dr. an hour away, but knew they would be able to get his blood without difficulty. We went to lunch, came home, he had a seizure, turned blue, threw up, passed out, had a seizure, turned blue, threw up, passed out, had a seizure, turned blue, threw up, passed out. His DAN Dr. just happened to call to check on him in the middle of this and told us to get him to the hospital before he had a heart attack. We went to the ER...

And so the story goes every seven weeks TO THE DAY, seizure, turn blue, vomit, pass out, seizure, turn blue, vomit, pass out, admitted to the hospital where he was pumped full of drugs for hours to try and stop the seizures, and they ran the same tests over and over again. The hospital didn't think he had Lyme even with a positive test and thought that seizures every seven weeks to the day was a coincidence, although, they could still not offer any explanation.

We tried treating him with ABX that the LLMD prescribed. One teaspoon and he had a seizure, turned blue, threw up, passed out, had a seizure, turned blue, threw up, and passed out. This time the Valium I administered did stop the seizure cycle, most likely because it was induced from the ABX and not part of his regular seven week seizure cycle. He had multiple mild seizures every day for two weeks from that one-teaspoon.

Clearly, ABX were not going to work. I emailed with a woman who coauthored the book, "The Lyme Autism Connection" and tried the homeopath that she used down in San Diego. This was definitely working with detoxing, but it wasn't helping with the seizures. He went from seven weeks to the day to three weeks to the day. This treatment was working on opening Jordan's detox pathways so his body could rid itself of the Lyme. I liked the idea of treating this way, but the process could take four years. I didn't want Jordan having what the neurologist told us were life-threatening seizures for four years. I was desperate to find something to help him.

We knew what was wrong, but needed something safe to treat him. Nothing was covered by insurance and we were running out of money. I had lost hope. Every treatment seemed to make him worse and I couldn't bear to see my boy suffer the way he had been for the past six months. I didn't know what to do.

I, literally, got on my knees and prayed for help every night. In the same week, a woman who attended the same Son-Rise® start-up emailed me about a newly discovered treatment she was doing. I had signed up for a Lyme conference that mentioned the same treatment, and I had signed up for an autism telesummit that unbeknownst to me had Kerri Rivera as one of the speakers. (Kerri is the woman who discovered this treatment for autistic kids.) I emailed back and forth with Kerri, I posted on the FB group, trying to get all my questions answered. I was terrified to treat Jordan with anything given his seizure history.

Then, he was hospitalized again for uncontrollable seizures and I realized I couldn't let fear get in the way of helping him. I started the day we were home from the hospital at a really low dose that Kerri recommended. She has held my hand through this process to help prevent him from having any seizures.

Since we started in May, he went 10 weeks seizure free and had several mild seizures that he brought himself out of without any extra medication and NO hospital. He is currently at a record-breaking 15 weeks seizure free.

Through this treatment we have learned that in addition to Lyme he has three different visible parasites. He is loaded—he passes more parasites than most of the teenagers in the FB group. It scares me to think what would have happened to him if we weren't led to this treatment. Thank God for Kerri Rivera sharing what she has learned and being so gracious and generous with her time.

I'm incredibly grateful we attended the Son-Rise® Intensive before all of this began. His team of facilitators created a base for him that continued to blossom even through this tumultuous year. Coupled with the parasite treatment, Jordan has gone from 20 to 90 words—he's picking up new words almost daily. His balance is amazing, his muscle tone is getting better, and he understands everything. Even more exciting, he's playing interactively with his sister. He is on the road to recovery.

We are finally able to start picking up the pieces of where we left off back in December. I felt stuck; I had PTSD; I needed help believing we can move past (what I had deemed) the horror of this year. The first thing I did was turn to Son-Rise®; I started having monthly dialogue sessions with Bears (Barry Neil Kaufman)—the co-founder of Son-Rise®, which has been incredible. This is one of those times that happen in life that can make you a better person or break you. Bears is guiding me to be better. I just arrived back from another Son-Rise® training where I realized that staying in fear and being nervous about getting excited or anxious about feeling hopeful again will prevent me from being the bridge to healing that I want to be for Jordan. I felt a relaxation that I haven't felt all year. I've been wound real tight, waiting, being on the look out for that next seizure.

This year has had a huge impact on Kaiyan as well. She'd see her brother sick and then her mommies would disappear. I'm noticing she's wound pretty tight as well. Her favorite moments are when the entire family is together. I'm hoping talking with her about what happened and spending more one on one time with her will help. She asks daily is Jordan throwing up, is he having a seizure? She doesn't really know what it all means, but is really aware it's not good. She, recently, said she wanted to have autism. After I explained to her that autism is why Jordan isn't talking or riding a bike, she decided she didn't want autism. She wants to be a boy and insists on wearing Jordan's clothes almost daily. I think it's her way of healing and feeling included in the process.

We've been doing Son-Rise® again and it feels great. I do feel like we have some time to make up for since this year has been spent dealing with health issues rather than cognitive issues so we are working up to having a full time program, having quarterly consultations, and doing another Intensive.

Son-Rise® and Kerri's protocol's are not only bringing our son back, they're bringing me back.

---

75. Healing From Autism

Hospital birth, bottle fed, fully vax until age 4. Digestive disorders beginning at age 1. Low tone, speech and language delay. Mild early education interventions. GF since age 2, GF, Soy free, sugar free since age 4. Majority of autism symptoms presented in 2013; in the fall of 2012, our son did not qualify as being in need of special education, and thus, could not attend school in our district at all.

Long winter days in a tiny home had me sending him out to play, in our tiny backyard, which had a patch of grass and a bush, under which small animals and birds lived. In his boredom, he sprinkled the dirt all over himself; his head, face, clothes, shoes, on several different days.

Later in the early spring, the symptoms of autism appeared more and more obvious: disobedience, disinterest in sitting for a story or coloring, lost interest in puzzles of more than 24 pcs, jumping on and off furniture for hours, despite scoldings and time-outs. Sudden relapse in bedwetting. Then by summer, the symptoms were very obvious: longer tantrums, rages, anger issues, hitting, fighting, a mean spirit; running out of the house without permission, with no respect for danger or regard for safety. Weepiness, hypersensitivity to touch, suddenly repeating the same phrase, over and over all day. Lost balance and coordination, bumping into walls and furniture, stubbing toes. Shoulder shrugging, all day, but not able to stop or say why he was doing it. Lost dexterity—could not put cards in a box. Lost organizational skills—could no longer put toys or clothes away. Extreme nighttime drooling and bedwetting. The need for sameness, and to have all food served cold. He frequently did not seem to be in his right mind.

In desperation, I asked a group of special needs moms for advice, and ordered a handful of books on Autism, including Healing the Symptoms of Autism by Kerri Rivera.

It was the best money I ever spent.

I read the book thoroughly, ordered the supplies and began the CD Protocol on July 8, 2013. Starting ATEC: 46. We ramped up slowly on drops, serving doses 8 times per day. My son has had two low dose/partial PP's, to minimize the emotional meltdowns, the gas and discomfort. I did not realize how very deficient in minerals he was, and did not give him enough ocean water. Now I order the big 10-liter jug of ocean water, so I am not tempted to be stingy. He needs more than 100 ml ocean water per day for his digestive system to handle the parasite dumping during the PP. His previous digestive trouble was unexplained chronic constipation, since age one, and that is really linked to his high need for the OW. Interestingly, his doctors had all said to keep giving Miralax, and that he might possibly need that laxative every day for the rest of his life. We stopped the laxative when we started the CD program, and began the enemas right away. When I sifted the stool and saw the number of parasites, I understood finally why he couldn't poop well on his own for the last 4 years, despite diet interventions. We are looking forward

to PP #3, in which I hope to ramp up to full dose on all components.

Poop sifting revealed what 6 pediatricians and 2 GI specialists could not tell us. Our son is infected with at least 6 different kinds of parasitic flukes and 3 kinds of parasitic worms. His stool has had a very large amount of sediment, with odd, tiny, but defined shapes. A search for "rodent and avian parasites" reveals photos of very tiny creatures.

I just completed his ATEC at Kerri's request: November 12, 2013: he now scores a 10, with a 1 in language, 2 in social, and 7 in health.

What does his recovery look like? We enrolled our son in a small private school this fall, with one teacher for 6 students, no aide. He now memorizes poems, Bible verses, and songs. He sings, knows his alphabet and all the sounds of the letters, and can count to 47 with precision. He shows kindness to others, is mindful of safety, and has glowing reports from his NT school. He sits with me for stories, and brings books to 'read' to his baby sister. He is not literate quite yet, but enjoys word search games, where he can complete levels and advance to more challenging puzzles. Twice now he has played the word search game on Leap Frog for 45 minutes. He has regained his balance and coordination. The rages, anger, and shoulder shrugging disappeared within the first 10 days on CD. He identifies printed numbers and letters, and does well in math, phonics, penmanship and reading class. He is learning to write numbers and letters in cursive, and follow directions on drawing worksheets. He operates the TV and DVR unaided, recording and watching programs he chooses.

He is happy; he has a patience and joyfulness about life that was previously lacking. He tells me jokes, and now has the coordination to operate a hand puppet while speaking for the puppet!! He is thoughtful and obedient. He has regained fine and gross motor skills, and motor planning skills.

There are still improvements we hope for: further speech, language, and vocabulary improvements. Social graces. More improved digestive health; I can see that he still has parasites in his stool. We will continue the CD Protocol, and we look forward to further healing. Thank you all for your support and encouragement.

The CD Autism Program has done more than cure our son of his brief affliction with Autism; it addresses the pervasive, underlying gut disorder and parasite issues that have plagued him all his life. Where complex testing in expensive medical centers has failed, a simple home health program succeeds. Thank you Kerri Rivera!!

76. Well...we too did an ATEC! Our son was 11.5 when we started the CD Protocol July 2012 First fully loaded (All PP meds on board) was November 2012

    VERY First ATEC: Jan. 2006= 124

    ATEC in July 2012: 64

    ATEC August 2012: 52

    ATEC Oct. 2012: 48

    ATEC Dec. 2012: 45

    ATEC May 2013: 40

    ATEC August 2013: 39

    ATEC NOV. 2013: 33

    I actually did one myself as I have done throughout all the previous, but I had hubby do one and combined and divided by the 2! Resulting in the 33! Oddly, it's the "SPEECH" that remains consistently around 14 & 15 throughout ALL of these! All the others continue to go down! We've had some ups and downs, but with continued evacuation of some MIGHTY big worms...we continue to see major gains!

    This is the ONLY Protocol that has EVER given us the progress we've seen in one year's time let alone in 6 months! Thank you Kerri Rivera and especially Patrick Rivera for being such pioneers in this journey to recovery! You are SOOO loved and appreciated beyond words! Thank you for never giving up! Thank you for giving so much, and bringing healing to our son! He's come a long way, but we have a ways to go! But with the progress he's making...I honestly feel it will seem like nothing from where we've come!

    Again THANK YOU! XOXOXO!

77. We had a great day today. For the first time, he joined me in throwing something at a target (blocks at carpet circles). He laughed and smiled and pulled me to play with him better than he has in weeks. I heard a lot more sounds and approximations today. When I couldn't figure out what he was saying, he kept trying until I did.

    My favorite part of the day, and I know this is odd, was when his head collided with my mouth. I exclaimed in pain and he was clearly worried/empathetic. He kept trying to get close to see my lip and giving me kisses. I've seen him concerned before but never that clearly empathetic.

78. Just wanted to share that on 21/8/13 my sons ATEC was 46, just redid because we're at the start of our first pp & his score has come down to 31! The big improvement came after introducing CD enemas 3 weeks ago. Although he's been on oral CD for about 2 months, it was always the case that if I missed a dose within 1/2 hour he'd be sensory, inflexible, super-anxious, shouting, aggressive etc & I'd have to syringe it down him but within 10mins of dosing the lightswitch would flick on & he'd be in control & a calm, loving boy again. Since the 3 enemas I gave him 3 weeks ago (only 3 because then his brother had one, panicked, screamed & totally freaked out my 4yr old who up til then had said he liked them bc they made him feel good afterwards) his personality has been shining through again, there's less panick/anxiety, less sensory issues & there's no 'reaction' if I miss a dose or more of CD. I've seen more improvements this week, on Monday he decided to sit down & colour & proceeded to colour neatly,

inside the lines - he was so pleased with himself! (He used to colour so neatly but about 6 months ago his colouring became scribbly & he frustrated that he couldn't do it neat anymore). Then tonight, when I asked him to hop out of the bath, HE DID! He stood up, stepped out & as I handed him a towel he took it & said 'thank you mummy' and wrapped himself in it & walked out - all completely relaxed - like it was usual!!! WWWOOAHAHH! Yes! He has never done this, it's always tantrums, always arguing, needs to bathe longer, has to be made to get out, refuses to step out, has to be lifted, needs me or hubby to wrap & dress him, & usually all while panicking, crying, demanding, arguing or screaming because it's cold, different, he doesn't want to, it's not right etc. I just can't believe what happened tonight! I'm still astounded. It's like the Finlay we 'know' isn't Finlay & now we're beginning to see who he really is!

So I'm REALLY excited about our 1st pp. We're already seeing full moon behaviours & although tough it's been great to see them because it's a reminder of what Finlay was like every day until 3 weeks ago!

He's already healing. It's soooo exciting! Thank you Kerri - may God bless you & all the children on this protocol. Healing, here we come!

---

79. *True Hope by Maggie Kaye*

Most people don't know that babies are born with about 100 million brain cells. That is more cells with more connections than there are stars in the galaxy! This is difficult to picture when you consider an infant's brain only weighs about 12 ounces at birth, about 25% of it's full size. But, there is a logical explanation for this: Brain cells; like the brain itself, have yet to grow. As neurons (brain cells) mature, they become larger, stronger, and form tentacle-like branches that form synapsis (connection and communication) with other brain cells. Brain growth is directed by neural activity. The neural activity of the cerebral cortex (the largest, most complex part of the brain) molds the way a child will think, behave, and acheive.

Conventional wisdom long held the belief that the human brain cannot change… that it is hard-wired at birth. Scientists today have proven that this is not the case. They have found that the brain is malleable. It has the ability to change shape, size, number of branches, number of connections, and even the strength of it's connections over time. The potential growth, or neuroplastisity (neuro means neurons or brain cells, plastic meaning changable) is far-reaching. At birth, the brain is simply a blueprint of what it will become. No one can predict the amount of growth that a brain has yet to acheive.

For the parents of a child with Autism, the diagnosis can be devastating. But, the biggest and most harmful blow can come from the prognosis: There is no cure. Kenn and I were given a diagnosis of an Autism Spectrum Disorder for our son, but we were not given this prognosis. In fact, the word "Autism" was avoided at our son's diagnostic evaluation until the therapists heard us say it first, and realized we were comfortable with the word. For many parents, a diagnosis is the end all, be all. For far too many parents, the words "No cure" are scary and harmful. We did not hear these words nor would we have accepted them as truth if we had. We do not want to change our son. We want him to be his best self. We are not looking for a cure. We are in search of treatment and *healing for his symptoms. We know and understand that a Therapist is not God. A Therapist cannot predict the future for our son. He or she can simply assess where Gunnar is developmentally and give us options for a treatment plan for a healthy, successful future. Our son's diagnosis was not an ending. It was simply the begininning of a journey through a world of strength, challenges, support, opposition, and the love of a parent that cannot ever be fully defined.*

Our son, Gunnar was born with an Autoimmune disorder, Hypothyroidism. He was tested at birth, was diagnosed, and has been treated by an Endocrinologist since he was three days old. We were not upset by the Hypo diagnosis, but rather ready for the course of action to regulate all of Gunnar's bodily systems. What did surprise us was the constant shrugging off of our concerns over our son's developmental delays and gastrointestinal symptoms over the last few years. We were continually disappointed by the compartmentalization of our son's physical and mental challenges by every Pediatrician and Specialist we saw. To us, Gunnar's symptoms all had to be as connected as are all of his body parts. But, we were treated as if our concerns were dumbfounded...as if digestive, behavioral, and physical challenges were not intertwined.

Let's be clear...The brain does not function in isolation. It is a team player. It needs vital nutrients and informational input to perform at optimum levels. To fill these needs, the brain relies heavily on complex interactions between the immune, endocrine, and gastrointestinal systems. Gunnar, like so many other children on the Autism spectrum, suffers from gastrointestinal issues uncluding chronic constipation, diarrhea, and abdominal discomfort. Scientific studies and countless parent reports are pointing to gut inflammation caused by casein, gluten, and soy in our foods. Gunnar has shown clear physical and behavioral reactions to these foods, and improvement in these areas with the removal of Gluten, casein, and soy from his diet. This is not an allergy from the perspective of a traditional allergist. This is what is called a T Cell Inflammatory response.

The use of a gluten, casein, and soy free diet as a means of treatment for Autism symptoms has gotten mixed responses. Many parents and doctors who deal with Autism, Immune, and Endocrine disorders rave about it's benefits, including me and my husband. Still, others call it "junk science". Clearly, if someone is looking purely at one body part at a time, they will not be open to the truth that the body and brain are codependent. I, personally, have been challenged by the choice to follow this diet for my own thyroid disease and for my son's Autism. I was even told on an online support forum that the GFCFSF diet is "fake science" and is causing "false hope" for parents of children on the Autism Spectrum.

False Hope?

This may be one of the biggest oxymorons I've ever heard. This ranks right up there with "God Hates". I cannot say what causes people to be so oppositional to our choice to follow this eating plan. Perhaps the resistance to this way of eating is due to a simple misunderstanding of the leaky gut syndrome that plagues so many children on the Autism Spectrum. This leaky gut syndrome does not cause food allergies. It causes food sensitivities.

In food allergies that many parents are famililar with, the symptoms arise immediately in the form of hives, watery eyes, sneezing, or difficulty breathing. They can even produce life-threatening anaphylactic shock. Only about 10% of autistic kids have this type of allergy. Some 85% of children with Autism have food sensitivities. Rather than immediate physical symptoms, these sensitivities produce and inflammatory response that results in more subtle mental and behavioral symptoms that can take anywhere from 6-72 hours to appear. The brain's primary fuels are oxygen and glucose which are manufactured from nutrients in our food supply. It only makes sense that we get out of our brains what we put into our bodies.

When it comes to the treatment of any neurological disorder, many parents and doctors focus solely on the obvious cognitive impairments and fail to realize that correcting their child or patient's underlying intestinal imbalances can; and often does, lead to significant overall improvement. Leaky gut syndrome which is so prevalant in children with Autism Spectrum Disorders causes a long list of vitamin and mineral deficiencies because the inflammation process damages the various carrier proteins normally present in healthy GI systems. Our plan is to treat our son from the inside out; Reduce the inflammation, test for vitamin and mineral deficiencies, provide necessary supplements, test for toxin poisoning and remove if necessary, provide therapy as needed, and set Gunnar up for the best possible outcome. When you feel better, you perform better. Who can argue with this rationale?

Many people have differing opinions on what does and doesn't work for families facing Autism. There is a saying in the Autism community, "If you have met one child with Autism, you have met one child with Autism" There is a broad spectrum with severe to mild physical and behavioral symptoms. One person's treatment protocol might not work for another person. I am not judging what others choose to do to treat their child, I am simply sharing what has worked for us thus far. I am not searching for or promising a cure, I am finding a treatment for and healing the symptoms that affect our son. Whether or not you agree with how my family and I choose to approach this journey does not change the outcome. If we have helped one person understand this complex neurological disorder, we have helped spread understanding, and that makes us happy. And, if you are a family facing Autism and don't know which avenue of treatment to pursue first, our advice is: Go with your gut.

---

80. Recovery #107

Having a sick child is a full time job. Even when they are well, your mind is filled with ways to keep them from getting sick again, ways to improve their current state, ways to help others who were where you were just a short time ago. It is my hope to do all three.

Autism entered my life a few years ago, but I didn't recognize it. My son, Gunnar was three when my husband and I realized he wasn't progressing as he should. He wasn't asking why, what, where, or when questions. He wasn't growing. He was lining up his trains and cars, screaming if we touched one of them. Gunnar was oppositional and refused to go into a crowded place. He didn't look anyone in the eye, and it seemed to make him uncomfortable to try. He had several sensory issues such as covering his ears when music played, even when the volume was low. He had an aversion to touch and would often yell, "ouch!" when someone touched his arm softly. He was constipated. He smeared his feces on the wall. He often woke in the middle of the night screaming. My husband or I would find him in the fetal position and he couldn't or didn't respond when we asked what hurt. Gunnar went ballistic when we tried to wash or cut his hair or brush his teeth. He was indifferent to me leaving for work, and what was most painful for me, he ran and hid when I returned. He didn't much care for his own mom and that was heart breaking for me.

We also noticed some regression. Gunnar stopped showing interest in potty training. He went from saying, "Gotta go pee pee!" to not even recognizing he'd soiled his pants. He started refusing foods he previously enjoyed. He went from using several words in succession to not speaking more than two words strung together. He started to be extremely picky when it came to the foods he would eat and spent most of his time at the dinner table staring out of the window. We were losing our son.

Our son was born with an autoimmune condition, Hypothyroidism. He started taking medication just three days after he was born. Initially my husband and I interpreted some of our son's Autism symptoms as side effects from his medication dosage fluctuations. After all, we voiced our concerns to his Pediatric Endocrinologist, and she assured us he was fine. She said the medication was likely making him lethargic. She said boys took longer to potty train. As time went on, Gunnar's symptoms multiplied and worsened, and other caregivers took notice and shared their concerns. At our son's next Endocrinologist appointment, I insisted on a referral for a developmental evaluation.

Our son was diagnosed with an Autism Spectrum Disorder in January of 2013. He was 4 years old. I immediately went into research mode reading everything I could get my hands on that was related to healing Autism. Two weeks after his diagnosis, we started a gluten, dairy, soy free diet and saw digestive issues disappearing. The night-waking was going away. He turned toward us when we called his name. He spoke in short sentences, requesting to watch a movie or eat a snack.

A month after Gunnar's diagnosis we had further testing done to see where he was on the spectrum. When we showed up for the appointment, the diagnostic team was impressed with our son's progress. He responded when they asked him to point to specific items, and he had no trouble matching items together. I remember thinking he was much smarter than I'd realized. Clearly the problem with our son was physical.

The test results showed Gunnar's speech and language to be at a 23 month old's level with his gross and fine motor skills not much further along. We were determined to heal our son and scheduled an appointment to have all kinds of testing done including food allergies, comprehensive stool analysis, and genetic mutation tests. These results showed that our son was sick with food allergies, leaky gut caused by an overgrowth of bacteria, and pathogens. We knew what we were up against. We were on the right track with diet, but had to find out how to get rid of the bacteria and pathogens. In my research, I stumbled upon the CD forum. It was the first treatment program that made complete sense to me.

We received the book in June. It was the first book our son ever showed interest in. He kept saying, "This is it!" and, "This book is the best!" He didn't want to put the book down. My husband and I looked at each other with tear-filled eyes. We knew Gunnar was right; this was it.

We started the CD Protocol immediately...just five months after our son's diagnosis. His starting ATEC was an 80. Immediately we saw regular bowel movements, diminished dark circles under his eyes, and healthy skin coloring. Gunnar began to sleep through the night. Four days into the protocol, our son started taking turns and sharing with other kids. That night, he danced at a graduation party. Every day, his vocabulary improved.

Four weeks into the protocol, our son no longer needed his thyroid medication he'd been on his entire life. He started using the bathroom unprompted. He dressed himself unprompted. He brushed his teeth on his own. Gunnar didn't mind getting his hair cut. He began to engage in reciprocal conversation.

Seven weeks into the protocol, we saw so many behavioral improvements; we decided to take the ATEC test again. Gunnar's score was a 40. It was cut in half in seven weeks!!! Eight weeks into the protocol our son celebrated his 5th birthday. It was the first time he showed anticipation for a party. He was excited to open his gifts and thanked everyone individually. Normally, Gunnar would run and play by himself when guests came over. He had always covered his ears and yelled, "Stop singing!" at previous parties. Gunnar was happy when everyone sang Happy Birthday to him. He was healthy and present. It was one of the happiest days of our lives.

Twelve weeks into the protocol, our son started mainstream preschool. All previous attempts to take him to school resulted in anxiety and complete meltdowns. He started speaking in complete sentences and his speech was relevant to the situation. He started showing interest in books. Fifteen weeks in, our son read his own bedtime story with no help. He picked out his own Halloween costume. He brought home his artwork and proudly showed it to us. His teachers continually voiced their pleasure at his progress. His speech therapist said he was at age level for speech and language. (that's 3 years worth of progress!)

Twenty-four weeks into the protocol, our son's ATEC score is a 10. He continues to go to mainstream preschool and is interested in learning. He is reading a variety of books. He is counting in English and Spanish. He knows his US geography, and does puzzles that are advanced for his age. He asks questions. His speech is appropriate and relevant with continued improvement in vocabulary and articulation. He loves to sing, dance, and paint. Our son is smart, funny, and very affectionate. He spontaneously hugs and kisses me and tells me he loves me. And the best part of all? When I come home from work, Gunnar yells, "Moooommmmyyyy!", runs up to me, jumps into my arms, and wraps his little arms around my neck. I have my son back.

I could never sufficiently thank Kerri Rivera for all of her selfless help. She and her team of parents give freely of their time and energy to bring kids and their families out of the depths of Autism. It is my hope to pay it forward. All children deserve a healthy childhood. If you are holding this book, you are likely in the position my family was in just 10 months ago. This is the way to turn your feelings of desperation into determination. This is the way to change the future for your family. This is the way out of Autism.

—Maggie Kaye

81. *Ok, my brother is 17 and started CD at the end of october. We are on 9 drops as of today. Non verbal. My mom called me crying and my brother said "I want snack please." My mom asked if he wanted something and he "no, no, no." He got his yogurt (df) out and said "thank you." This is just so amazing. Thank you God for putting us on this path and around so many amazing warrior parents to help us with our journey. Happy healing to all!!!*

---

82. *At the age of 3 our son was absent. He talked a lot... to himself. Scripting. It was almost impossible to get him to look into our eyes when we spoke to him. He almost never answered back, and when he did, it was scripting again (from a show on TV or a movie he was into.) He played by himself. He refused to potty train. He would wake up in the middle of the night crying and holding his stomach but was unable to tell us what was wrong. He stopped eating whatever we put in front of him and seemed to only want fruit snacks, American cheese, hot dogs, chicken nuggets and fries. And thats it. He didn't seem to be growing anymore, both physically and mentally. He seemed to be slipping away from us. You could see it in his eyes. Those eyes that were pointed off in a different direction. It was gradual...hard to notice right away. But definitely a change, and not one we were happy with.*

Up until this time he was progressing like any other child. He ate well. He slept well. He played well. Was even starting to potty train. A typical child. But not anymore. Then there was the diagnosis. Autism. No parent wants to hear that, but we knew. Every parent knows what I mean. You just know. And at this point we (as parents) have to make a choice.

We can choose to do nothing. Just live with it. We can listen to our doctor, or a specialist in the field. You know, someone who claims to know everything about you and your child in the 5 minutes they spend with you. Or you can talk to other parents. Parents that spend every moment with their children. Not just a few minutes every six months. You can network. You can research. Ask whats working for them, or more importantly what's not.

We chose the latter, and because of this our son is recovering. He looks into our eyes. He asks questions. He sleeps at night. He's potty trained. He sets the dinner table with his older sister and asks to be excused when he's done eating. He's in pre-school now and plays with all of the other kids. He calls them by name. He draws. He paints. He reads books. He does all of the things a typical five year old does.

Our son is recovering, and I need to give two heartfelt thanks for this. The first to my wife for the countless hours of reading and research she did immediately following our sons Autism diagnosis. She is an incredible woman who refuses to give up on anything. Ever. She refused to believe that we had to accept what was handed to us. She knew in her heart and mind that we could make a difference. We just had to do it. Because of this determination, she found Kerri Rivera, whom is the next person I want to thank. She is a true pioneer, someone who refused to keep thinking inside the box, someone who is helping families like ours all over the world.

"We have the world at our fingertips. Every book, every encyclopedia for us to read at our local library, in our own homes, and now on (most) of our cell

phones. It's a beautiful tool for us to use. Use it. Do your own research. Talk with parents. Find out what works and do it.

The only thing I really have to say about Kerri's book and the protocol it explains is that it works. We have our son back.

—Kenn Kaye, Father of Gunnar Kaye

---

83. Last night, my 19 year old son came out into the kitchen, picked up a purple straw from the dish drainer, and pretended to play it like a clarinet with great enthusiasm. Pretend play. For the first time in 19 years.

---

84. We've been playing the "healing game" with my son for some time, (7 years 11 months old) but we've never really healed anything. To be honest we've never known what we were up against...until now. Like everyone here, my child is very sick. He doesn't grow, he has maldigestion and malabsorption issues and he's chronically constipated. His history of constipation is long and extensive. ANYTHING that disrupted his gut flora would result in this extreme constipation; whether it was a cold, a new food, treating the GI. To say he has leaky gut is a tremendous understatement. So, when we started Kerri's protocol 6/15 my biggest health markers for initial healing were growth and for him to poop daily on his own. With his history being what it is I wasn't surprised to see he was instantly constipated. How could he not be? We are killing pathogens and parasites like gang busters. We started enemas on day two and have done them daily. But, an amazing thing is happening! He is healing. He has grown two inches in these last three months and he starting to poop on his own. BTW, these aren't just lame little poops they are total TROPHY poops. They are soft, formed, have no undigested food and there is lots (I'd show you a picture but we barely know each other)

Yep... It's taken 3.5 months to get here, but his little; fragile and damaged body is doing what it is supposed to do.

Trust the process... It's not easy; it's not always fast. There will be ups and downs. But, my gosh, watching the body heal is an extraordinary thing. It's nothing short of a miracle.

---

85. Hi Kerri,

I started my son on the CD last night. I'm taking it with him.

Well, I for one, feel fabulous. My lungs are clearing up, the low-level depression I felt is evaporating. Wow!!!

I've noticed some subtle changes in my son. He is more "with us" in the world and not looking out the window at cars quite as much. Also, a little less flapping his hands.

He and I have been doing a ketogenic version of the GAPS diet (no sweet vegetables, no dairy, no sweeteners) since January of 2013, and I think that's why we've been so successful with the CD! :)

I was thinking of upping it to two drops per 8 oz bottle--one for him, one 8 oz bottle for me.

I am hoping that Sulfur is Ok to still give him. We used to cut it with Kombucha, but that is now a no-no.

Thanks and Huzzah!

86. Ryan is the first of our 3 children to recover. Ryan was not considered autistic by most standards but did score a 19 on the ATEC test prior to starting the CD protocol. He is 9 years old and has been in mainstream classes without an IEP. We did hold him and his twin brother back one year prior to starting kindergarten so they could have more time to heal from Lyme Disease which we had been treating since they were 4.

Ryan was a healthy baby but I did notice after saying his first words at the appropriate age, he stopped talking a few months later. (I now know that is a symptom of autism!) And both he and his brother were very late with language despite knowing their alphabet at a very young age. Ryan did eventually talk but was often hyperactive and had a hard time sitting still in class or at the dinner table. It was often hard to get his attention and to get him to listen to requests. He was constipated since he was a baby and was a very picky eater. I dreaded mealtimes because it was so hard to get him to eat. We often had to spoon-feed food into his mouth even when he was 7 years old. Treatment for Lyme Disease helped many of his symptoms but he still had some remaining symptoms such as weakness, stomachaches, seeing orange and blue spots at night (more noticeable in the dark), nightmares, bedwetting, difficulty falling asleep and early awakening, and overly emotional and irrational behavior. These symptoms worsened dramatically when our house well water became contaminated with parasites and bacteria. It took us two years to figure out that the water was the cause of our deteriorating health. During this time, Ryan became unable to play sports or have play dates without melting into irrational tantrums when things didn't go his way. When playing mini golf, he refused to finish the round after getting a score of "10" on one hole and had a crying tantrum. In tennis class, he would sit down on the court and start crying if he didn't get to hit as many balls as the other children on the court with him. We didn't even attempt to put him in team sports for fear that he would melt down and storm off, refusing to play the rest of the game.

Then we discovered CD and Kerri's protocol, and his and our lives changed forever. Within three weeks of taking CD, Ryan's ATEC dropped to an 8. This improvement was the difference in Ryan being able to play sports. He was able to play on a baseball team and while he did get angry if he struck out or made an error, I was there with a dose of CD and that would keep him from a complete meltdown. As the season continued, Ryan's emotions became more and more stable and normal. His energy increased greatly and now after 6 months on the protocol, Ryan is playing three different sports, taking piano lessons and excelling in above grade level reading and math. His ATEC is a 3 but we will continue until it is 0. His first report card since starting the protocol was the best of his life. We were most excited to see that his scores for behavior and attention were above expectations. Last year, these same scores were all below expectations because Ryan was so hyperactive and unable to focus due to the parasites. Ryan still sees a few orange spots at night but they are diminishing and we know they will be gone so long as we stick with this protocol until he is completely healed. We are so grateful that Kerri blazed the way for us all by developing this protocol. I have been searching for the past 7 years for a way to fully heal my children and the CD was the last but most significant piece of the puzzle for us. We will be forever thankful to you Kerri!

87. I first heard about CD, then called MMS, to treat autism in May 2012 and wanted to try it out with my then 10-year-old son. I bought supplies, and did the then-current protocol for a few months, but then school ended and summer vacations started and I put CD on the back burner or did it very sporadically. My son was verbal and high functioning, but still had lots of autistic behaviors. His ATEC score in 2012 was 27.

I started reading about CD again in the summer of 2013. This time there was more information out there. Kerri had written her breakthrough book and lots of facebook friends in the autism community were mentioning it. I bought the book and dove in, first using my old supplies (CD with citric acid) then buying HCl and trying that. My son did very well with the new protocol, starting low and getting to full dose around the time of his 12th birthday at the end of August. I started seeing worms before we even started our first Parasite Protocol! When I started the Parasite Protocol and added in ocean water, things kept getting better! No set-backs or regressions. School was seemingly much easier for my son. He was in a mainstream class with resource room help for reading and writing for the second year, but this year, math homework was no longer taking several hours, but 20 minutes! His reading comprehension was improving as well, and more importantly, I didn't worry about hearing about behavioral issues anymore!

I wanted to complete three months of CD before I took another ATEC. When I filled in out in November, at the start of our third Parasite Protocol, I was shocked to see a score of 7! My son had dropped 20 points from his 2012 score! Seeing the single digit score was so amazing! My son had been diagnosed with autism at age 2 ½ and there were no options given to me at the time. An early IQ test given by a speech therapist had shown he was mentally retarded and that was that. However, I looked into everything I could, and was not going to give up on my son. So glad I didn't! Nine years of autism, but the beginning of his 12th year marks the end of it! I know his ATEC score will be 0 soon!

---

88. "thank you for your help in recovering me"

This is what my son just typed to me this morning on his iPad with the app we use for supportive typing!

Thank you Kerri & Patrick for all you have done and continue to do!

Without you BOTH, we would NEVER be in the place we are right now... HEALING & RECOVERY!

Just know you are LOVED!

—Melissa in Indiana

---

89. Sophia was born on March 9, 2006. She was a typical happy baby who slept well and seldom got sick. She met all of her developmental milestones and laughed and made great eye contact. When she turned one just after her vaccines she became violently ill and vomited with fever for 2 days straight. After that she was never the same, her smile was rare and words were gone. When she was nineteen months after more shots, we took her to an ear doctor out of concern that she was not responding to her name or speaking clear words. Her hearing was tested and we were told she was fine and to give her time. After a few months of no change her pediatrician determined that she was developmentally-

delayed and had all the symptoms of Autism. We were stunned and unprepared for this news. I went into warrior mode and ended up with a DAN dr, who started her on lots of supplements after initial lab results showed heavy metal toxicity and high amounts of intestinal yeast. We followed the program and advice of this doctor for the last 4 years with the only change being dietary fluctuations. Sophia did improve but hit a plateau where no new gains were made in the last year or so, so in May 2013 her DAN doctor suggested that we do another round of stool testing after a urine acid test showed bad bacteria overgrowth and terrible mito issues. Her comment to me was "this kid's DNA is so messed up, I haven't seen a test this bad since the 1990's." This was after thousands of dollars and too many supplements to count. I was done at that point. There were no answers there obviously. I came across this protocol on a Facebook page for autism parents and purchased Kerri's book in September 2013. I immediately knew that this was the answer for my daughter. I had a gut instinct that she would be healed . We started the diet immediately and CD just after. My daughter had been a juice addict before this and I was worried about her taking the CD and being able to drink the water. This was only an issue for a day or so. I have not missed a day of giving her 8 or more doses. We get up very early and dose her ocean water and 2 CD doses before school. On weekends we are doing 16 doses/day. In the second week we started seeing some herxheimer/die off, very sleepy followed by fevers. This is when the transformation started! I followed the fever protocol and did enemas and she got better. She also had an episode around week 7 of very red throat and fever which we double dosed for and resolved. We have seen a withdrawn, self -focused child with little interest in the world outside of herself disappear and turn into a child interested in friendship with peers, reading books and understanding the story (huge!), and having relevant conversation with great eye contact. She gets all A's at school and has made a complete turnaround with behavior. We have so much hope for her future and she is blossoming into a beautiful, happy girl!

90. Here are a few of the emails I mentioned from my son's therapist in regard to what's happening at therapy! :)

This is an email from the exact day I restarted the CD, which was August 21 of 2013.

We discovered a new game today. He was being a turkey and running up the hall to try to get around me to get places he wasn't supposed to go. I started singing (to the tune of rolling down the river) about whatever he was doing "walking, walking, walking down the hallway" "jumping, jumping jumping down the hallway" climbing, climbing, climbing up the ladder. He thought it was hilarious, especially when I'd change in the middle of a verse "running running, jumping down the hallway.

—Your son's therapist

Great day today! Vail seems to be understanding first, then sequencing and I think I finally have a bribe for him--he loves our fish.

Also, he made a friend today. One of our other pt's was playing in the gym and he was watching him, imitating him a little and said his name 2x!

—Your son's therapist

We tried to play the game and he wasn't interested. Instead we ended up pushing the fisher price horse, sheep, goat, and cow off the treehouse. He would "randomly" produce sounds which we took for requests for the animal associated. Then we would give him the animal "requested." Reviewed his sound cards and he produced the /n/ and /h/. Coulda sworn he said go a couple of times, and mom said she heard a whispered "home." Listen and be watchful for whispers! Oftentimes children with apraxia can get one system working but not the other, ie. articulate with no sound, or vocalize with intonation and no articulation, like when he says "ah uh oo" for "I love you." Yep, he does that! Cheers!

91. Hi had to share this moment today, just wish daddy wouldn't have missed it!

Well, we were seeing daddy off for work this evening, when Vail decided that he wanted to go run around in the grass. I told him we needed to put on socks and shoes and then we could play outside. He walked straight to the door, we walked in, I pointed at his socks and shoes, and FOR THE FIRST TIME EVER (always knew he could, just to stubborn to do it unless he really wants too!) he promptly walked over, picked up his socks and shoes and turned and handed them to me!!! (all the while doing it with an attitude!!!"lol)

This is Just from MOM to therapists. :)

CD and Kerri have been life changing for our entire family. We now can give Vail choices, usually of two items. For example I showed him two pairs of pants and asked which he wanted to wear, and he grabbed one pair and started to put them on even though he was still in his pj's. I showed him two shirts, and he picked a shirt. Same thing with his shoes and socks, he is able to choose now on his own. I look forward everyday to him doing something differently or completely new, and he almost always does now!!! This was not possible for CD!!! THANK YOU KERRI !!! WE LOVE YOU FOR SHARING AND FIGHTING THE FIGHT!!!

LOVE,

—The parents of Vail

92. Best day of the entire school year! My son initiated verbal interactions 5 times today and responded to his teacher in a group over 5 times, WITHOUT A SINGLE PROMPT! Most days his TA is poking him to pay attention and ask other kids for directions, rather than an adult, all day long! She is tracking these interactions as they are his IEP goals.

93. Casey is a young man who is 17 years old today, and the estimated ATEC score from 2006 is from when he was 10 years old. Proving once again that recovery is possible at any age.

Casey H. ATEC History	ATEC Estimated 10/12/2006	Start CD 5/6/2013	3 months 8/6/2013	6 months 11/6/2013
I. Speech/Language/Communication	6	1	1	2
II. Sociability	14	11	3	0
III. Sensory/Cognitive/Awareness	25	13	6	5
IV. Health/Physical/Behavior	39	28	8	5
TOTAL ATEC SCORE:	84	53	18	12

94. Daniel - beginning ATEC June 2013 - 101. Today ATEC Nov 12, 2013 - 44! We are thru our 3rd PP and starting speech supplements. Speech, by far, has been the hardest thing. In all other areas he is under "10" on the ATEC! Kerri Rivera words are coming. This week alone he is saying "Hi" and "Bye" and trying to say others. I can't wait to hear "I love you Mom"! You are the Bomb Diggitty Kerri. We all love you!

    UPDATE: December 3rd, 2013

    I officially want to tell the world that my son, Daniel, who has autism is nonverbal no more! He is starting to talk. Praise God! This battle has been the struggle of my life, but i have learned to trust God, be patient, and enjoy the journey! Where some take a lot for granted regarding their children, I have been waiting almost 7 yrs to hear his beautiful voice! And thank God he has one! Autism is treatable and there is hope!

95. We had a super exciting trip, we went to a therapist on the 28th who teaches Rapid Prompting Method. We have tried since by daughter was diagnosed to get her to speak, but haven't had any luck yet, she is now 11. We thought we would give RPM a try to see if the therapist could get her to communicate.

    We not only found out that she is able to make correct choices, but can actually SPELL! Her very first word that she spelled was CLOUD!

    Later on in the session the therapist asked her what her favorite color was... she spelled out PINK!

    I was sitting on the floor in awe... For the first time in 11 years, I finally know what my girl's favorite color is... it was surreal... it was amazing... she is so smart, but had no way of letting us know... I am soooooooo proud of her!

96. Diagnosed at 20 months old in August 2011

    Started supplements under Dan in September 2011

    Started CD / PP on July 1, 2013, after seeing rope in stool

    Starting ATEC on July 1, 2013, was 46

    Present ATEC 22

    Gained 5 pounds from July 1st to present!

    Too many improvements to list!!!!!

    Also doing GcMAF which has also helped......but, I believe GcMAF may have helped more with the viral load. I suspect this because we actually started IV GcMAF in January 2013, before CD . Huge gains with GcMAF but after 35 shots, her gut was still a mess and GcMAF definitely didn't help with the gut. Found Kerri in July 2013, and began our healing journey.

The following lab results are proof of just how well the child described above is doing since starting the protocol. Here is what her mom had to say:

> "The original test was taken last August of 2012, which showed a deficiency in almost everything despite the fact that my daughter had been on supplements for over a year at that point. The re-test was just taken October 2013, only 4 months after CD / PP and removal of ALL supplements. Wow!"

You can see in the second test that her high viral titers were reduced as well.

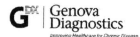

Genova
Diagnostics
Improving Healthcare for Chronic Disease

83 Zillicoa Street
Asheville, NC 28801
© Genova Diagnostics

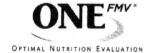

ONE FMV *
OPTIMAL NUTRITION EVALUATION

Patient: B
DOB: November 18, 2009
Sex: F

Completed: August 27, 2012
Received: August 21, 2012
Collected: August 13, 2012

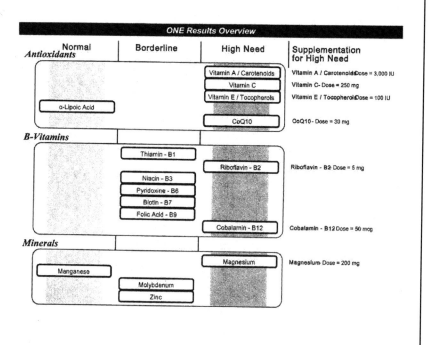

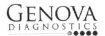

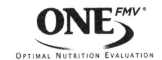

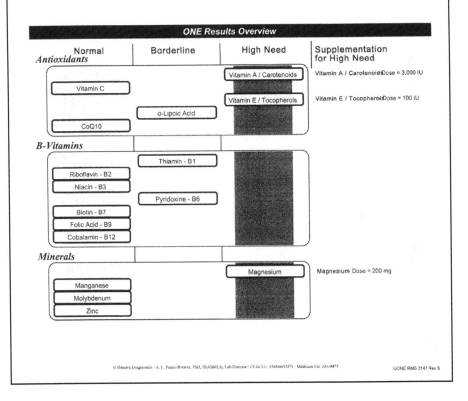

Patient Copy

63 Zillicoa Street
Asheville, NC 28801
© Genova Diagnostics

OPTIMAL NUTRITION EVALUATION

Patient: B
DOB: November 18, 2009
Sex: F

Completed: October 28, 2013
Received: October 18, 2013
Collected: October 17, 2013

ONE Results Overview

Antioxidants

Normal	Borderline	High Need	Supplementation for High Need
Vitamin C		Vitamin A / Carotenoids	Vitamin A / Carotenoids Dose = 3,000 IU
	α-Lipoic Acid	Vitamin E / Tocopherols	Vitamin E / Tocopherols Dose = 100 IU
CoQ10			

B-Vitamins

Normal	Borderline	High Need
	Thiamin - B1	
Riboflavin - B2		
Niacin - B3	Pyridoxine - B6	
Biotin - B7		
Folic Acid - B9		
Cobalamin - B12		

Minerals

Normal	Borderline	High Need	
		Magnesium	Magnesium Dose = 200 mg
Manganese			
Molybdenum			
Zinc			

© Genova Diagnostics - A. L. Peace-Brewer, PhD, D(ABMLI), Lab Director - CLIA Lic. #34D0065571 - Medicare Lic. #04-8475

UONE RMS 3147 Rev 5

LabCorp

	Patient Name						
B.C.							
	Patient ID	Control Number	Date and Time Collected	Date Reported	Sex	Age(Y/M/D)	Date of Birth
			08/21/12 11:21	08/25/12	F	2/09/03	11/18/09

TESTS	RESULT	FLAG	UNITS	REFERENCE INTERVAL	LAB
Zinc, Whole Blood	478		ug/dL	440 - 860	01

Anti-DNase B Strep Antibodies

	<71		U/mL	0 - 77	01

Results verified by repeat testing
Limit of assay detection is <71

Rubeola Antibodies, IgG

Rubeola Ab, IgG, EIA	4.33	High	index	0.00 - 0.90	02
			Negative	<0.91	
			Equivocal	0.91 - 1.09	
			Positive	>1.09	

Presence of antibodies to Rubeola is presumptive evidence of immunity except when active infection is suspected.

Human Herpes Virus Type 6 IgM

	<1:10			Neg:<1:10	04

Results for this test are for research purposes only by the assay's manufacturer. The performance characteristics of this product have not been established. Results should not be used as a diagnostic procedure without confirmation of the diagnosis by another medically established diagnostic product or procedure.

➤ **HHV 6 IgG Antibodies** (7.66) **High** ◄ index   01
			Negative	<0.76	
			Equivocal	0.76 - 0.99	
			Positive	>0.99	

Results for this test are for research purposes only by the assay's manufacturer. The performance characteristics of this product have not been established. Results should not be used as a diagnostic procedure without confirmation of the diagnosis by another medically established diagnostic product or procedure.

Antigliadin Abs, IgG

Deamidated Gliadin Abs, IgG	15		units	0 - 19	02
			Negative	0 - 19	
			Weak Positive	20 - 30	
			Moderate to Strong Positive	>30	

HSV Type 2-Specific Ab, IgG

HSV 2 IgG, Type Spec	<0.91		index	0.00 - 0.90	02
			Negative	<0.91	
			Equivocal	0.91 - 1.09	
			Positive	>1.09	

➤ **Rubella Antibodies, IgG** (58) | IU/mL | | 01
			Non-immune	<5	◄
			Equivocal	5 - 9	
			Immune	>9	

Quest Diagnostics   Page 2 of 4   10/17/2013   04:07:42 PM   **Report Status: Final**

Patient Information	Specimen Information	Client Information
B.C. DOB: 11/18/2009 AGE: 3 Gender: F Fasting: U Patient ID: NG	Collected: 10/07/2013 Received: 10/07/2013 / 21:37 EDT Reported: 10/17/2013 / 14:42 EDT	

Test Name	In Range	Out Of Range	Reference Range	Lab

A positive result indicates that the patient has
antibody to CMV. It does not differentiate between
an active or past infection.

RUBELLA IMMUNE STATUS   QHO
→ RUBELLA ANTIBODY (IGG)   (3.13)
```
                      Value          Interpretation
                      -----          --------------
                      < or = 0.90    Negative
                      0.91-1.09      Equivocal
                      > or = 1.10    Positive
```

The presence of rubella IgG antibody suggests
immunization or past or current infection with
rubella virus.

EPSTEIN BARR VIRUS VCA   QHO
```
  AB (IGG)                    < OR = 0.90              index
                      Index          Interpretation
                      < or = 0.90    Negative
                      0.91 - 1.09    Equivocal
                      > or = 1.10    Positive
```

DNASE B ANTIBODY   <95   < 251 U/mL   SLI
MEASLES ANTIBODY (IGG)   4.09   index   QHO
```
        Index          Explanation of Test Results
        ----------     ----------------------------
        < or = 0.90    Negative - No Rubeola (Measles) IgG
                                  Antibody detected
        0.91 - 1.09    Equivocal
        > or = 1.10    Positive - Rubeola (Measles) IgG
                                  Antibody detected
```

Positive results suggest recent or previous infection
with Measles (Rubeola) virus and imply immunity.
Patients exhibiting equivocal results should be
retested in one month, if clinically indicated.

HERPESVIRUS-6 ANTIBODIES   XE
  (IGG,IGM)
→ HERPESVIRUS 6 IGG   1:80 H
→ HERPESVIRUS 6 IGM   <1:20
  INTERPRETATION   PAST INFECTION

```
    REFERENCE RANGE:  IgG  <1:10
                      IgM  <1:20
```

Human Herpesvirus 6 (HHV-6) infects T-lymphocytes,
and has been identified as an etiologic agent of
exanthema subitum. Rises in antibody titers to
HHV-6 have been detected during infection with
other viruses. In seroepidemiology studies of the
prevalence of exposure using serum screening
dilutions of 1:10, the detection of IgG antibody
in a mid-life population approaches 100%. Due to
this high prevalence of HHV-6 antibody,

PAGE 2 OF 4

Testimonials from the First Edition Continue Here...

97. *Meeting a Rescue Angel*

  The way OUT of AUTISM

  My 5 year old little daughter, Anna's story has been long and paved with lots of suffering and doubt, compared to her age, but prayers have always helped us in our journey. We are aware that it may take years to get out of the dark depths of Autism but now we know we are going in the right direction. Finally! Thanks to Kerri Rivera, the Rescue Angel of so many suffering children. She showed us the way out!

  We have wasted so much time by trying to face the fact, that unfortunately there is a problem with our perfectly healthy-born daughter. After the consultation with many doctors, they first suspected a hearing problem. As the result of this, she went under many surgeries and antibiotic-treatments, which made her state worse mentally and physically as well. The medical professionals could not find any evidence of physical abnormalities, so they choose the easy way out, the one word diagnosis of Autism! Dear Mom, please accept it, you cannot do anything about it. Try some developmental therapies, but do not put your hopes high!

  It is very hard to accept the unexplainable. What does autism mean? If you google it, you will find the verdict immediately: "Autism is a lifelong developmental disability characterized by impaired social interaction and communication, and by restricted and repetitive behavior" How is it possible that a perfectly developing child changes overnight? She stops saying the words she said before; she stops paying attention when called by her name and simply forgets some of her skills she knew so well before. How can one accept that? For us, it was impossible. We took up the gauntlet!

  We spent so many sleepless nights on the Internet searching for solutions, to be shortly shocked to learn that in the US, there is a totally different concept and approach to autism. A group of medical professionals and scientists are proving the crucial role of environment and vaccines in the rapid rise of autism, accepting genetics as not the single cause but a factor of susceptibility to the disease. More and more so called DAN (Defeat Autism Now) clinics and practitioners are treating children on the spectrum all over the world with different biomedical interventions with various success rates. Whichever method one chooses in their realm, the base line to all is a strict diet, especially free from gluten, casein and sugar. There is no way out without eliminating these from the diet of an autistic child.

  We immediately changed her diet from a bread and butter with chocolate milk style to a much stricter one. The first items to remove were sugar, gluten and casein, but these were shortly followed by potato, rice, corn and all artificial additives. We slowly changed to SCD (Specific Carbohydrate Diet). A few days into the diet and Anna slept through the night, and what's more, the painful eczema spots that had been on her face since she was a baby have shortly disappeared. Parallel with the diet modifications we also started the DAN interventions. We spent a fortune on lab testing, supplements and to see a DAN practitioner in Germany. Unfortunately none of these brought us significant improvements.

  But I knew and believed that there has to be a solution.

And yes! I cannot keep it to myself and I would like to spread the word happily, powerfully and self-confidently, that there is a solution! This year in August, I have found the presentation of Kerri Rivera on the internet. Autism is preventable, avoidable, treatable and curable."

At the beginning "Kerri Rivera rose against the wind rather than with it when, after a frustrating slew of hits and misses, her youngest son, Patrick, was diagnosed with autism nine years ago. He was two at the time. Surrounded by literally no local expertise or any type of peer support circle, she did what most mothers would do: She became informed and involved in the biomedical community. It was through the Autism Research Institute (www.autism.com), a non-profit organization dedicated to autism research, diagnosis and treatment for the past 40 years, that she learned about a specialized biomedical protocol involving a special diet and supplements, physical therapy, applied behavioral analysis, chelation and hyperbaric treatment. There was light for Patrick, Kerri's son at the end of the tunnel."

But Kerri did not stop here! As she told me, she felt that there was a missing piece to the autism puzzle. A huge piece! It shortly turned out to be the MMS piece. She developed MMS protocol which can be done at home. Following Kerri's protocol, 68 children lost their autism diagnosis in the past two years! This result is outstanding, considering the fact that this is said to be an incurable disease.

The day I saw her presentation I e-mailed her and I got an answer within a half an hour. Kerri Rivera's MMS protocol is the missing piece of the puzzle to cure autism, ADHD, asthma, allergies, seizure disorders. Even mothers of children with Down Syndrome have reported improvements with this protocol.

My whole family was in Mexico in August. We spent two months with the person, who is also a mother of a child with autism, who sacrificed part of her life to help others. For free, out of faith, humanity and love. Approximately 8-900 children are following Kerri's protocol currently all over the world. The protocol is available for everybody and can be done at home (www.mmsautism.com).

Anna is getting better every day. Although we have heard very promising sounds from her, speech is not developed yet. However she has improved a lot in the last 3 months in many other areas like mood, communication, learning ability, focus and attention span are all better and she started pointing. There were no signs of these at the beginning of the summer.

We are fully aware that there is still a long journey ahead of us, but now we know we are on the right track. Thanks to God and Kerri Rivera to guide us to recovery!

---

98. Hi Kerri,

    PLEASE use our testimony. MMS kept my daughter's PANDAS under control after switching from Silver Hydrosol BUT the biggest is the PP's (parasite protocols) in combo with MMS. She began sleeping through the night, THEN, sleeping in her own room after sleeping in our room for 9 months. THEN she began putting herself to sleep for the first time in 7 years. We always laid with her--her WHOLE life--I KNEW it was NOT "behavorial", knew it was due to something going on interally, AND NOW, we read, kiss, and WALK OUT of her room! It's SURREAL really. Seriously SURREAL!

Also, she was a chronic chewer, nose picker. Almost GONE! Peaks at new and full moon, BUT goes away. She was chewing about 20 straws a day before PP! Mangling them! UNREAL! I have pics of the straws... cant even recognize them as a "straw" once she was done with them. CLEARLY parasites. CLEARLY on the right track. NO other interventions. Except for how the MMS PP protocol is outlined MINUS Rhompe etc.. and Neem. NO sleep intervention supps etc.. None.

---

99. Favy is my God sent angel. He is 4 years old and since he was born he came to change lives, to make families stronger and to help others forgive. As many of your stories, everything was "perfect" (besides of milk intoleration, delay speech and sleeping problems) the rest was great, milestones on time.. Then gradually after 13to 18 month something was clearly wrong, we loose him and then the bomb!: diagnosed in Puerto Rico by a developmental pediatrician and a neurologist as PDD-NOS on December 6, 2010.

We moved fast and start the diet GFCFSFYF no sugars.. Etc Thanks to CEA non- profit organization who help parents with kids with autism. Soon we saw positive changes, then probiotics and a natural anti fungal. Difficult days... But always seeing little good things. On march 2011 I met an angel: Kerri Rivera and we start MMS protocol!!! Then we start to see the light! We moved to FL and they diagnosed him (now I know he was having a die off when reevaluate) he was diagnosed as Autism. For me , not a big differences, still in the spectrum and he still sick!!! We need to cure him!!!

After MMS the big changes came ,and still coming!!

first from 2 to 4 hours straight per night to 6to 9 straight during night plus a nap during day!!!!! Eye contact was much better and he had less tantrums. He learned fast 3 signs to communicate. He was more happy. I didn't see more great results because I was using Mms incorrectly for almost a year (with juice, antioxidants and vit c) When a couple of months ago I started doing it right (just water and no vit c nor antioxidants etc) he started to improve again and better.. After a lot of efforts, dedication, patience and hours of hard work, with Kerri Rivera MMS protocol Favy to improved in many areas.

This is all he have improved:

Educational:
*   Respond to his name when called and say his name when ask.
*   Recognize people: Mommy, Daddy, Sister, Teachers, Therapists, friends
*   Name and identify some body parts: eyes, nose, mouth, ears, belly, feet
*   Recognize some animals (Ipad application or tv) : cow, horse, duck, chicken, zebra turtle.
*   Recognize some colors: blue, yellow, purple, red.
*   Recognize and count 1-10 (can repeat 11, 13)
*   Recognize and/ or use some common objects: plate, spoon, fork, bottle, chair, pants, shirt, shoes, backpack, lunch box, blanket, pillow, tv, books, some toys, ball, cars.
*   Stack objects like blocks, books

* Match pictures, objects or things.
* Color independently but refuses, he can trace but hand over hand.

Social / Emotional:

* He enjoyed for the first time his birthday Party, he was happy! He opened his presents and show emotions!!!
* He is beginning to interact more with others.
* He can follow direction of 1 step and some cases of 2. (clean up your plate to the sink and push your chair.)
* He is affectionate : kisses, hugs, eye contact is better.
* Wave and say bye.
* Greet with a good morning or good night.
* Play around and with others: chase, tickles, peek-a-boo,
* Dancing and imitating some song rituals like: The wheels on the bus, If you are happy, head shoulders knees and toes, and some in Spanish too.
* Throw, push, blow, pull, jump, run, walk, go up and down stairs, climb, open, close, zip, unzip,
* He can watch an ABC DVD seated or lay down , dancing or repeating.
* He can be seated for almost 5 to 8 minutes with his favorite books.
* He enjoys to go to playgrounds, go up and down slide or swing.
* He enjoyed the trick or treating this year, going house to house picking candy and wore all night his costume.

Comunication:

* I think this is the area of more improvement. From 0 to almost 35 words and different ways to label, request, interact and communicate!
* He can answer questions with yes or no (yeah- nah)
* He signs (modified) more, all done, juice
* He can use 3 words at a time (mommy water please, mommy come here, I love you, mommy ipad please, mommy hungry, eat)
* Say independently—not all of the sound clear but very similar sounds.
* Mommy
* Dadda
* On
* Yes(yeah)
* No (nah)
* Please (peas)
* All done (ah dah)
* More (mor)
* Water (at-ter)
* go
* Four
* Three
* Tickles

* *Zebra (eebah)*
* *Turtle (totlo)*
* *Uh oh!*
* *Oh No!*
* *I Love You!*
* *Under*

When Prompting or Repeat:

* *Tv (tetete)*
* *Dvd (dededah)*
* *Off*
* *Come (she)*
* *Itch (each)*
* *Scratch (ach)*
* *Bubbles (babah)*
* *Bye (bah)*
* *Swing (win)*
* *Push (pah-sh)*
* *Five (hi)*
* *Nine (nun)*
* *Ten (ttn)*
* *Baby*
* *Ble (buh)*
* *Purple (por-po)*
* *Yellow (ye-yo)*
* *Chase (ch sound)*
* *Play (ay or pah)*
* *He can imitate some animal sounds like tiger, horse and wolf.*
* *He make choices between to objects . (playing, dressing, eating)*
* *Independent Functioning (he needs some prompting)*
* *He eats independently with spoon and clean up after finished.*
* *He can drink of a regular cup.*
* *With pictures or social stories he can transition to different activities.*
* *He is showing understanding of routines and rules. (dvd or toy stay home, 2 minutes and we are all-done)*
* *He can pull up and down his pants (multiple prompt)*
* *He can put his shirt on but need assistance to take it off.*
* *He can pick up and put on hamper his clothes.*
* *He can put his shoes (crocs) independently and cooperates with other type.*
* *He move furniture to reach what he wants.*

Health:

Favy still in the Gluten, Casein, Soy, Yeast, Antibiotics and Hormones free diet. He is trying new textures, flavors and consistency in a variety of food allowed.

He is drinking more water. MMS help us every time he have a cold, a mosquito bite aor nasal allergies. Is the best product we can ever find!

We are excited about all he learned, do and know during this last year because of the use of the protocol of MMS. We are proud of his efforts, but we still have areas to improve. We will continue with MMS, diet and wil start the parasite protocol with faith because MMS Rocks!!!!

We love you Godmother Kerri! God Bless you and your Family.

---

100. Conversation at pick up:

    Aide: "What did you spike his breakfast with this morning? I've never seen him like this!"

    Me: *smile* "Oh glad he had a good day"...in my head...'three doses of MMS before drop off'...

    This child is going to figure out he has wings and start to SSSSOOOOAAAARRR!!!!

---

101. I have a 4-year-old son on the autism spectrum and MMS has been the most effective treatment we have tried for him. He had bad eczema on his legs for over a year that I was never able to get rid of. We tried diet, medication, cream and nothing seemed to clear it up. Within 2 weeks of starting MMS it was completely gone and has not returned. My son has made great strides in the past 5 months of being on MMS and the parasite protocol. He is more interactive with all the members of the family, talking more, and becoming more successful with his OT goals.

---

102. Kerri; Thank you all for your great job. Because through the Webinar—Autism and MMS—the information has come to me and gave me the strength to start a treatment.

---

103. Hi Kerri,

    My wife and I did an ATEC on 8 year old son and it came in at 7. Wow.

    We're learning so much from you about how this whole recovery thing works. The child's health takes three steps forward then two steps back then three steps forward then two steps back...but over time that one extra step forward seems to slowly add up. His pee is smelly again but, as you taught us, it's pee-tox and this is a good thing. His focus is still a bit of a challenge at school and he still won't shut up :-) but we are feeling that he truly is slowing getting better.

    We've got a ways to go yet but we feel that we are truly moving forward. Thanks so much for all of the help you've given us and any help you might be able to give in the future.

---

104. My son is 19 years old. We started MMS in July. For 2 months my son did not sleep. The end of August at full oral dose we started the baths. At night you could see he was uncomfortable. I don't know how we did it but we talked him into doing enemas. My husband does it. They induce him to have a bowel movement.

    Before enemas my son would have nights where you heard him walking back and forth from his bed to the toilet. In the morning I would say you had a bad night *last night, what was your problem? He would spell constipation. He doesn't seem to be doing this since the enemas.*

On Saturday 11-10 our son went to the first day of the season Special needs Ice Hockey. He is just learning. There were no problems with him about anything. In fact for the first time he put on his hockey gloves without objecting, which we have been trying to do the last 2 years. He followed directions from a volunteer on the ice, using his hockey stick to hit the puck back and forth to him and towards the goal. When hockey was over we went outside and hung out at the car and did nothing for about 20 minutes and had a dose of MMS. He did not care one bit. He entertained himself by watching the sea gulls. He was not impatient.

Next we walked over to the bowling alley, which is next door to the ice rink. He participated in special needs bowling. They have the bumpers up so the kids don't get gutter balls. My son actually threw some balls that didn't hit the bumpers. There were times in the past where every ball he threw hit the bumpers. Again there was not a single problem, incident, or signs of agitation from him while we were there. This is the first time in his life where we were able to go from one activity to another and not have an upset. He enjoyed himself.

What was really interesting was that he usually stims with a container of pumpkin seeds when he is in the car or at the bowling alley. This Saturday he left the container of seeds at home and not once did he even ask for them while we were out.

My son asks for a heating pad, which he has been doing for years. We wonder is it worms that have been causing all this pain for him? We would love to eliminate the pain, the repetitive behaviors, and the prompting through self-help and activities. He does lay around a lot. Everything he does is at a slow pace. He lacks stamina and speed for appropriate activities.

---

105. *Hi Kerri, my daughter's first atec was 85. We just did it again and it is now 55! :) :) (approximately 2 months on MMS)*

---

106. *Hi Kerri,*

I just wanted to let you know that we are up to 30 drops per 8 oz bottle and now I'm seeing some new things. He used future tense this morning (he sticks larry boys super suction ear to his window and waits for him to fall) This morning he said "Larry boy will fall." Usually when he falls he says in his high pitched voice "are you ok". Today when Larry Boy fell he said in a deep 11 year old voice "ouch". I just burst out laughing.

---

107. *Dear Kerri,*

In the spirit of giving thanks, I wanted to say how deeply grateful I am to you and your amazing work with mms and recovering children. I have never felt such hope for my son and such joy sifting through poop!!!

What a truly tremendous gift you have given us all...

Sending love and Thanks

---

108. *My son is getting tiny bit more normal every day!!! I could kiss you!!!!!*

109. There was once a day not too long ago when all my son would do is scream and cry. No words at all. No communication. Today he asked me "mommy who holds up the clouds so they don't fall?" :) xoxo love that question! It means so much!! Autism is big. But God is bigger!! Don't give up ladies!! God led us to mms & to Kerri for a reason!!

110. Kerri is fabulous. She is very loving and supportive and will do anything to help our daughter recover. Using her MMS and parasite protocols have resulted in our eleven year old girl's ATEC scores dropping by half in less than sixth months. She is fully connected and much more responsive and affectionate. She herself is now motivated to succeed! We look forward to full recovery through Kerri's guidance.

111. I think we are over the initial die off hump!!! We are getting good reports from school about better focus and independence. Also, my son shampooed and combed his hair independently this morning. He even used a Q tip in his ears! I only asked him to try and shampoo by himself. He rewarded me with the combing and Q tip! Awesome mms!

    Thank you again!

112. I am so grateful to have found you!! MMS here in our house is a MUST and my boy gets better by the day because of it.

113. 6 months ago, my son was on antibiotics for PANDAS, he was suffering with OCD and anxiety, as well as completely distracted - like a zombie.....his teachers came out one day with tears in their eyes because my son said he feels like monsters are inside his head and they are scaring him! They were so worried about him, as we all were!

    We started MMS in April. My son got up to full dose relatively quickly and we added in MMS baths and MMS enemas and then I pulled the antibiotics—cold turkey! I was emailing Kerri at the time and was afraid to stop the antibiotics. She guided me and gave me the confidence that was needed! As suggested by Kerri, we also did night dosing of MMS. This really helped my son. Keeping a constant flow of MMS was the key.

    My son is flourishing!! He is HAPPY and confident. His focus has increased greatly! Since the start of the new year, he has had great day reports everyday in school! SO many gains in all areas! His coordination and strength have improved - he can do 11 sit ups (In June he couldn't do 1) He was chosen as Student of the Month in his Tae Kwon Do school (he is now a purple belt). The best news to report is his ATEC is now a 10!!!!

    Our family is so grateful to Kerri!!! This protocol has made the BIGGEST impact on my son's recovery!

    Thank you so much Kerri - My son's Fairy Godmother!!!

    Xoxoxo

114. I was praying for a new direction to go in to heal my boy. I literally woke up the next morning with a link to Kerri's presentation in my inbox from a friend whose daughter is making beautiful gains with mms. We are on day 3 here and things are going great, I am so excited! Thank you!!

115. Yes, my son is making real progress - slow and steady but real progress. The MMS & Parasite Protocol has been very beneficial for him...that's why I am trying to stick to it very closely. Also, I have wanted to tell you that one of the best things that we have ever done for my son is the enemas!!! He is a gut kid with chronic constipation and your enema program has really improved his daily life.

Thanks again for all of your help and guidance—always truly appreciated!

116. Hi, I'm the mother of Lizbeth Hernandez Saray Miramontes and I want to share my testimony in case it is useful to you.

My 13-year-old daughter started The Diet in January 2012, in June the full moon protocol to deparasite and withinin two months, she expelled a worm. This helped her regain 8 kilos of weight. (She was 10 kilos underweight when beginning the protocol) Her attitude has changed completely, from being very passive and low energy, she began to smile and be more active.

Thank you and God bless!

117. From the ATEC at www.autism.com

Total Score: 5

I. Speech/Language/Communication: 1

II. Sociability: 1

III. Sensory/Cognitive Awareness: 2

IV. Health/Physical/Behavior: 1

Started at 56 score in March.

I´m still having problems in environmental awareness, because in his mind sometimes he is Super-Hero (he wants to help to all the people in disasters, his own words). Sometimes he is eating portions like me, not such big portions but he is burning calories in the swimming classes. His meals are so healthy.

So, my homeopathic doctor told me (and recommends me) to wait until January next year to start the PP. He wants to see the effects of MMS, Probiotics and some homeopathy that he will provide at the end of this month.

We continue using as I said MMS, Theralac, GFCFSF diet, NAET and A.B.A therapy. I am so happy to share it with you.

Hugs my dear God Mother

118. My daughter is doing well on the MMS. Her ATEC went from 53 to 26 in three months. The special education teacher at her school was very impressed with how well she is doing. She told me to keep doing whatever it was that I was doing, because it is working!

Thank you for your help.

119. Kerri, good day

I want to tell you about the progress of my child, the treatment began in July and the progress that we have seen is:

-He has gone from not wanting to eat ANYTHING, TO EATING BY HIMSELF, SITTING DOWN he grabs his spoon and he cleans his mouth every time he gets dirty

  * He has stopped wearing a diaper, and goes to the bathroom by himself, almost like any other typical child.

* *He lets people other than my wife and I hug him.*
* *He now gives hugs and has started imitating a few other things.*
* *He can now obey simple instructions that he couldn't before.....no, pick it up, get down, get up, give me your hand, etc.*
* *At the institute where he receives therapy they have told us that they are seeing great improvement in his eye contact, as he now focuses his vision more clearly on an object.*
* *He still will not play with other children, but at least he is where they are.*

Thank you for everything and we are together in this fight day after day, winning small battles everyday to win the war.

God bless

---

120. *My son was a non responder. We worked with a DAN! Dr. for 14 years. We did the DAN! protocol tirelessly with very, very little gains. Did 3 years of ABA and 2 of SonRise. Did the diet. Still do the diet. We started the MMS protocol in April of this year. My son has had more gains since April of this year than with 14 years of DAN protocol combined. My local children's hospital specialist told me to put my son in a home and forget I ever had him. What a jerk. We pressed on and I could write a book about the gains since April. My son's Dr said he had two near impossible "tough nut kiddos to crack open...one being my son." Well, MMS works. If my son can improve I know yours can too. Whatever you have to do to do enemas, and get him to drink it...do it. My son is drinking 35 drops a day. Trust me, it is yuck. But he understands that if he drinks it, it makes the autism go away and he slams it down and says, "yuck." He totally knows I am helping him and cooperates. Be encouraged.*

---

121. *Hi Kerri,*

We're now at 1/4th of a drop per oz and today my daughter for the first time EVER answered a 'Where is...' question. I was putting out the garbage and when I came back in I remembered I had forgotten to put away a black marker

and when I found it was missing, I could only hope the property damage would not be too bad this time. I checked the living room and the kitchen but could not find any traces and meanwhile my daughter had taken the photo camera

and was taking pictures of herself in the mirror. Amazingly she seemed to have a way better understanding of the thing. I asked her twice where the black marker was, and after the second time she pointed towards the kitchen and said "There."

SHE HAS NEVER DONE THIS BEFORE! I checked the kitchen and found the black market next to the fruit. The pears, melon and mango all had black circles and stripes. I was a bit overwhelmed I should say.

Thank you, thank you, thank you for never having given up your search!

---

122. *My son Fernando Latin is 8 years old and was diagnosed at age 3 and half. When I started this struggle with autism all the relevant studies were performed. We visited a neurologist, psychologist and a gastroenterologist, he began taking the supplements according to DAN! protocol, but the list of pills he was taking was increasing and my boy was restless. Then I went to a homeopath,*

the treatment worked a little but it was so expensive I couldn't continue, it is needless to say how much money and time I spent on appointments and tests, plus the hyperactivity problem was growing each day. Until God put in my path an extraordinary friend MARIA CAMPERO and she talked to me about a foundation in Port Ordaz "VENCIENDO EL AUTISMO" FOUNDATION (Carolina, Yamileth and all that beautiful team) they brought Kerri Rivera to lecture here in Venezuela, on 04/02/2011. I will never forget these words AUTISM IS PREVENTABLE, TREATABLE, AND CURABLE. A new hope that a mother's heart never looses... In that conference she also talked about MMS and its benefits I was lucky Kerri evaluated my child, I started giving him MMS plus some supplements and have won this since:

* Better pronunciation, for example he used to say Dowg and now he says Dog.
* He obeys orders.
* Spends more time sitting.
* Evacuates normally with no bad smell.
* He stopped biting his clothes.
* He stopped making noises like: wiiiii yiiiii.
* He stopped playing with his hands.
* We go somewhere and he is relaxed.
* If we take a picture, he looks at the camera.
* He is more aware of his environment.
* He is improving a lot and really fast with his ABA therapy

These are all the benefits I've seen with my son after starting with the MMS, I know there is a lot to do but know a have real hope. Some advice for parents that are starting this road: please accept what is happening, inform yourselves. I always think that to get your children through this you need the four-legged table:

* Diet
* MMS, Supplement treatment
* Therapy
* Help at home

I've always asked God to give me enough wisdom to help my child and to put me in a direction were I could find people that can help me, and believe me he has listened: Venciendo al Autismo Foundation, Kerri Rivera, my sons therapist Milagros Alcanta, Danny her teacher-shadow, Maria Campo, a woman not only committed to her son but to all of those who she can help and guide me, including Marilyn Aparcedo and her team. All of them are my bases to keep going and as Kerri and Carolina say: This is an endurance test and there is no giving up!

I have nothing but thanks these wonderful and professional people, Thank you!

Norkis Pinto, El Tigre—Venezuela.

---

123. Alexander was a normal baby until he was 6 months old, after that he suffered a change that, when we got home from work it was like no one came in, he was very uneasy, we talked to him but he didn't seem to care, first we thought that he didn't listen, the pediatrician and neurologist recommended hearing tests,

we did them and his results were normal. The pediatrician also recommended a psychiatrist but I thought it was very early for that so I took him to a psychologist, but he didn't diagnosed him, instead he referred me to a psychiatrist specialized in autism, and with a simple test he confirmed the suspicions: your child has autism and this has no cure, take him to special classes and therapy. I quickly signed him to a special camp and school, but they they just took my money and my sacrifice to travel 60 kilometers daily, they didn't do what they promised, they charged me triple just to give me a diagnosis and I believe he didn't even receive therapy. In my despair I went to the internet, I made an email account, a facebook page and started to look for parents that were going through the same things I was, then I contacted a Dominican mom living in Puerto Rico and she told me about Kerri Rivera and the diet. She told me that Kerri was the person to go to about this and Kerri answered immediately and asked me if my boy was on the diet and I said he was only 50% and she told me that if I wanted my boy to get better I had to do 100% so I wrote her back when I was doing the diet entirely. She gave me the first three supplements MMS1, THERALAC AND QUINTON WATER. Everything has been so difficult to get but if you persevere you get want you're looking for. I got the MMS1 but I was scared because of the strong smell of chlorine but I gave it to him with faith, I took it and my youngest baby girl started taking it. She had had a cold for about a month and it disappeared, Alex started to get better in every aspect but the biggest changes began 15 days ago, since I give him his MMS1 treatment. I start at 3 o'clock and finish at 12 at night. On weekends I start at 1 and I complete 12 doses of one drop mixed with citric acid and give him that daily. My 3 year and 4 month old baby boy is saying his first words. He is more connected, pays attention, he is aware of what happens to him and he is more loving than ever. I am so happy; I thank God, Kerri Rivera, Zeneida, Cynthia. But I mainly thank MMS1, because with a supplement so cheap, I'm getting my son back, the one that Autism wanted to steal from me.

---

124. Juan Eduardo is 9 years old and he was diagnosed with Autism at age 2. It has been a long road in which we have tried everything. 7 years after trying and failing, in April of this wonderful 2011 we started in the right way. MMS came to our lives. Juan Eduardo was a self-centered boy and with a lot of fixations to objects. His improvement in school has been slow, but in 5 months he has improved what he improved in 5 years. MMS in our lives has been wonderful, despite the hyperactivity and lack of sleep at the beginning of the protocol, the life of Juan Eduardo and our lives have changed drastically in a very positive way. He will start regular school at the beginning of next year. He is a happy boy, he sleeps all night, he talks a lot more even if there is a long way to go, his quality of life is so much better. He shares with whoever is around him, a lot of times he surprises us with his qualities. He has adapted to the MMS in a great way. We took the panel viral test and the results were amazing, there was no virus. When I saw the great positive effects the MMS has made, I started to do protocol 1000 for maintenance with 100% success. Last year I suffered from several episodes of flu in which I had to take antibiotics, but this year I feel excellent, Thank God and Kerri and MMS I haven't been ill. I thank God, Kerri for putting you in our lives; I'm sure he has given back everything you selflessly have done for everybody. The smiles and looks in our children's eyes are priceless. Thank you Kerri and Jim Humble. A big hug.

---

125 Yes, I have increased the drops. Honestly, since we last spoke, he has had some of his best days...super happy. He actually read a book on his own on the way to school this morning. Seems very calm. Thank you.

---

126. Hello Kerri! I have not written you in some time. I must tell you I have already been using MMS for two months. We have seen a lot of improvement. He suddenly speaks, says single words. If I sing a song or the vowels, he tries to imitate me, although it is still not very clear. But he tries to imitate. He smiled back at me when I smiled at him. And so those are several things. Tantrums are also less.

127. She is doing excellent! Every day we see small but important progress. I am not sure if she has noticed the changes in herself, the best will be when she starts school and classmates and teachers can give me their opinions. Family members have also commented on the changes we have seen in her.

She is also answering questions about what she wants... With yeah, nah or the sign for all done with and then says dddon!

Now she wanted to see Mickey and told me tttttiii and I showed her the movies and she said "ickey!" ;) We are communicating!!

128. We are a family that lives in a country where living is not easy at all. The maternal death rates and child deaths are very high, and there is hardly any chance of getting access to special medical treatments and therapies. Our son started to show signs of autism since he was 2 years 8 months old. He had begun speaking but at that moment he stopped talking, he started to show no expression with his eyes, to roll around trees, to scream and to tantrum, and to not allow contact with anyone. Little by little he started to be very hyperactive and to have serious sleeping problems (he didn't want to wake up and he could not go to sleep at night).

The start of my son's autism went along with colds, severe coughing and infectious diarrhea. Our son's teacher had always had excellent reports about our son's behavior, but since this severe cold with synovitis in his hip, the transformation begun. Since then, the awful diagnosis and the absence of guidance led us to an abyss. Our son presented total absence of self, almost no language, hyperactivity and many sicknesses. 6 months went by in which he met with a real parade of doctors and therapists that gave us bad treatments, bad diagnoses and almost no information, our life became a living hell. We went into a state of denial in which we didn't want to see anything on the Internet regarding Autism. In that time our son had been diagnosed with severe sinusitis, complications with his adenoids, and limitations that he developed because of his hearing capacity.

By the end of the year 2007, I alone broke the pact I had made with my husband, and started to search the Internet and found Yeroline Ruiz's page where she commented about the biomedical protocol through which she had gained her son back in months. Little by little I tried to convince my husband, who at the beginning was completely reluctant to the possibility, but by December 2007 we made our first order of supplements and quelators (magnetic clay from the United States). The supplements took forever to get to us and when they arrived we gave them to our son without any clue or guidance and hardly any diet. The results were horrible, he got worse and worse, and this lasted about 8 months. During this time the therapists gave us a terrible prediction about our son's future. Our family problems were also getting worse and the only guide we had was Yeroline and the Curando el Autismo foundation. Thank God we didn't give up and we passed the hard times.

We eliminated some of the food that is forbidden in the protocol and we started to use Enzymes. Our son started to improve, his health got a lot better and we stopped visiting traditional doctors and I decided to take care of his treatment, the process was not easy because there aren't even the basics for the protocol in my country, from the flour to the milk, everything is really hard to get. Obviously a DAN! doctor or supplements are unthinkable. However even if his health had improved, the Autism symptoms were still present, the speech therapy did not help and sometimes even made it worse. With a lot of effort we brought Rosa Dominguez (Tomatis Therapist) and we begun applying this technique to our son. The economic effort was very big but the results were worth it, he was more in control of his body, the clearest sign of this was the control of his sphincter that happened almost magically. His language also improved even if he still didn't use it socially, but little by little we verified that our son had no sign of retardation compared to other kids his age. Even with the improvement, the tantrums, frustration and limitations of his language remained, we decided then to make a new effort and traveled to Panama to the Stem Cells Institute to make a stem cell transplant.

Our debt was huge, and despite the effort our baby showed two contrary signs: a positive one that was that our boy was completely connected to his environment (he is never outside of the world anymore) and a negative one: he became aggressive. He had never shown aggression, auto-aggression or violent behavior, but from the moment the anesthesia was applied these began.

Our child started hitting himself when things didn't go his way and he bit other people out of frustration. We remained on our path with despair because we could not see the light. We tried hyperbarics for 70 days in a row, eqinotherapy, and others. In 2011 we came across Puerto Rico's CEA conference and we found Kerri's topic and the SCIA topics very interesting. We decided to do the SCIA tests and we confirmed that our boy also had virus and an inflammation even though his immune system didn't seem very affected. Because of our country's limitations we couldn't complete the SCIA tests but then we had a lead on how to start a new journey. All we needed was a doctor that could apply the SCIA protocol.

But then there was a miraculous day in which we saw Kerri's talk and hope grew inside us, we contacted her immediately and she answered immediately too, with good will and all the indications as to how give him MMS and how to apply the protocol. After two weeks we started seeing a change in our son. Eye contact was way better; he speaks fluid sentences and gives structure to his words.

We are now three weeks into the protocol, we can see almost no aggressions and tantrums, we teach him letters and he recognizes them, reads and writes his name (he does it with some difficulty) his receptive language is %100 active, he is very loving, specially with me. (His mom), he hugs me and kisses me and tells me he loves me. We know we still have a lot to go but I'm certain that we will make it. My son has now Borderline Autism; his connection with the world is total. We are still thinking about doing all the SCIA tests but just to find out our child is cured. The light and hope that Kerri and the MMS have given us does not compare to anything. Thank God! Kerri is a blessing in our lives!

129. *This email was after an ATEC drop of 64 to 44:*

    This is truly AWESOME!!! He lacks in the "Speech/Language/Communication" area the most!!

    I honestly thought when I was filling this ATEC out that he would have regressed because I just thought he might have...it seems everything else we have EVER done it is always too good to be true! It actually is not this time!! Praise the Lord Jesus Christ! \o/ I even had my oldest daughter give her thoughts on the questions too so that I doubled checked myself regarding his behavior etc...you know to make sure I was not out of touch! :)

    We definitely have a ways to go, but I have never had my son at this level of 'awareness' before! We are doing RDI (Relationship Development Intervention) and have been since Feb. 2011...he's made great gains with it, but he is FLYING now only because of the MMS!!

    ~Melissa, IN, USA

130. *Hello, my name is Silvia and I have a 5-year-old son named Ricardo who was diagnosed with Autism 2 ½ years ago. From that moment he has been on a gluten and casein free diet and a therapy routine that help him day by day. Three months ago I met Kerri Rivera and the Venciendo el Autismo Foundation, and started giving Ricardo MMS. From that moment on he has improved significantly, his language is better and his behavior is a lot more controlled, plus with the biomedical treatment he goes to the bathroom regularly, this makes me very happy because he was always constipated.*

    Silvia Morales — Caracas.

131. *Since I was a baby I was a very sick child ... I remember I had many gastrointestinal problems, I made my mom's life miserable with all the diarrhea and vomiting ... I couldn't gain weight and I had no appetite. All this accompanied me for many years; the diarrhea became chronic constipation, fluid retention and dry skin.*

    All of this without knowing I had a serious problem, until I gave birth to my first child. The constipation was a nightmare, my baby got ill, when I fed him breast milk he would get a rash, and then he had convulsions for about 20 seconds, when I fed him again the same would happen but now the convulsions lasted for nearly a day. The doctors didn't know what was going on either. In one of my researches I ran into a page that talked about Autism and Candida being one of the main causes, this is when I find out that my son had chronic candidiasis and that he got it from me when I breast fed him. I tested my child and myself and we both had Candida, and I have had it since I was a baby.

    One day I heard about the existence of a woman named Kerri Rivera who is devoted to helping children with Autism and I contacted her and she gave me all the help to treat my child. I will be forever grateful. She talked to me about the MMS and how to give it to my son. I also started taking it and in a matter of days I had a white layer in my tongue, it was the Candida getting out. I have gained my energy back, the headache I had in the mornings is gone, I feel vivid and almost all the Candida is gone. I've been with MMS for a month and I've never felt so satisfied with a treatment. This simple and yet powerful remedy has given my health and family back and with this I can assure, by my own experience that MMS works.

132. Hi Kerri, I want to tell you that Erik has started with the speech therapist, and psychologist, when she finished the session with Erik, I asked if she thought that Erik could still be diagnosed with autism. She looked me in the eye and said, autism? Are you sure that he was correctly diagnosed? I found her the forms and she told me today Erik has eye contact, he socializes, and is cooperative. She said he does seem small for his age, and that we were going to have to work on strengthening the muscles of his mouth and the tongue as well because they are very week. She said that not chewing would affct the development of one's language, and Erik has only been chewing for 8 months, which started after we did the chamber with you in Mexico. That was the answer she gave me, and that's something, the fact that she told me that this is not autism is really something, even though she doesn't want to contradict the diagnosis they gave two years ago. The truth is, I am so glad he has come to improve, and that is since you KERRI have started to help my child. It's been a year since we started with the MMS protocol and the improvements have been incredible, he still lacks language as he mispronounces many words, but the worst is over. You can publish this if you want, thank you very much for all your help.

    Kisses

133. We had first formed stool at 4 drops. It was so inspiring. Since then somedays we have formed stool, some days we have loose stool but I relate this to detox - I can clearly see his gut healing. His expressive speech hasn't changed yet but he obviously understands much, much better and is able to follow complex comands like "come and give me one teaspoon from the drawer" or "go and put this in the dishwasher" or "wait for daddy to get out the baby from the car and then you can lock the door and put on the alarm". Things like that, that were unthinkable before. I hope he will go beyond his few words soon and will begin to talk.

    Although speech is the thing that interests me most of all, perhaps the most impressive thing that MMS brought to us all of a sudden is the sense of smell - our boy never seemed to feel any smell, good or bad, in his entire life. He got this sense a week ago. We are thrilled - something is waking up in his brain, perhaps some pathogens in some part of his brain or in his nose or whatever died and now he is able to sense a smell. Things are getting moved.

    Thank you Kerri.

134. My son is 8 1/2 years old. I have spent six years and well into six figures to help my son. While I would see gains, nothing was really moving him forward. Three months with MMS, DE and ocean water; the junk that is coming out of him is both horrifying and thrilling. I think he is finally starting to feel better, and because he feels better he is more with us. He is trying so hard to speak and everyday he is saying at least four new words. He also watched a movie and laughed at a funny part!

135. We started MMS 68 Days ago and my son's ATEC has dropped from 50-23... Now that's a MIRACLE!!! He is So much more "with us" and I'm seeing improvements daily. He is just so much more fun to be with now:) He did have a plateau, but is back on track. We have only done 4 enemas to date, but they made a big difference! Baths do as well:) I can't wait to see what he is like on his 4th birthday (still 39 days away).

    Kelly, CA, USA

136. Is it just an amazing day or is the MMS already working? Its just day 1! I know people say that once your child starts talking, they never stop, but holy cow... Today in the grocery store, it took me 3x's longer to shop because he was talking about everything he saw around him and needed a response on all of it from me! So unlike anything we have ever experienced with him before. Could it really be the MMS already? Also, potty training has been going well (slow & and steady), but today, he didn't need much prompting! Many times, he just stopped what he was doing and ran to the bathroom to go all by himself! This is amazing, because he never stops a preferred activity to go potty! When i thought it had been too long since he went last and said "its time to go potty." he just ran in there and peed, washed hands etc. No tantrums or weight dropping, he just ran in and went! God is answering my prayers! :) I'll keep you posted on what happens tomorrow!

137. You know Kerri, I had to email you directly I waited until today to retake my son's atec...just did his first Parasite Protocol and did the 72/2 hr this weekend, so waited a few days to pass by before we did...so this atec was based SOLELY on this past monday, tuesday & today. I got an 11, hubby got a 13. so average: 12. (he was 32 before MMS, then 27 after 3 weeks of MMS...now 12) I had to email you to thank you b/c well...because. What is there really to say :) cant think of the right words really :) thank you?? not really enough if u know what i mean :) ...But to think i was going to skip your presentation at A1 b/c I thought it's too good to be true. But you caught my attention when you started tearing up as you got up on stage :) you were the only person/speaker to show emotion like that. AND have NOTHING TO SELL ON YOUR TABLE :) You were there only for our children...getting nothing back in return! :) I know I've been emotional, but I'm prego and my sons getting better so cut me some slack :)

I'm SO grateful for all you do Kerri. If there is something I can do in return, Please let me know. I know you have a lot on your plate. You have a heart of gold; such a giving, compassionate person. a "rare-ity" (this word is in my dictionary!!) You & Patrick are always in our prayers. I seriously want to go visit you in Mexico w/my family so my son can meet you when he's recovered. I told my hubby & he's up for it hehe :)

Anyways, long email but really just wanted to let you know how well he's doing and to 'thank you'. It blew my mind after I got the results. He still has issues in socialization and getting his vocab/speech up to his 4 year old level. I think much of that will change as he learns English better: he'll interact better with his peers.

Thank you Kerri from the bottom of me & husbands heart :) You are loved & covered in prayer. :)

138. We started to see a setback in January with our 1 year 8 month old girl. Until this date she had had a normal development, like her sisters (she is our third child) but then, she stopped talking, she just screamed and twirled. She would twirl like 20 times a day for no reason until she got dizzy and she fell to the ground. She didn't look at anybody in the eyes and could be behind a curtain hours comparing her toothbrushes; she wasn't hungry nor asked for her milk, we had to push the food into her mouth so she would eat it. I was desperate so I went in to a forum and a friend from Venezuela told me to look for Kerri Rivera in my country so I did. She immediately answered and gave me hope, since the

three doctors I had seen before told me that Autism had no cure, that all we could do is to teach her how to survive and be a little bit more independent.

I found my hope in Kerri, I read the testimonies on her page and sent her a message that she answered right away. She told me to do the diet, remove milk and everything else, I went to her clinic and within a week of the diet Abby could look at me and smile (she had stopped doing that long ago) When I went to her clinic Autismo2 in Puerto Vallarta she looked at Abby with all the patience in the world, she gave me MMS, the supplements and all the hope in the world. Everything was new to me but I had faith that I was in the right place and from that moment on, while always counting on Kerri's advice, my baby girl started to get much better. Her first ATEC was 95 and a year and a half after it's a 15. My girl now smiles, talks, dances, she obeys and stopped screaming, her only tantrums are of a normal girl her age. I did hyperbarics and am still doing MMS, supplements and deworming her. She is now diagnosed with Pervasive Developmental because the Autism symptoms are gone. She doesn't run from one place to another, she plays, looks for other kids to play with and has friends. The only thing left is for her to establish a conversation, and to put together the words to make sentences, but I know she is going to make it.

Once she sat down on ant hill and a bunch of ants bit her, we had to go to the hospital and the doctors gave her cortisone and she was seriously ill, now when a bug stings or a mosquito bites she tells me where it bit her, and she asks me to apply a calendula ointment that I use for the mosquito bites. She sets the table and can eat by herself, she doesn't use a diaper anymore, we can go shopping or to parties and she is well behaved, there is no more tantrums or fixations, this is wonderful! I know there is a long way to go, I've been in this fight for a year and a half, but with KERRI RIVERA'S HELP I will rescue my baby from autism, even though some say that Autism has no cure I know it does. Kerri has been a blessing for our lives and I thank God for putting her in my path.

Thank you Kerri, I have no way to repay what you have done for Abby.

139. Our 10 year old son, Ben, showed symptoms of autism since he was an infant. Until he was 6, he never connected normally with family or peers. As his mother, I ached for a hug, to be called "Mommy," or for a lingering look of love. I never got them.

Until he was diagnosed with autism at age five, I was utterly befuddled. What had I done? What was wrong with Ben? Why didn't he want to play with other children? Why did he drool endlessly, laugh constantly for no reason, and bolt from play dates and parties with no warning? Why was he constantly lethargic, to the point where we called him "the playdough boy?"

Ben was always happy, dwelling far from us, in his own perfect little heaven. My husband and I were depressed, even despondent, despite attempts at gluten-free, casein-free diets, ABA therapy, and many supplements, because we saw no substantive and lasting changes in our child.

Finally we found the Son-Rise Program®, which brought Ben back to us. After three-plus years of a mostly full-time Son-Rise Program®, Ben became highly interactive, engaged, and interested in his peers. That alone was a palpable miracle. As we say in Hebrew, Dayeinu! That would have been sufficient. But we constantly experienced regressions back into autistic symptoms. For no apparent reason, and despite endless biomedical interventions, including the DAN!

protocol—to the tune, I might add, of tens of thousands of dollars, multiplied over four to five years—Ben would suddenly revert to autistic behaviors, and we would lose contact. He became once again non-responsive, uninterested in family or peers, and seemingly unable to connect. Only the day before, he had been totally connected.

After being on the SCD and GAPS diets, and finding even them ineffective to alleviate these regular and devastating returns to autism, we were advised by Dr. Campbell-McBride that it sounded to her as if Ben had parasites. A friend of mine who was also a Son-Rise mom had mentioned to me that she and another Son-Rise mom friend of ours were trying something called "MMS." When I heard the words for which the acronym stood, I gave an internal scoff. "Master Mineral Solution? Is this a joke?"

I can tell you, in all seriousness, that now, five and a half months into our MMS autism protocol, MMS is definitely no joke. Since starting MMS, we have seen nothing but progress in Ben. We are still doing GAPS, but avoiding foods we know Ben cannot yet digest. Ben's ATEC score has dropped from 43 when we started MMS to a startling 20. We are seeing sustained, natural, unsolicited and consistent eye contact, like never before. Ben is consistently responsive, certainly on par with most 10 year old boys. He is playing hockey in our driveway with friends. He is solicitous of others, and compassionate when others are hurt in any way. He is funny, expressively loving, and eager to please and be loved. It makes me cry to write this. I wanted this so badly, and now, with MMS leading the other interventions, I have what I prayed for.

We are not perfect on the MMS. Ben is in his first year of school post-Son-Rise, and dosing during the school day is not easy. But we are tremendously hopeful and excited.

I truly believe, as Kerri Rivera has often said, that parasites are the missing piece of the autism puzzle. Like so many other warrior parents, we have done everything. But everything minus one was not enough for Ben. Now, I think we truly have the tools, and it is only a matter of time, faith, and love, to fully and permanently recover our beloved Ben.

---

140. Caitlin has been on the MMS protocol for 3 months now. Caitlin is now off her 100 plus supplements a day that were the glue holding her together so to speak, with no regression. She is happier, more affectionate and focused. She no longer has a distended belly. She used to have terrible smelling gas on a daily basis and very foul smelling bowel movements. This is gone! She has increased muscle tone (has a diagnosis of low muscle tone and bilateral hip anteversion). She has been seizure free as well! She continues to make slow but steady gains in her reading and math skills at school. She isn't conversational in her speech yet but can comment on things and express her wants in longer and more elaborate sentences. She is falling asleep faster and sleeping longer.

---

141. Eczema!!

At last my son (4 yrs) is living now without eczema, he was born with severe eczema all over his body, we used every allergic cream and med and even the magical Dead Sea Clay but it didn't work, but now after using mms and pp (parasite protocol) for 2 months... ITS GONE!! Thank you MMS!!"

Thank you!

---

142. *This is the story of our son who is 4 years and 9 months old today. Our story is a desperate struggle to defeat Autism, the same struggle that a lot of families are going through to free their sons and daughters. Guillem started to have ear inflammation and laryngitis when he was a few months old and we medicated him with antibiotics, he had his vaccines according the vaccine calendar, and by the time he was 9 months old he was showing signs of Autism. He would put his fingers in his throat until he choked, he would hit his head on the wall and he was always mad, his tantrums were frequent, longer and more intense, he started to look at the lights and to twirl with no sense, he showed less interest in people day by day and he would get really mad if someone said anything to him. He was hyperactive, couldn't stop running and going up and down the stairs. The nights were terrible too, he didn't sleep well and woke up screaming as loud as he could plus he could not say a word.*

My father and my brothers blamed me for this; they said that my boy wanted to dominate me and to get my attention. I had a hard time recognizing that it wasn't this, that my boy had something else. Once I accepted it I spent hours and hours reading on the Internet, and I read about the gluten-free diet and that was our first step. When Guillem was 2 and half years old we changed the diet and it worked. Guillem started to respond to orders, there was less screaming and his first words appeared. Three months into the diet we contacted Kerri, this has been a key moment in our history, because she has been our guide to get our son out of this long tunnel. The first thing she did was to check what our son was eating, I thought that I was doing a perfect diet but I wasn't, there were some foods with sugar, soy and additives, the next thing we did was to talk about the supplements and MMS, but I was very scared to use it and it wasn't until three months later, the day Guillem turned 3 that I started giving it to him. Now we have been using MMS for a year and 9 months. We give him MMS daily and every weekend we can but minimum one weekend a month we do the 72/2. His improvement was amazing, his language got better, his dressing skills, he learned how to use the bathroom, his sleep was normal, and the screaming was almost gone. The next step was to start with the MMS enemas, every enema made Guillem more alert, more present, we started with the enemas 4 months after starting with the MMS. We saw that the enemas expelled a great amount of biofilm and the more he expelled it, the more abilities Guillem gained back, I saw the importance of healing the intestine and that has been my obsession since.

The next important step was the sessions in the hyperbaric chamber, his first sessions were at age 3 and 9 months, and the changes we saw were mainly in the obsessions he had, he paid much more attention to everything, his social skills were very affected but after this he made his first friend. Now we do hyperbarics with seawater every three months. Another piece in the puzzle were the parasites but with Kerri's help we've been on the protocol against parasites for 7 months and every deworming cycle our son improves. I know that we have to keep fighting but I also know that we are closer to the exit. Now Guillem sings, he plays with his brothers, we go to the movies, we do puzzles, we paint, and he is very happy, he has learned to spell his name and he walks joyfully down the street telling you about his day. He goes to school, plays football and more importantly, we are a family again.

For all of this we are deeply thankful to Kerri, because she has always been there for us, without Kerri and MMS our story would be completely different, so we owe them EVERYTHING. I know that we will someday say Guillem is cured, and all the other children with Autism can say that too.

UPDATE: As of December, 2012 Guillem no longer has a diagnosis of autism, here is an email his Mother sent to Kerri when she knew he had recovered:

> *KERRI!!!*
>
> *My son has an ATEC of 10!!!!*
>
> *I have it repeated several times because I did not believe it...*
>
> *I have copied it below...I'm going to have it framed!*
>
> *The truth is that this Christmas we have enjoyed our whole family, we've been to the Zoo, to the fair, and during family meals he was very well behaved and enjoyed the Magi and the magic of Christmas. Christmas last year was totally different. For all this we give infinite thanks! There are not enough words to tell you how we feel! Without you our story would be different. We will continue working to get to zero!*
>
> *A big hug!*

---

143. I started with MMS on April 2012, I was afraid but had a lot of faith. I did the ATEC for my son and it was 92. He could not use the bathroom alone nor say a single word. The day I started I thought there was nothing different, but when we were at the beach on vacation I noticed that when I called his name he would turn, and come to where I was. All this with one drop! Before that day I always had to stand up and find him so he would pay attention to me. He wouldn't look at me but he would listen to instruction. Days went by and when we came back from the beach he went straight to the bathroom... I couldn't believe it; I sat down and asked my self WHAT IS THIS? What happened? And I silently thanked God and Kerri. This was decisive for me to continue. After this he improved day by day, after 5 weeks his ATEC had gone down to 76 points.

     I made a few mistakes at the beginning because I didn't know the protocol very well, and wanted to rush things. Again, Kerri with her infinite patience and love for others led me to the right path, and I started to see more, way more.

     My son started writing, he knows his letters, he reads some words (he has memorized them) he is great in the bathroom, he listens, his eye contact has improved significantly, his last ATEC was last month and it was 60 points. I know we have a long way to go, but I every month there is improvement and even though there are some bumps and setbacks the good things overcome the bad.

     My son has also started saying words, names of movies, he can say over 100 words (names of movies or things he likes). Some will think it doesn't mean anything to know the name of a movie but for me, it is to know how my son's voice sounds and that, is priceless. Now my next goal is to hear him say "MOM"

     ~Myrna Sterling, Mother of Gianmarco, age 5.

     Myrna is the president of the GM foundation for Autism

---

144. My wife and I have always been fond of traveling, getting to know different cultures and people, this is why we had our little one we decided t o keep traveling but to adapt to his rhythm.

     When he was 9 months old he went on his first international journey. Everything was perfect, he was the happiest baby on the plane, he played with the people in the seats behind us, the stewardess wanted to stay with him to play, all the plane ride went along perfectly.

Something happened between his 15th and 18th month, his smile was gone, we no longer had happiness in our home, only nerves and less language. Maybe the excessive vaccines were destroying his immune system and leaving the door open for parasites to take hold.

When he was 18 months we went on a second trip and it was an absolute nightmare. He wouldn't stop crying and screaming on the plane, he didn't want to play with anybody. We spent a few days getting to know this new place while our baby fell further into this abyss in front of our astonished eyes.

Something was wrong, and after an episode of auto aggression we knew that this was not normal. After watching a couple of videos on the Internet we started to understand, and we went to a psychologist who didn't give us a diagnosis because our son was so young.

Later on we went to a neuro-pediatrician who also used the excuse of our son's young age to dismiss us, and finally a last doctor who didn't explain anything either.

Not even our family listened because they thought we were exaggerating. We were left alone and our biggest ally was and still is the Internet.

After the medical failure and their "anti-diagnosis" we took the best and most important decision of our lives, that was not to listen to any of the diagnoses, or to wait another 6 months to be called by the neuro-pediatrician again. We started down this road without an official diagnosis but with all the symptoms and behaviors that define autism.

We started with the casein, gluten and soy free diet with no experience on how to do it and our baby suffered awful withdrawal symptoms. We couldn't believe what we were seeing, his nervousness and aggression took us to our limits. After a few days on the diet his tantrums went down little by little until he was stable. But we needed something else because everything was out of control; this is when we went back to the Internet.

After three months of false doctors and pseudo medical experts we found Kerri Rivera.

She gave us hope, and filled us with confidence, but most importantly she was clear with us from the beginning. Everything she told us was logical and everything made sense as to why it was done so we trusted her without a moment's doubt.

He got better and better everyday. Kerri told us how to do the ATEC and what it meant. Our first result was 57 points when he was 2 years old, which was very high for us because of his young age. We have been doing everything Kerri suggests, improving the diet, and using everything she recommends, and the results have been spectacular, right now he is 2 years and 10 months old, his ATEC is 8 and he is doing great. Our goal is to have him at 0, and I'm certain that once we free his intestines of all the parasites, he will be a strong, healthy and happy boy.

He doesn't have any behaviors like the ones he had one year ago, now he smiles again, he talks and asks for things, he plays a lot and he is happy.

This was possible thanks to his Godmother Kerri.

Kerri, you have done and given us everything in exchange for nothing, and that is your defining quality as a human being and as a person.

Every day you give hope to all that YES WE CAN defeat Autism and now we have a lot of puzzle pieces to complete our puzzle. We may find a new one soon because there are a lot of people investigating and that makes us feel alive, to fight against the entire circus that has sprung up around this problem.

I would recommend that if anyone is not seeing progress in their children, to come to Kerri, and try everything she says word for word. She has done it all and has the best investigators and doctor on her side. The ones that aren't intimidated by the absurd laws of the upper echelon, those who only want our children to be sick all their lives so they can sell medicine to us.

We will keep up the fight.

---

145. Hi Kerri, I just got the third MMS Autism newsletter, and I tell you it couldn't have arrived at a better moment. For the last few days my nephew has had a strange infection, he was hospitalized and the doctors couldn't figure how to fight it because it was resistant to many antibiotics. I told my brother-in-law about MMS and he started using it. After two days my nephew was healed, the doctor asked me for a little so he could examine it, and his answer was that the way MMS functions is amazing, he couldn't believe that such a simple and powerful product hasn't come out to the public eye.

---

146. My husband and I were on the couch having our morning coffee and my son came bolting out of the room and ran up to my husband's face and said..."Oh Hi Daddy, I'm back!" And then ran back to his room...this is our once in a while "word" little man. After 3 non-progressive PPs (parasite protocols) the 4th one was a charm. A nightmare, but quite an eliminator... Lots of Worms Gone! And he is slowly coming back...we are seeing it in fact he is even reassuring us that he "is back".

~The previous email was accompanied by an ATEC drop from 95 to 35 in 6 months.

---

147. Dear Kerri,

It's a pity I don't speak English and that's why I can't write you on my own. Currently, a lot of good things are happening to my son (31 years old). I have followed all your advice and as a result he has completely calmed down. I have learned to prepare CDS at home with the help of Jim Humble's video. The CDS is a 600 ppm solution; my son drinks 30 ml per day with the feeding bottle method. I suppose this is the daily dose for a person of his weight. We are past the third PP and preparing for the fourth one.

Unfortunately I won't be able to attend the congress in Prague, since I can't find anyone to look after my son. If it were in the summer I would risk going by car and taking him with me.

I am very grateful for your attention to our life and progress and for your help in curing my son. God bless you for helping children with autism by sharing your knowledge and experience with the world. I will try to give a regular account on the progress of my son. I have no doubt he will be cured, too.

148. *Three more tiny little gains on our step by step path to recovery....yesterday Nick got a haircut and did not cry at all AND was relaxed enough that it was the first time it wasn't like a sheep shearing, he actually got to get a little style (so cute!). Also, he was doing some pretty terrible screaming in the car in the parking lot at Whole Foods while I tried to find a parking space (I wanted to scream too) and I let him know he scared me. When we got into the store he spontaneously said "I'm sorry" -total first! Lastly, He has requested a hug from me three times recently - HUGE new thing and I love it. Thank you MMS and Kerri.*

149. *Thank you Kerri. For all of your help, answering my emails, and for all that you're doing to help all of us, help our kids!!! I was at a breaking point. Nothing was helping her anymore, her organs continuing to get worse, hadn't grown in 4 years, and had become Jeckyll/Hyde this past 4 years...A violent, raging Hyde being increasingly present more and more each year, each month. I knew something had a hold of her all these years. And it amazes me how 2 endocrinologists, 3 pediatric GI specialists, and many other doctors had no clue.*

    Thank you for ALL you are doing to get the truth out there. You are an angel!!!

    Merry Christmas - xoxo

150. *Puerto Ordaz, November 4th, 2011*

    My name is Carolina Moreno and my husband is Rafael Colmenares, we are the lucky parents of a little 6 year-old whose name is Ana Victoria, she came to this world to give us the world's greatest lesson, through her we have learned the real value of life, to be steadfast, and brave. We learned that it's our job to fight for our dreams if we want to accomplish them, and over all we've learned that God is who holds us up and gives us the strength and tools to move forward.

    My journey with Autism began the 27th of march of 2007, my daughter Ana Victoria was 23 moths old, her initial development was normal, but little by little she stopped talking, she didn't understand anything, she didn't miss her parents, she didn't play with other children or even her toys, she didn't like to be kissed or hugged, she acted as she was deaf but we didn't know that all this were symptoms of autism. It wasn't until the day that we went to a neurologist in our area, that someone told us that this was Autism, an incurable condition, and that our daughter would have it all her life. It was a very hard moment for us; all of our plans to be a happy and healthy family went down in a matter of hours.

    As parents we didn't want to give up, after recovering from the horrible news, we began looking for information on how to help Ana Victoria. In our country of Venezuela there were 4 specialists in Autism and they were all using the gluten and casein free diet, vitamin therapy, as well as expensive tests performed in the United States to check candida and bacteria. Thanks to them I learned how important the diet was to get Ana back from Autism, without it, recovery would be impossible.

    We did some testing through Great Plains labs, and the results indicated candida, bacteria, inflammation and much more . We started with Ketazol and Flegyl. My daughter was taking up to 400 mg of Ketazol even though she was barely three years old. Now with everything I've learned I can not believe that a physician could prescribe such a high dose to a child who is only 3 years old and weighs only 16 kg. That alone should be punished and criticized

However, I felt that I wasn't doing the right thing, years passed, Ana Victoria was 5 and her comprehension and attention levels were very low, my husband always thought there had to be something else we could do!

One day my dear friend Carolina Garcia talked to me about Kerri Rivera's blog, she told me that it explained the reason for the supplements and the hours they had to be taken, for example that the antifungals had to be given away from food and the pro-biotics worked better if they are given at night. After I read her blog and visited her website in July 2010 I called the Clinic Autism02 and Kerri Rivera herself answered me. I explained my daughter's case, and she asked me to give her an opportunity to help, and if in 2 months we didn't see anything different with our daughter we could continue doing what we always did. I told my husband and we agreed to try. I felt a great sense of peace when when Kerri told me, "I'm here, and I promise I will walk with you until we recover your daughter"

In August Ana Victoria was on Kerri's full protocol and in November God gave me the opportunity to go to Puerto Vallarta, México. An entire month in this city were my daughter received the hyperbaric chamber treatments, we started with MMS, plus we got together with Kerri at her home every night with pen and paper, she explained to us step by step how we could heal our children. From that moment a beautiful friendship was born between Kerri and I.

This is when I understood that Autism is caused by a weakness of the immune system and this brings as consequences; viruses, bacteria, candida, intestinal and brain inflammation, food allergies and contamination with heavy metals, and that it is necessary to attack every aspect to be able to heal autism.

The 23rd of November Ana Victoria Started to take MMS and in 30 days of treatment we noticed the firsts changes. My daughter's stools were consistent; there were no food residues or foul smells. When I came back from Vallarta I was full of new knowledge and a lot of MMS bottles, Ana Victoria had already a very well defined protocol and the best thing was that it wasn't a long list of supplements, only 7, MMS and Theralac. Everyone in my family noticed a great change in our daughter, better eye contact, controlled hyperactivity, she started saying her first words with sense and purpose; I want park please, I want food please, I want to sleep. She was doing much better in therapy and at school. Anita had begun her way back to the world she left when she was 1 and half years old.

When I saw this improvement in my daughter I decided to share my experience with other members of my community and it was there with my dear friend Yamileth Paduani and her husband Alejandro Teran that Fundación Venciendo el Autismo was born. Mr. Alejandro asked if Kerri could come to Venezuela and talk to parents in a simple way so everyone could understand that Autism is curable. Kerri was delighted to accept the invitation and in only 7 moths of work we had 2 conferences and many evaluations and nowadays there are 700 kids on Kerri's protocol that is: casein, soy, gluten and sugar free diet, some supplements depending on every child, MMS and Theralac. The results are very positive and there hundreds of families that have started with their children's recovery.

Then came the great discovery of the parasite protocol, for me, it was the missing piece in my daughter's puzzle. The first few months of the PP were severe (fever, laughter, hyperactivity) and many worms in her stool. However, after all these worms came out out I saw how her mind cleared, and month by month we waited for the full moon to deworm ...

Ana Victoria is now improving very quickly, she is a girl that enjoys being with her family, the park, a day out, she goes to school and she says to me that at school she now does her work in silence without crying, when I arrive home she greets me with a smile, she runs to me and calls me Mom, she tells me what she wants and what she doesn't, she can use the computer like an expert, she takes her own shower and dresses herself, she even picks out her clothes, she knows when Christmas is coming and that there will be gifts. Her therapists and her shadow teacher are really happy to see how Anita is progressing day by day.

Yesterday we were all at the table eating lunch ... and she points with her finger ..."Papa's food, Mama's food and Ana Kikota's (Victoria's) food...yummy... heeheehee. My husband and I were laughing with excitement and happiness. Some time ago we felt that speech would be nearly impossible for Ana Victoria.

My advice: do not be afraid of MMS ... be afraid of autism; that which is unforgiving and has the power to destroy lives and families if we don't attack it on time.

We are grateful to God because He has never abandoned us and has always given us the strength and tools to fight and to believe that it is possible to recover our children. We thank God for putting Kerri in our path and we ask God to bless her everyday for having such a big and noble heart, she who is always helping others in a selfless way. We also thank Jim Humble and Andres Kalcker for helping us find the missing piece in this great puzzle that is Autism. We can do it!!!

To all of you, many sincere thanks for helping the children in my country.

Blessings,

Carolina Moreno, President of Fundación Venciendo el Autismo. (The Defeat Autism Foundation)

Venezuela.

---

151. Good Day, first of all I want to thank God for giving me all the necessary tools to be able to help my son, Jesus Soto who is 8 years old today. Jesus was born normally with no complications, loved by his parents and family, everything was going fine, but when he turned 18 months old he became ill; laryngitis, and fever, amongst other things.

He was diagnosed with Autism at age 3. As a worried mother, I took him to the psychologist because I observed several behaviors that were not normal. After the terrible diagnosis we started to take him to a specialist after specialist, they were all very good doctors, his DAN! doctor in Venezuela, and my sons gastroenterologist were very helpful. I met a very special friend Mayerling Aparcedo who brought the ABA method to Venezuela. My son had many improvements but we still felt that we needed something else. I spent my time on the internet finding out as much as I could until I found Kerri Rivera that without even knowing me helped me via Internet, talked to me about MMS and about the supplements and how to take them. My friend Carolina Moreno had the joy to travel to Puerto Vallarta and wrote to me from there, telling me that MMS was helping a lot of children. The 14th of December I ordered my first MMS and the 27th of January it arrived to my country, from that date on my son is taking MMS.

The 2nd of April Kerri arrived to Venezuela and I went to see her, I took all the tests I had and she checked them, after only two months of taking MMS his viral load went down to near normal levels, and his liver profile showed no problems. I made some adjustments that day and I continued with the treatment seeing a lot of improvement in his language, socialization, understanding of things, his hyperactivity has gone down and the laughter for no reason stopped. I'm very happy with the results and now all the family is taking MMS.

I'm very grateful to God for putting my husband in my life, as he has been a very special part of this battle that we are winning, I also want to thank our family, Kerri, Carolina, Yamileth, Mr. Alejandro and everyone from the Fundación Venciendo al Autismo.

Yours truly,

Maria Campero

---

152. My baby girl Yuliangel Nazareth Quijada Montero was diagnosed with autism when she was one and a-half years old. From that moment she was given a treatment to allow her to sleep and to control her tantrums: "Risperdal" which had absolutely no effect, I gave her up to three pills before bed and even them nothing happened, I was just damaging her brain. She didn't sleep night or day, I was worried because she screamed all the time and she hit herself.

The 2nd of April 2011 I attended the conference of Fundación Venciendo el Autismo, where I heard for the first time that Autism had a cure. Kerri explained in a very simple way how I could cure my girl, even though I didn't have all the economic resources necessary for her treatment, the Foundation helped me with a part of the treatment, MMS and multivitamins. From there I started noticing changes, with a lot of sacrifice and effort my girl was on a strict casein, soy and gluten free diet. When I started giving her the MMS I would give her 72/2 on weekends and then I noticed that there was a lot of mucus in her stool, from there she started talking, she slept the entire night, and took naps in the afternoon, she pays attention, she knows how to count and all the colors with only three years of age. For me MMS is a miracle, since I started giving it to her she is a very healthy little girl, with no colds or any of the diseases she used to have, she is now considered to be very high functioning (14 pts. on the ATEC scale) with MMS, Vitamins, and the diet my child is getting out of the Autism spectrum. She does not go to therapy because of my finances but my sister Yenitze Montero interacts a lot with my girl, and her grandparents Raiza and Julian help me a lot with the diet, my nephews Jesus and Luis are also helping me with the home therapy and of course her dad and me fill her with love and care. My daughter is healthy, she has meaningful speech, she recognizes herself, she sleeps well with no pills and we are all very happy with the results. God Bless the entire team at Fundacion Venciendo el Autismo, especially Kerri Rivera for bringing MMS to my country, it is absolutely miraculous. Blessings.

Yurliana Montero and Jonatha Quijada

---

153. Martin is 6 years old, weighs 19 kilograms and is diagnosed with severe non-verbal Autism. He was diagnosed when he was 2.

He almost made no progress with therapy, when he turned 4 everything seemed to be lost, but when he was 5 we tried a new therapy and he started to say a few words. He also got very sick almost everyday, he coughed a lot, had an ear inflammation and fever, he couldn't go to school.

He started taking MMS the 29th of June 2011, when he was only taking two doses of one drop and two drops every third day has intestines were not moving and he had a psychotic attack (something that I've never seen before) and this lasted 2 hours.

Children with Autism are severely intoxicated so his reaction to the MMS was very clear. After 15 days of taking 8 takes of a drop a day Martin stopped coughing, he is more alert, connects all the time, his expression changes, he started to make friends, he starts to play with the computer, I hear from school that he'll be a preschooler because all the improvement he has had and that he didn't have all year. (I was almost going to get him out of school) he was attending school with a shadow teacher but had no apparent social communication or increase in cognitive capabilities.

This past October, in a meeting with his team of therapists, I asked them all what they thought about Martin's improvements and they were very happy, I asked 2 of his speech therapists who have worked with him for more than three years, "Did Martin have severe autism?" "Yes." They both responded. "And now?" I asked them. "Noooo" they both agreed. The rest of the team, who have only known Martin for a few months looked at each other, and said that they could not imagine Martin like that.

The path out of autism is scary, but MMS is giving us great joy and hope.

Martin has not been sick anymore, the last time he was sick, before MMS, we had to admit him to the hospital, his cough was so bad that he was vomiting non-stop.

First off we give thanks to God, we thank Jim, Andreas, my dear Kerri who guides me with all her love, and to every single mother that is in this struggle. I also thank Mr. Luis from Buenos Aires, Argentina who has made it easy for me to get MMS; he is a wonderful human being who helps those in need.

We are on the way to full recovery for Martin, I'm sure of that.

154. So I just redid my daughter's ATEC. She was a 71 a month and a half ago and is now a 60!!! I thought she was making nice improvements but it really set in when I saw her score. Some things that have changed for her are now she is pooping on the toilet every day and telling me. She used to just go every few nights in her diaper. There's no more diarrhea, she's not constipated, she's sleeping great. She is just starting to show signs of imaginative play and a big one for us is that she just learned to blow. She couldn't blow no matter what we did to try to teach her. Now she's got it. Hopefully more good things to come.

155. My now 8-year-old daughter was dx with autism at 18 months old. Started GF/CF diet and started with a DAN! She slowly made progress with speech, had a few words, a few 2 and 3 word sentences, and despite having autism, she was always a happy, calm, sweet little girl. Shortly after her 3rd birthday, she "changed." She became more of a Jekyll / Hyde personality, and all progress in speech and improvements in eye contact and sociability started to fade. Seemed like everything we did was just like yo-yoing back and forth between improving, and then crashing yet once again.

Last year at this time, we had just left the doctor we had been taking her to. For years she was on antivirals, antifungals, antibiotics on and off, SSRI's, Tenex, and when her violent SIB had become so bad the second year into treatment with him, he put her on Abilify. SSRI's and the Abilify did nothing for her except make her behave worse. Neither did any of the other things he had her on. The first year she was doing pretty good, but possibly because the antivirals were acting as an anti-inflammatory. She always had chronic constipation with loose stools/diarrhea. Nothing helped that either. We finally left that doctor who yelled at us in his office for 20 min straight, in front of my daughter, because he did not like that I had been challenging him on all of this for the past 6 months. I was no longer going to let him put the blame on us and everyone else... that her ABA and speech therapists didn't know what they were doing, and telling us she acted out this way because we didn't know how to give proper time outs or how to correctly give "pep talks" at bedtime. I was convinced that she had PANDAS/PANS and/or parasites that were causing her ever increasing SIB, loss of all progress she had made in speech over the past 4 years, and the fact that she had not grown in 4 years...did not gain 1 pound, feet did not grow at all, and she only grew 1/2 inch in height in that 4 year span. We had taken her to a very well respected endocrinologist the previous summer who ran all the tests. Could find nothing wrong as to why she wasn't growing. But he decided to put her on HGH anyway. Thankfully, we left and decided not to give her the HGH. We also took her to one of the best Ped Psychiatric doctors at UCLA who specialized in autism that summer. He observed her, her SIB happened right there in his office for him to see. He said her SIB is coming from pain, discomfort, something medical going on inside, most likely stemming from her gut. He suggested we get her scoped upper and lower. So we did. The only thing that came up was on the upper endoscopy, and that was that she had esophageal gastritis. So the GI dr gave her Nexium.

All the parasite stool tests we had done over the years had always come back neg except for one at age 3 came back with Giardia. But that was it. So last January, when we had finally left that her doctor of 3 years, her liver AST and ALT were at 130 and 135, her Creatinine (kidneys) were severely elevated at a dangerous level, she now had hypothyroidism, and after testing her cortisol thru blood and saliva we discovered she was barely making any at all. She had dark circles under her eyes, grinding her teeth for 3 years now, and agitated beyond belief ALL the time. Mind you when we started with him 3 years prior, her thyroid, liver, and kidneys were all in normal range. She did have dark circles, many many food allergies, some SIB, but nothing compared what we were dealing with now, or what was to come.

So now, what to do. We took her to a very highly recommended Pediatric GI in Los Angeles who was very nice. Listened to what we had to say. Ran the most sensitive and comprehensive stool analysis. Came back with nothing at all. Then took her to the head of pediatric Infectious Disease at Cedars Sinai. She obviously had her mind made up before she even walked in the door. She saw the word AUTISM on my daughter's chart, and that was it. I showed her every blood and stool test, explained the not growing at all for 4 years despite all the endocrinology labs said everything related to growth was in normal range, her severe SIB. She said to us..."I know you want to help your child. You want to find something "medical" that has caused her autism so you can fix it. But the truth is, your daughter has autism. You need to accept that, and take her to a pediatric psych dr who can help her with these SIB's. There are lots of meds that can help her be calmer." Had she not listened to one damn word I told her!!! All the meds we had tried in the past did nothing, already took her to a psych dr who specialized in autism telling us something internal was wrong. She would not run any blood tests, or any other kind of Infec Disease tests. So with that, my husband, my sister, and I completely dumbfounded started to walk out. The dr then had the nerve to say..."She hasn't been vaccinated since 18 months (she was 7 here) Let's get her caught up right now before you go. I can give her 6 vaccines today." I looked at her and said you have got to be crazy! I am not giving my very sick child vaccines full of the poisons that did this to her."

So a month later we started with doctor who "gets it." Who listens, and treats parents with respect. Values their opinions. And the networking I had been doing for the past 6 months on a few different bio-med autism groups with other moms was paying off. The moms are the ones who KNOW!!! That's how I found my daughter's current doctor and how I found Dr Maile Pouls last June to help her with nutritional and metabolic healing. Dr Pouls ran a $100, 24 hour collection urine analysis, and we found out she had severe malabsorption, Ph was too Alkaline, she was catabolic, extremely electrolyte and mineral deficient, severely Vit C and D deficient, and had severe bowel toxicity. Working with Dr Pouls and her new doctor lead them to suspect parasites/worms. I was encouraged to look into mms, but of course I had heard nothing but bad things like it's bleach. I was very hesitant to try it, but I researched it, and sought out other moms on Facebook who were doing it. The toxins from the parasites had completely taken over her body and brain. She was SIB almost all day, every day by now. It was pure hell. We thought we were going to lose our minds it was so bad. We had stopped taking her anywhere but school and dr's appointments for the past 2 years because she would just suddenly out of nowhere, for no reason, violently freak out and there was no way to help her calm down. Her doctor said she's so toxic, and her body is so sick that she can't detox. That the mms will not only help kill, but will neutralize the toxins and help her calm down. So we started mms, and I could not believe how much calmer, happier, and more present she was in just a week. MMS is literally saving her life, and bringing her back to us. Before starting mms, we did just parasite meds like Alinia and Mebendazole. The parasite meds alone did not help her, even though she was dumping worms, but she was still completely psychotic, and getting more crazy and manic every day. Since starting mms she has dumped hundreds of worms, some 10-12" long, ascaris eggs, TONS and TONS of the shedded skins of the worms, tons of liver flukes, and hundreds of tapeworm segments. We had not done any PP yet. This had all been with MMS only! We actually started Albendazole for treating tapeworm about a month ago and saw immediate improvements with it. It really seems like this is her biggest beast right now to deal with.

These are her labs from before MMS, and after starting MMS:

2/7/2012 - one month after leaving scumbag dr of 3 years

AST = 79 ALT = 108 Creatinine = 1.24 EOS = 11.2 Sed Rate = 9

~ Started MMS 11/23/2012 ~

12/4/2012

AST = 73 ALT = 64 Creatinine = 1.32

1/15/2013

AST = 61 ALT = 60 Creatinine = 1.30

2/27/2012

AST = 51 ALT = 42 Creatinine = 0.92 EOS = 5.1 Sed rate = 12

Ref Range for AST is [15 - 46] ALT is [3 - 35]

Ref Range for Creatinine (kidney) is [0.60 - 1.20] Shows how well kidneys are working. Anything close to or over the 1.20 is considered to be of serious concern

Ref Range for EOS (eosinophils) is [0.00 - 3.0] * High EOS are always seen with parasites

Ref Range for Sed Rate (marker for inflammation) is [0 - 10]

Her doctor said her Sed Rate is likely high because when killing off pathogens and detoxing, inflammation will go up temporarily.

So I say never give up. Don't listen to doctors who don't listen to you. Kerri, thank God you saw those bottles of MMS at the clinic that day and asked what they were. And that you bought some out of curiosity and tried it. And that you selflessly have taken what you've learned and experienced, and shared it. Given so much of your time to help others, to help heal and recover their kids. You are truly an amazing person. We finally have the answers to our daughters autism after almost 7 years of numerous doctors and specialists, so many tests, so much money and valuable time wasted... and now we finally have real hope...real results. We know without a doubt she is going to get healthy, which will in turn give her the happy joyful life back that she once had before she got "autism." ~ xoxo

---

156. Today was just wonderful! We have been on MMS since 12/11 and this is our second round of Ivermectin from our Dr, just started today. My son has been very rigid lately, but not today. For the first time in over 6 months we went to the park and had a great time (no stimming), then we were able to run an errand and pick up books from the library. (he usually gets upset unless we do one specific route in the car). Felt like a regular mom running kids to the park and one errand. So lovely!!!

---

157. Just a testimonial to MMS. For those of you new to the group and still unsure of MMS protocol I wanted to tell you about us. I was afraid at first, but we decided to try MMS. Within 3 weeks my son went from an ATEC of 36 to 18! That was amazing. Then we were afraid of the enemas. We said no way, we would just do oral MMS. of course after seeing others progress here we decided to do them. He would calm down! Then for months we agonized over the PP. We were afraid of it. We were scared of the meds, everything. Finally we decided to try it too. We are in the middle of our first PP and our son, who used to hit, kick, bite and scream at me over the smallest things all the time, has now been a perfect joy. When he gets mad it is over quickly and does not escalate into world war 3. Also these bumps he had on his face have cleared up along with his attitude! So if you are unsure of MMS like I was, here is one more testimonial of just how good the protocol really is.

    Thanks Kerri, all the other moms that came before me!

---

158. Dear Kerri and the readers,

    I would like to say that we started giving MMS to my son Filip, autistic/PDD NOS, when he turned 5 years old, after having tried lots of things (diet, many different supplements, HBOT, some sort of behavioral therapy Teach and ABA), we have seen enormous changes already in the first month.

    I had heard about MMS from a mom of an autistic child. I started reading about it, but was not impressed by the comments I read on the internet. I contacted a few mums that I knew from the Son-Rise programme in the US and they have reassured me that it works miracles.

I was however very sceptical of MMS, as I have read so many "negative" comments on the internet. This is why I decided to start it myself for a few months to see what would happen to me. Also, I had to figure out how I was gonna dose MMS 8 - times a day, when I am working 10 hours a day and Filip is going to the kindergarden.

In fact, I was just feeling great when I started using MMS.

I wanted to start with my son when on holiday, but my husband displaced MMS bottles by mistake. I was so mad. I have only found them the last day when we were returning home. I have immediately decided to give one drop to Filip before we started to drive. I need to underline that my husband was very sceptic. Filip would at that time speak, but it would mostly be scripting and rarely would he say things in context. Otherwise he also had other autism symptoms- tantrums, no friends, low muscular tone, no drawing, obsessive occupations (in Filip's case watching cartoons and reading books), no sense of danger, wandering out, nose picking, scratching but, toe walk etc. But suddenly Filip started commenting everything in the car, asking questions, observing the things he would see from the car etc. Me and my husband looked at each other and my husband commented " Maybe it is working after all".

Filip's ATEC was 48 at the time we started. At start, my mother-in-law helped out in dosing and we were able to dose 8 times a day. Filip's ATEC fell to 32 the first month. Unfortunately, my mother-in-law read some horrible stories on the internet and the FDA's advice was detrimental for her decision to stop dosing Filip, even though she was seeing wonderful results, she was scared and said that she is only believing the official medicine, admitting that the official medicine has nothing to offer our son.

I was very disappointed, but continued to dose as much as I could, however not reaching the recommended 8 times a day. I was therefore only able to dose 4-5 times a day. I started telework on Friday's in order to at least get 8-10 doses in on Fridays, Saturdays and Sundays and 4-5 doses the rest of the week. My son was great in November (the volunteers working on Son-Rise with Filip were commenting on unprecedented success), but his ATEC only fell to 28, I would say due to low dosing the progress was slower. Filip was having some hard times in January, when he was more hyperactive. At that time we have also introduced the GcMaf injections, which could have added to Filip's hyperactiveness.

But since two weeks now Filip is back to his shape. He is so communicative, uses unseen vocabulary, amazes us every day, he started drawing without being prompted, communicates with everyone, was invited to a birthday from a girl at the kindergarden, started to dress without prompting, started to tell me: " Common mummy, hurry up, let's go." or "Where are you mummy? What are you doing?" or when he occasionally wakes up during the night " Is it day already? or " I should not go on the street, because a car can hit me" or " Daddy, you are not sad, you look angry" or just yesterday when he draw a picture in the kindergarden he said to his teacher " I want to show it to my mum". The list goes on and on and every day I have to thank the all mighty for having led me to Kerri and to the MMS protocols. I know we are on the right path to recovery and I am not scared of the future any more. And, finally, i just did his ATEC to check out his ATEC- it is 16!!!!!! LOVE IT! LOVE IT!!!!!!

Kerri, thank you!!!!!!!!!

159. My daughter has had really bad SIB for over 4 years. We've been in the ER for massive goose-egg bumps on head, and she always had severe bruising on her tailbone and spine from dropping herself down, butt first and legs in a "W" position, onto the floor, and then would fling and flail herself into walls, tables, furniture, bang her head on all of the above and the floor, a rage like she was the girl from the Exorcist. Nothing could stop it. It just had to run its course...like a tornado. Comes out of nowhere, and it will disappear when it's ready to. Nothing can stop it.

But after starting MMS, it was 80% better right away. Then after 3 weeks it started coming back. For a month it was really bad again, and we could not move up past 2 drops without her going crazy. Then after you had us switch to the HCl, she was remarkably better in about 5-6 days. She has had a few "episodes" in the past 2 weeks, but now they can last 30 min max, where before mms they would last anywhere from 15 min - 2 hours literally non-stop. The year before starting mms, there were times I had to lay her on the bed or couch and just sit on top of her, like on her butt so she couldn't hurt herself. I would just lose strength after about 30-45 min of trying to hold her.

160. Hey everyone! Just wanted to give a positive report about the HCl activator. My son is 12, non-verbal, very hyper and lots of food intolerances. I got mine in the mail today, gave a quick 3 drop dose to my son before he went out the door to school, noticed he was a bit more compliant and calm than usual after school. have given 2 more doses since coming home and he has been doing his usual, but he is much more calm today than he has been in months!!! I gave him a snack and he took it and started to eat and I told him: can you say thank you mom? and he actually responded with a sorta grumbled "graaaa mooooom" which was to me "thanks mom."

161. Thanking God for Kerri Rivera and happy here too. My 15 y/o is in the chorus of his HS play. He has to do 5 costume changes, his own hair and makeup and several song/dance numbers, which he did perfectly on opening night! He is not your typical MMS/autism kid. He was pretty much recovered, starting with biomed at age 2.5, until age 11 when he hit puberty and he started getting rigid and anxious. We had some supplements going and were starting to look at stem cells when we found Kerri. He is not on the strict MMS protocol but takes it when he can and does PP and enemas each month. He is so much better since starting this last August! So thankful for all the info and support from this group.

162. Hi Kerri,

Last week I contacted you regarding our 8 year old son and his focus issues and the disappearing act his mathematical skills have taken, and we've done our best follow through on your advice to up the number of doses to 16 per day. I visited my son's Integrative Medicine doctor this morning, who has been his biomed doctor for the last 3 or so years to do a live cell microscopy, and to see if he had any ideas about the focus issues our son has been having. I told my son's doctor in detail what we've been up to over the last 10 months (MMS Protocol, Parasite Protocol) and he took it all in.

When he looked under the microscope he was shocked to see that our son's nasty dysbiosis issues were gone! He told me that he's had almost no luck completely getting rid of dysbiosis in a case like my son's. The yeast beast is gone! He still has evidence of leaky gut but the drainage looks great. He was so excited, our 20 minute scheduled visit turned into 40 minutes as he wanted to know all about what we did so he can find a way to use it in his practice. He also remarked that you must be one bright lady to come up with the protocol, but we already knew that. :-) He had us fill out an ATEC when we first visited him back in 2010 and our son was at 55. He dropped into the 30's when we started him on Carnitine but the MMS protocol has brought him down to the 6. The doctor also noticed the distinct lack of autistic behaviours, so it's nice to get some outside feedback to help confirm what we are showing on the ATEC. I asked him directly if he thought we should change anything at this point and was direct...don't change anything keep going. And so we continue on our quest for the zero ATEC. :-) About two years ago we did a chelation challenge test (DDI) and found our son extremely high in lead and so we proceeded with IV chelation at that time. He ants us to do a chelation challenge test to check the metals status just to rule out lead and the possibility that metals might be still at the heart of our son's lack of focus and more ADHD like symptoms.

He wants me to send him some information on your MMS protocol. He attempted to use chlorine dioxide about 10 years ago and found that he couldn't get the results that you are getting. I'll send him to MMS Autism website but can I include your contact info (email)?

Thank you for being so patient with us and everyone. As you know full well when it involves your own kid the emotions come out and it's hard to remain logical.

---

163. Drum roll....

I have been dying to share...

Been off MMS for a few weeks...AND HOLY SMOKES we are ALLLLL GOOD!!!!!!!!!!!!!!!!

Summary...

My daughter—PANDAS—MAJOR sleep issues—fluctuate between diarrhea and constipation

Me—Acne—horrible—and nail fungus

ALL GONE. ALL.

NOBODY could EVER, ever, ever tell me why I broke out so much esp. with our squeaky clean diet.

First PP, OMG it was REALLY bad—worst ever—and became cystic—painful—so for SURE worse before better in my case BUT believed in protocol and KEPT GOING.

By month 4, GONE and yet to return

Fungus—gone in month 1, never to return

My daughter:

Well, you know, AMAZING!!!!!

YOU, Kerri, YOU helped me figure out FINALLLLLY after a zillion docs, WHY MY KID could NOT SLEEP! EVER! 7 LONG years... long long—exhasuting years—and it was PARASITES NO DOUBT in my mind! Month 1 of PP, literally like a light switch, SLEEPING —falling asleep ON HER OWN—(not with a circus routine to "get her to sleep") AND staying asleep ALL NIGHT LONG! UNREAL! This is HUGE!

AND bye bye PANDAS (Siver/Aloe nipped it, MMS maintained her gains,

BEAUTIFULLY!) SO I do believe in our Silver Aloe protocol for PANDAS, 100% worked for us! AND MMS. Both.

AND since OFF MMS, my daughter is 100% pooping NORMAL—OMG first time in her WHOLE LIFE!!!!!!!!!!!!!!!!!!!!!!!!!!!!!!!!!! (on MMS it was still fluctuating...)

AND she is eating things she would have NEVER ever touched! EVER! Raw veggies, nuts, trying EVERYTHING I make... unreal... this is HUGE too... the "healthier" you get, your tastes DO change... and one becomes less "picky"

I have learned that SOME probiotics can literally throw a child into a PANDAS rage--and also brought back MY symptoms—literally within 12 hours of consuming. (Like "Regarding Caroline" posted) This clearly happened to us. Mental note: NOT all prob's are appropriate for everyone. We react to fermented food—so I am going to experiment with no prob's and with THeralac __ONLY THeralac BTW

Now,

We are back to silver/aloe, daily, as prevention

We will still take DE (prevention)

Vit D3

Trace Mineral Drops

Enemas as needed

AND I am going to go BACK to the herbs for 3 months around full moon "just in case"—

I CANNOT WAIT to meet you in person, THANK YOU, and share our story with EVERYONE that will "hear me".

Again, my daughter did not have 'autism' per se, but autoimmune issues, meaning that, perhaps, her treatment protocol is 'shorter' then someone who is "more sick' etc. if that makes sense.

We also did a boat load of work prior to this. Meaning diet in place, for instance, for 4 years already—so healing began. This was the final layer for us. The frosting on the cake!!!!!

I have 2 brand new bottles of MMS in my cabinet :) AND will ALWAYS have it on stock!

With MUCH LOVE and respect to you Kerri.

-Jeni, IL, USA

---

164. My daughter was born Sept 9 2010 and she had pretty good health until she had 15 months, she was able to say five to ten words by then, she had all her vaccines on time as recommended by our pediatrician, and she was really lovely and happy but suddenly every start to change slowly, we noticed she start losing the words she had learned, she use to wave people saying hi, and suddenly she was not interested on waving anymore and she start to isolate herself little by little to the point she stop being a happy girl, she barely looked at us and we started to worry about it, anyway, I believe the first thought every parent may have think in this very same situation is that her personality is different than other kids and is something temporal.

When she had 18 months we went to the regular doctor check and they asked us to get the opinion of a development pediatrician since her social and language skills were behind the expected, and this started the worst nightmare ever.

It seems like every single development pediatrician has a waiting list huge enough to have more than a couple months totally scheduled, we called on May and the first available appointment was 4 months later, we called like 4 or 5 of the recommended pediatricians and institutions but it was all the same thing, but we finally got a pediatrician, not form the recommended list, but he made room for us in a couple of weeks and we were able to see him in a couple of weeks.

The diagnostic was mild autism, the recommended treatment was ABA therapy and the follow up was going to be 1 year later since he did not have may expectations of positive changes in the next 6 months, we were devastated by this, my wife was in denial, and I started our journey to recovery the very same day, I started researching and suddenly I found tons of information about autism and people who claimed to have recovered their children from autism.

I sent emails everywhere and I never imagined I would have such a great response from every person I wrote extending me a helping hand on all my doubts with the most sincere and honest recommendations, 2 or 3 days later I found Autismo2.com website and I saw all the videos available.

I bought 3 or 4 books on amazon, I saw many hours of recordings and seminars in Spanish and English, and I was amazed about some kids losing their diagnostic, but also about how they were affected by heavy metals, bacteria, viruses and all sort of things.

At the beginning I thought my daughter could not be sick, she has never had a single cold, how come? but a home heavy metal screen test gave us the first clue, and some lab tests confirmed the very same problems all our kiddos share, mercury levels on the roof, candida, yeast, you name it.

I started the GFCFSF diet the first weekend after her confirmed diagnosis and just one week later we started noticing changes, then I started with baths with bentonite clay, and noticed more improvements, we also started ABA on July, and little by little our daughter started to improve, later on we introduced MMS baths, Quinton water, DE, probiotics, and she improved every day.

I honestly believe that the early diagnosis and prompt reaction from our side played a big role on her fast recovery, It happened that we never canceled the first appointment that was made with the most recommended development pediatrician, by then we were looking for a second opinion and a new evaluation due to her huge improvements, we never imagined this pediatrician will say what.

Although my history with this disease or condition has been very short nobody knows how much pain, stress and suffering had caused to our family, we now enjoy our daughter more than ever when we see her playing with her old sister and taking away every single concern we had, we continue keeping an eye on her development but she is doing really well, I wish nothing more than every single mother I have hear on the discussion groups I follow have the very same results we have had with all the guidance from such smart and courageous parents like Kerri Rivera and many others that shed us the light on our darkest night.

I am more than grateful with all of those parents, I would do anything on my reach to help them, we need to help every single kid and family that goes through this disease to recover our kids.

UPDATE:

I'm very happy to forward the last ATEC from my daughter, today we came from her 2 year check up with the new pediatrician and she found her pretty well, she just told us" It's pretty hard to believe she was diagnosed with mild autism keep *doing whatever you are doing, since I would say she is acting like a regular kid for her age."*

I would say that keeping in mind that most of her ATEC score is on the Language section, for a 2 year old and from what we came from she is on her way to full recovery (Previous ATEC was 55, at this writing was a 23)

---

165. I found Jim on the Internet 2 years ago, and I immediately started Jim's protocol for MMS. Unfortunately we were so loaded with mercury, so when I reaches 8 drops of mms, and my son 2 drops (after more than 2 months on slow upgrading) we were really sick, again. All the heavy metals that where released with mms could not get out of us. That´s when I found zeolites, and that was our way back.

Now, two years later, my arthritis is gone, and now I know it was mms that killed the clostridium bacteria that I had been carrying since I was 13 (I am 52 now). 6 months ago my son fell off his bike and got an open wound. It was infected and some hours later the blood was black in his hand. Now I had a choice, to go to the doctor and give him antibiotics, which I knew would kill the bacteria but make him worse, or do it my own way. I gave him 2 x 3 drops of mms, and the blood was ok in some hours, I thought. Some days later he started to wave his hand. I thought he had eaten something else that he could not digest, but it got worse. After 4 weeks he was not only waving/flapping both his hands, but also his head. Then I started get suspicious. I tested him for bacteria (I use a Rayonex PS 10 for testing, bioresonance) and I found Clostridium botulism.

Now I had a choice again. I had a fully booked week, but his father came and took him home to his island, where they could use MMS every day and be in a calm environment. He got 2 x 3 drops of mms, for 6 days. After 3 days his father called and said "Eva this is scary, the flapping is getting worse". And I smiled and calmed him down, the bacteria are dying and the toxins are being released, I said. The zeolites took care of the toxins, and after 4 week he was ok again.

My lesson in this was, apart from the clostridium toxins, that I also found an imbalance in my son on Condrogenesis with the Rayonex. When I was 13 I stepped on a rusty nail. The blood was poisoned in the foot, but I did not dare tell my parents. After 3 days the whole leg up to my knee was black. I got antibiotics, of course. At 18 I was diagnosed arthritis in my knee. I think I had small amounts of bacteria left, as my son had, and the toxins from clostridium bacteria degenerates the cartilage near the infection. After some years one develop arthritis. I did, but it's gone now!

Eva, Sweden

---

166. Drum roll please.......my son is 17 years old. He's been on mms for 5 months now, I'm so excited I don't even know, could it be 6? I think we started late July. He started with a 63.......he is now a 7. He went from 63 to 25 in just a few weeks, then a 13 a couple months later, now a 7. I feel like I'm cheating every time. I go back and look, argue with myself, nitpick....but whether he's a 5, 7 or 9, it's nothing short of a miracle because just one year ago, he was WAY over 100.

The ATEC is not perfect, not even close. There are things that the ATEC does not show. All that is true, but this is incredible improvement that no doctor I know would have ever been able to accomplish. Been there, did that, spent the 425K+.

And no, it's not just MMS, but that has been the main treatment and everything else we do supports MMS and general health because I believe that in the end, it's a battle between your immune system...and all that's attacking it. We are winning and I sure do wish they would STOP CALLING IT AUTISM. That alone hurts so many.

Here's a little background on my son: Matthew was very high functioning from age 6-12. That was after diet since 3, floortime play therapy, some aba, AIT, IVIG, chelation for a year, OIG, years of infusions of glutathione, vitamin C, B-com, etc...immune stuff. Then he did very well GFCF ages 6-12, ran track (very well), 2nd degree black belt, boxing lessons, etc....Then puberty hit, and what I did not know about, Lyme and co-infections RAGED, and for around 3 years, I lost him cognitively, worse, worse, worse. At 15, he was like an advanced Alzheimer's patient, ADVANCED, he had lost ALL short-term memory, it was horrible, he struggled to think and could not.

He became more and more violent; choking me, kicking me, did I say he was a blackbelt? Even though he lost everything cognitively, like the ability to answer a question, those karate skills popped back into his head and he nearly killed me.... really close a couple times.

That was a year ago when his ATEC was over 100. So, here's what worked: 1. Low amylose diet helped with the constant urinating. (he acted like a diabetic and had 14 of 16 PANDAS symptoms so auto-immune) 2. Biofeedback helped calm him some. 3. Cholestyramine helped him psychologically - I could see him clear up mentally in minutes. (chemical/mold/dust sensitivities big time) By this time, his doc had him on Ketamine for pain. 4. PEMF (pulsed electromagnetic field device) stopped the pain in 6 weeks, got him off of Vicodin, which was not working anyway at double doses, and all the Ketamine. I hated drugging him. Got him off the psych drugs over 6 months time. Then he got a lot better but communication did not really come around until 5. MMS. BAM. Big improvements in communication and PERSONALITY. With MMS, even his laugh changed to a typical sounding teenager's laugh, and for the first time in years, he can sit still and stop pacing, pacing pacing....the parasites were eating him alive....and now more recently, I know 6. Hydro-colonics is taking us to another level of clear communication. Now there's lots of spontaneous language.

I write things on Facebook so that I can remember and maybe write a book one day. I don't care how bad things get, believe me, your kids can get better and it's amazing, they really do store up all this info that you didn't think was there. It is there, and they will share it with you one day.

I hope one day Matthew can share his perspective with others. It's just that it has taken a very long time for us to help him understand that the things he did back then were not in his control so I'm careful not to talk about it. For months he would out of the blue apologize and feel terrible, over and over. Then there's memories of his dad losing it also....protecting me.

Thankfully, Matthew has blacked out or forgotten a lot of it. He did say he remembers being locked in his room. We had to turn the lock around and sometimes lock him in there. Bad memories. We were all traumatized. But not anymore. He is a different person today but he's always been the sweetest boy I know. I knew that, even back then. One day, he'll probably talk more about it.

167. Hi Kerri,

First of all a HUGE big thank you for what you are doing with our children! My daughter has been on MMS two weeks now and she is like a different child!!!!!!!! Every day she gets better...By leaps and bounds. She WILL be one of your recovered ones ;)

UPDATE:

My daughter has now been on MMS for three weeks. ATEC down from 78 to 44. This IS a miracle. We have been in absolute desperation for almost three years trying to figure out what in the world is going on with our child. After hundreds of thousands of dollars, experts all over the world, LA, New York, San Fransisco... and nothing would work. Minor improvements but nothing that I could say really worked. Everyone always agreed that she probably does not have "autism" but what is making her behave that way?!?!?! So a long story short... If I could I would wrap my arms around all of you helping my daughter and so many others through MMS until I was sure you truly understand what your dedication means and that you are saving lives...literally <3 This is by far the biggest thing that has ever happened to my family. We are forever thankful.

UPDATE #2

I sent you my daughter's ATEC a week ago but redid it today. We started MMS in December and I decided I will do the test every month. Here are the results, 4 more points gone!!!! In 1 month from 78 to 40... Almost half off!!!!!! Her team is blown away ;) all we need now is that language score to come down... Kerri my goal is to have her recovered by A1!!!

Update #3

We are seeing such amazing improvements every single day. I think the true testament is the daily feedback from people working with her who do not know we are doing MMS. Here is part of a note from her SLP " her communication on the whole is truly remarkable- words, iPad, eye contact...everything is improving!!!!!!! So exciting. Has anyone told you lately that your daughter is a superstar? You should be so proud. :)" And I am...

Our main challenge has always been anxiety and today we had a breakthrough on that front. Instead of clinging to me for her dear life when I separate from her at school she took her friends hand, waived AND said goodbye and walked away... Here is the best part, she then turned her head, waived and gave me the biggest smile . Her face at that moment is forever engraved to my heart.

Also for the first time EVER my son was able to have a friend come over from school in our car without her having a major meltdown. Instead she shared her iPad with the friend to show him her program and use it TOGETHER!

Honestly I think our major challenge at the moment is for the rest of the family to heal with her... We had lost all hope and settled for life with Autism. We can now look at the future very differently and actually look forward to it! Love our new life

UPDATE #4

I have never really posted gains but this is too huge not to share. We started MMS 3,5 months ago and at that point I could hardly take my daughter to the grocery store. And even if I did it was a guaranteed meltdown. Well we just got home from a two week long vacation that included travel by air, time difference, different language, going from hot weather to freezing temps and piles *of snow, totally different foods, nothing but strangers to her, visit after visit to new places... The list goes on and on. The BEST part - the vacation was full of excitement, fun, laughter and happiness every single day   I have to pinch myself to believe this is my life after such a short time on MMS. Thank you all for your support and guidance   I have my life back and can't wait for the future now! We still have a looooong way to go but we'll get there.*

Today is a wonderful day already

168. MMS Works!

It's my number one pathogen fighter. Our family continually suffers from Strep, my son specifically from Pandas. MMS remains and continues to keep our strep symptoms at bay. I have used everything for our bacterial flares (Abx, herbals, supplements even homeopathics) and nothing has worked so effectively like MMS does for us.

Recently I changed over to the HCL activator and within in a few days we heard my severely apraxic son's first WORD "Mama" Its been just over a month on the HCL activator and he is now stringing two words together!! MMS is a huge part of our recovery protocol. I feel relief beyond measure that I found a post on MMS and decided to try it, and mostly I'm immensely grateful to Kerri for putting the MMS protocol together and for her love for our kids.

169.
We just had a good meeting with all of Amor's teachers and therapists. In the last few months there has been big jumps in Amor's cognitive skills.

I used to worry that Amor might have dyslexia. I never pushed her to read even if was behind her peers. I know frustration will only make things worse. Her 'x' and 'k', 'b' and 'd' were always mixed up. I have been observing this mix up for the past 2 years. Early this year, her speech therapist agreed that dyslexia might be an issue and we were ready to start studying dyslexia management.

However, Amor now shows interest in reading both phonics and sight words. She can answer letter names and sounds precisely. The same speech therapist now says that we shouldn't look at dyslexia anymore. It might have simply been a mix-up as part of early learning. Amor's dyslexia issues in 2 years all of a sudden went away in 2 months??

Amor is also doing well with number recognition and improving in one-to-one correspondence. This is something her former speech therapist (back in Japan) was working on for a year...with little progress.

All these seem so simple but these are great strides from someone who has vision issues. Amor also wears glasses.

If I were to plot Amor's improvements with time, the biggest jumped occurred in the past few months, which of course can easily be explained by MMS.

MMS clears the gut of bad bacteria, yeast and parasites. All these affect sensory processing thus inhibiting the child's ability to understand her environment and people around her. Clean the gut, remove autism...in Amor's case, remove GDD.

We are also running a son-rise lifestyle program. I.e. we don't put fixed hours into her program but use the son-rise attitude and son-rise her in the weekends.

170. Luca came into our lives July 26, 2010, he was premature, but all my kids were born in week 35, so I was not surprised. He was perfect, I have thousands of videos of him looking into my eyes, smiling, playing with his sisters, following daddy to the door when he was ready to leave to work and saying bye bye. He walked at one, and was a perfect little baby. It is hard to know exactly when he changed but I can tell you when I started to get worried, and saw him behaving differently. I had a neighbor the same age as my son, and when they got together to play I was surprised at how my neighbors son followed simple directions and looked into my eyes every time I called his name. When I had play dates with my friends all the moms were so relaxed, and while they were talking and kids were playing with toys, I was always chasing Luca and trying to keep him in the same room because he was not interested in toys or playing with other kids.

My first trip to the Zoo with my three kids was a disaster, Luca didn't want to move from the Monkey's area and had his first melt down, all over the floor screaming and crying. I remember seeing all the families with kids the same age as my son, and seeing how they understood, and paid attention to what their mothers or fathers were saying. For me that was enough to feel for the first time something was not right, and it was not that I was a bad mother, I knew deep in my heart it had nothing to do with discipline.

I enrolled him in a school thinking that would help. The first day when I picked him up the teacher said they needed to move him with the babies because he was not ready for the 2-year-old class. That day I came home just knowing - and despite all my family, friends, husband and Pediatrician thinking I was crazy, we got him evaluated and the rest is history. On November 15th, 2012 it was official and we got the papers. Classic Autism, by that time we had read so much, watched hundreds of videos and searched every day on the Internet for interventions, schools, therapy etc.

I remember I wanted to start ABA the same day that I got the diagnosis, but the waiting list was really long and we would have to wait. So we waited and started an early intervention program in the Kent District. Surprisingly, I think we took the diagnosis really well; we just wanted to help him as soon as possible.

After the first month I stopped asking for a miracle or cure. I even asked all family and friends to do the same. I needed to accept it!!! My miracle was already here. My husband wanted to do the Gluten free diet and I was not even 100% in agreement...why??? He is such a blessing; let our miracle eat whatever he wants!!! I agreed to do the diet anyway, but wasn't really interested. I just had the feeling my husband was not "getting IT" or accepting autism = our new precious miracle. Now I can recognize and see clearly I was in total denial too. I was so afraid to let anybody know, even myself, that I didn't want this for Luca. I tried and tried and tried, but a voice inside of me was not in peace. I spent a lot of time crying and looking for recovery videos on YouTube, imagining Luca being one of them, and was fascinated with those stories.

Then one day I found Kerri Rivera's conference in Bulgaria, it was a "Godcidence," (like my father always says) I wasn't looking for MMS, I didn't know anything about that. I remember I watched the conference 3 times, and I felt butterflies for the first time since I got the diagnosis. It was like that voice was finally quiet and listening to every single word! "I want this."

I did my homework and found a lot of negative information about MMS but I did not care...that voice was so strong that I knew, the same way I knew about

Luca being autistic, that this was something I needed to explore. I looked for her in FB and to my surprise she answered me in minutes, when I asked her about the testimonies she connected me with some moms with recovered kids, REAL moms that decided to believe too. After I saw pictures from before and after and reading about their journeys I felt Hope!!! I knew deep in my heart this was the way and the path we should take. So I got my case together and when I was ready I talked to my husband about it.

It was easier than I expected, we wanted so badly to recover our son!!! It was not an easy process but finally after almost 3 months I GOT IT...WE GOT IT...THERE IS NOTHING WRONG TO WANT THIS, that is ALL we want for Luca!!!! For the first time I recognized my kid's autism was not a blessing, he was sick; GI problems, extreme constipation, food issues, sensory problems... and that voice (God voice) sounds really clear and loud; I NEED TO HELP MY KID TO RECOVER!!!!!!

On February 18th we started a Dietary Intervention with all Kerri's recommendations, the one diet that we were doing was full of sugar and carbohydrates, so we started to be really serious about all the food choices. We kept a very detailed food diary and ordered the MMS. By March 12th when our bottles arrived at our doorstep we were ready to start Kerri Rivera's Baby Bottle Protocol. March 13th we did our first bottle and that same day I asked Luca to look for a ball in the other room, and give it to me, and he did.

It was like he was sleeping soundly, and then he woke up. He was extremely alert and he was looking in a different way. At first I thought I was crazy, but then my husband noticed it too and the changes keep coming. He improved dramatically in all his therapy sessions, his waiting time, sitting at the table, responding to commands, pointing, eye contact, everything improved!

Kerri recommended doing an ATEC when we started back on February 18th, so I did, his score was 64 points. By April 1st he dropped 20 points! He now follows simple directions, plays with his sisters, recognizes them by name, hugs me and says mommy and daddy, has close to 200 words, and every day is a surprise for us.

I'm proud to say my son is on his way to RECOVERY AND HE WILL RECOVER, HE WILL BE RECOVERED!!!!!!!! I'm loving Kerri Rivera's Protocol, I'm loving my kid dropPing 20 points in his ATEC in a month, I'm loving searching his diaper, and inspecting his poop finding parasites, I know it seems impossible but I truly get excited! (Probably some mothers would understand) I'm loving this side of the picture FULL of hope. HOPE. I don't think I can leave this road now, I don't think I want my son to live in his "perfect" world and not in mine... I'm a fighter and thanks to Kerri I'm a believer ...THAT... is the blessing right there HOPE AND FAITH IN GOD IS ALL I HAVE AT THE MOMENT... Luca is really special, but it's not the autism that makeS him special, autism sucks!!! Overcoming it and all the obstacles he encounters every day, and doing what he is doing now is what makes him THE MOST SPECIAL KID ON THE PLANET, HE ALWAYS WILL BE SPECIAL TO ME NO MATTER WHAT, AUTISM OR NOT....I see it in his eyes now, he is a fighter like me, he is telling me what to do, recovery is soooooo in the picture!!!!!! I can actually see it!!!! I'm a HAPPY Mom!!!!!!!!!!!!!!!!!!!!!!!!

-Alma

171. Today is a wonderful day already. My daughter got up to her alarm, took a shower without help, got dressed, packed her lunch, woke up her sisters, and is now getting breakfast for everyone ready. It amazes me how independent she is becoming, and how much our life is changing because of her new independence.

    She is 10 and we started MMS in Sept. She had done 5 PP and following the PANDAS protocol the last week after emailing Kerri Rivera last weekend with concerns about eye fluttering. She is also on Fish oil, garlic, Magnesium, and GABA. Before she was very hyper, spacey, a lot of language, but not using it correctly. She was extremely impulsive, and would fixate on object to play with and ignore others. Now she does reciprocal play, she talks back and forth with her friends, she cracks jokes that are now actually funny. She is focused with her school work and not hyper - except in typical situations.

    This week my husband forgot to pick her up to take her to therapy and she came to my classroom to tell me how irresponsible he was, and that she was disappointed in his inconsistent behaviors. I had to laugh, but at the same time I was so proud as I explained to her the whole situation because we where having a fabulous discussion about life. She is doing so well. Thank you to all of you who have restored some of my hope that there is a cure.

172. We are now in our 7th month of using MMS (CD) and in our 4th year of treating B.D., our son, who was diagnosed Autism. Our first week of MMS (CD) brought on a skill that we had spent years trying to accomplish, over night potty training. Week 1 of MMS (CD) and B.D. was out of pull-ups and in underwear. We weren't even close to full dose and already seeing positives. We knew we were on to something big at this point. One month later, we all witnessed my son blow out his birthday candles and open birthday gifts. Probably the first time he knew this event was a birthday and it was meant for him. As a gift to him, we took a trip to Disneyland. Not only did B.D. walk the entire park at our side, but he never once cried, whined, or objected to anything on the trip. Prior to this, he had to be in a stroller or wagon at all times.

    B.D.'s skills continued to flourish over the next few months. We enrolled B.D. in swimming lessons hoping he would feel comfortable without a life jacket on and clinging to an adult. This hope turned into a major accomplishment. B.D. has passed all Beginner levels in swimming and is now on to Intermediate. He is now swimming unassisted in the deep end of the pool! I used to hold my breath during his sessions hoping he wouldn't do anything that would scare the other kids in the pool. I still hold my breath, but now I'm at the end of my seat recording him as he's giving every single bit of effort to learn from his instructor and pass another level!

    Just the other day, we went to a birthday party that was held in a warehouse full of screaming kids, loud music, inflatable jumpy houses and slides. This place can over stimulate just about anyone! In the past, my son would vocally stim, cover his ears, run behind the jumpers where the generators are (trying to turn them off) and require me, or his Dad to keep him engaged with the rest of the kids. Well, not anymore! He blended right in with the rest of the kids! Not a single stim, didn't cover his ears, stood in lines, listened and followed the rules and instructions, stood in lines and PLAYED with the other kids. His Dad and I were able to hang out with all the other parents, watching him run and whiz by with all the other kids as if that is how it has always been. Only it hasn't. He has come so very far in the past 7 months. We have a 6 year old son who no longer has sound sensitivity, loves to eat whatever is placed in front of him, DRINKS tons of WATER, has manners, shows empathy, is careful and aware of other kids (especially babies and toddlers), making progress academically, and so very affectionate. B.D. isn't recovered... YET, but we expect it to happen now more than ever. We have to put our shades on because the end of the tunnel just got closer and brighter!

173. My husband and I were told to come to the 2nd grade assembly this morning. They gave awards to 2 kids in each of the 4 second grade classes. One was for outstanding in academics, and the other was for most improved in Self Control, which is the "character trait of the month" for the whole school. Kayla was given the award for most improved in Self Control in her class! She walked up and got her award and stood up there with the other kids holding theirs. Up until a few months ago, she would have violent, self-injury tantrums at school every day... throughout the day, lasting anywhere from 10 - 90 min. She could never get through a class singing performance without losing it and tantruming, screaming through the whole thing. Her teacher came up to me on Wed. and said she just can't get over how happy my daughter is lately, and that all the teachers and staff in the school have really noticed too. FUA!!!! I'm so proud of my girl!

174. Our third child (K) was diagnosed with moderate autism at 21 months of age. K was very ill. He suffered from vomiting and diarrhea mixed with severe constipation for years. At first, we began every intervention we could afford. The first step was removing all gluten, caseine and soy. We saw a decrease in stimming behaviour and an increased ability to learn. We implemented many vitamins and B12 injections, cranio sacral therapy, anti-fungals, HBOT and an even stricter diet removing all artificial colours, flavours, preservatives and most sugar. Our son was making slow but steady gains. ABA therapy continued from when he was two until just this past March (4.5 years). K was seeming much better but despite these gains, was never close to "normal".

In July of 2012 a friend suggested MMS. I did my research and so it began. In three days K started to sleep through the night. After less than one week at a very low dose, K stopped the constant verbal scripting and obsessive speech- his most evident sign of autism. In that same week he began dressing himself independently. In the coming months, K's ATEC began dropping steadily. He began to make jokes, initiate social interactions, show empathy, cope with noise and busy places and best of all- understood safety. The risk of him running away was a memory. We could go places and he would stay near us. Teachers and Educational assistants were raving about his progress, unaware of the protocol we had begun. His most significant changes happened after a three months of the Parasite Protocol, using mms, Vermox, rompepiedras, neem and diatomaceous earth. Through enemas, he expelled worms as long as 24 inches to my husband and family doctor's disbelief. What K expels in his stool now looks normal and ordinary.

His ATEC in July 2012 was 46. Ten months later he has a score of 6.

He is undecipherable within his classroom and amongst his peers. He laughs, plays and acts like any other child his age. His academics are at par with his peers.

Our son does not appear to have autism anymore and only a trained eye would suspect that he ever had it to begin with. We thank Kerri Rivera, her Facebook group for all their support and MMS for being the final, and most significant leg in our sons' journey to recovery.

Maria A., Ontario Canada

175. My severe autistic boy has been now doing wonderful!!! This protocol has completely changed my life!! He's been dumping tons of parasites since we started MMS about three months ago we're now in the second pp...he's now much calmer more happier!! His ATEC dropped down from 80 to 48 in three months only...that was truly amazing he is now gaining weight, I feel like I'm getting my child back to normal again!! I wish I could tell the whole world how Kerri Rivera has changed thousands of people's lives!!! God bless u Kerri for all your hard work to help others!!!

176. My son Nick started MMS just after his 7th birthday. Within 6 months he had cut his ATEC score in half from 66 to 37. Nick showed speech gains from the very first drop of MMS after having made no changes in speech for two years. Really, Nick hadn't made any improvements at all for two years. He was in a total stall until we began MMS. We raised Nick's oral dose of MMS very slowly taking two months to get to his target dose and never experienced die off that was unreasonable. Three significant changes are obvious in Nick's health at this point; he has been off of his Mitochondrial cocktail (for several years he has had blood labs pointing towards Mito dysfunction) for over 8 months and we haven't seen any of the lethargy that used to concern us so much, he was able to wean off of his seizure medication for his absence seizures and we haven't seen any return of seizure activity, and his thyroid appears to be beginning to shift from his long standing diagnosis of hypothyroid. The nicest changes we see are in the vibrancy of his health and how happy he is! His eyes sparkle and he has lots of energy for the day. He is no longer sitting on the couch staring out the window waiting for someone to figure out how to help him feel better. Since beginning MMS, every day Nick shows us just a little bit more of the boy that he is underneath the veil of autism and sickness. He tells us what his favorite things are, what he wants to do, and his sense of humor is coming shining through. MMS has given me a ton of hope that we just might get our boy back!"

177. After 7 years of biomedical treatments, numerous therapies, and more doctors than I care to think about, our son, who was diagnosed with autism, could speak a full sentence, was potty trained, and could finally go to the mall and movie theater without screaming and putting his hands over his ears.

Victory??...yes...however, we knew we had so much farther to go. You see, as your child gets older, you realize that he is missing the key things in life that are crucial for independence. Our son had become "stuck" if you will, he was not socially maturing, and still lacked empathy, mature connections with peers, and proper communication with teachers and the other adults in his life. He would still yell when he didn't win a game, and he did not always react in an age appropriate manner, if something did not go his way.

My research went on as always...searching, searching, searching...we were not getting anywhere with his current doctor, and I knew that we had to change our current plan for treatment.

A good friend of mine called me to tell me about a new product that some of our warrior mom friends were trying. The letters MMS were spoken to me for the first time in March of 2012. My son was 11 years old and I was desperate for help. The first thing I asked was, "How much does it cost?" $25.00...what?? It can't be! We have spent our life savings, and now I am looking at something that cost less than a night out for dinner?? I decided to check it out!

I emailed Kerri Rivera and told her that I wanted to start the MMS autism protocol, and I'll never forget her quick response..."YIPEE", she said, let me know if you have any questions, I am here for you.

I read, studied, and called my friend about twenty times over the next couple of days, and then we began the next chapter in our journey.

About three weeks into the protocol, our son seemed calmer, as well as aware of others on a more mature level...we were excited! Once he was at full dose, we began, baths and enemas, and he continued to improve. Our next move was to try the 72/2 protocol, which is giving MMS every two hours around the clock for 72 hours.

Well, it was as if someone had kicked our sons maturity clock into high gear. We saw HUGE gains!

"Hey mom, I like your dress...you look really nice today"....WHAT??

"I'll try that new kind of chicken for lunch"...WHAT??

"I feel like I'm beginning a new life"...WHAT??

"It's OK that I didn't win the race, I had fun"...WHAT??

I wanted to call the Good Morning America Show and say, LOOK AT WHAT MY SON IS DOING!

He also began to grow and put on weight for the first time in three years! He put on 10 pounds and 2 shoe sizes in about 2 months!

The gains continue to come, and our boy is coming alive...recovering...finally it's here! My eyes well up with tears as I write these words...the words I have dreamt about for eight long years.

He celebrated his 12th birthday on January 3rd, and has told us that 2013 is going to be the best year of his life...YES...it is!

He is our angel, our fighter, our miracle. Thanks be to God for MMS!

We are blessed and forever grateful~

178. Once upon a time there was a little boy who had a strange mind, he hooted and he danced and he did not learn like the other children around him. So, he was sent to a special school. For his whole educational life he was separated, because he could not express correctly the answers put before him.

As he grew older he seemed sad and very much in pain. He appeared to try to stop the pain by clawing at his face and arms. He also stopped talking. We, his mom and dad, were very sad.

Then an angel came into our lives and told us of a magic potion.

"But" said the angel. "You must give him the potion every hour of the day and night for him to be better."

So the little boys' mom and dad have been doing that now for 9 weeks and 4 days. Every hour.

Now in those hours the mom and dad still cry. Some, because the little boy has been hurting for so long, and..... now they know why. But they also cry because they see that their little boy is not hurting like before. They are happy for his healing, and that he does not claw at his body any more.

And they are also happy because their little boy is talking again. And he is laughing. And the things that he knows surprise them. We thought he was not learning...turns out he was.

179. Feeling really good still about my Natalie's progress from the combination of anti-parasitic medication, the supportive components of the PP and CD (HCL version). Natalie is about 63-64 lbs and she takes 2 drops of CD an hour both at home and at school. We don't wake her for CD in the middle of the night; but if she wakes for the restroom or something, then we give her another 2 drops (we just keep it pre-mixed in the bathroom near her bedroom). CD has been the single most important catalyst to Natalie's improvements/healing over the past 10.5 months; utilizing all three modes of delivery (oral, baths and enemas). Kerri having escorted CD into the ASD community is like a Miracle, in my opinion. Sorry... I don't mean to be corny nor impose my Beliefs on anybody else; but I sometimes find it hard to contain my Joy now and I get chills just thinking about all of the children now feeling better and/or beginning to feel better and better with CD. Before CD, it was hard to feel Hope for my special little Natalie; who was formerly suffering very extreme PANS flares and re-flares monthly as well as rapid-onset grand mal (tonic clonic) seizures every 2.5-3 weeks on top of her ASD and global developmental disabilities. Now Natalie's PANS 'flares' if/when they occur are waaaayyy less intense and better-controlled/'snuffed out' with CD than the former roller-coaster of oral antibiotics that her Drs had tried for years, her seizure activity is decreasing significantly and we've even begun a slow reduction in her anti-seizure med Lamictal ODT. We're optimistic that Natalie will be able to remain stable on less and less of that med, as we feel it might be causing her some nasty side effects. Our Hope for her is that she might even be able to come fully off of Lamictal ODT, as we continue CD and PP for her. Time will tell. While she's still a 'work in progress' [Note: She's 14 years old and been ill since infancy and it's a bit harder to heal longterm infection(s) and/ or infestation(s)], we do see lowering ATECS in Natalie's future and brighter and brighter days. Patience is a virtue. So Grateful. Thank you Kerri and all you supportive Moms & Dads. More and more healing to come to ALL of our children!

---

180. Hi Kerri,

Thank you for helping my daughter, age 15, recover from Autism. Thank you for the MMS/CD program and the support to carry it out. Here is a summary of her recovery:

June 19, 2012 Atec=52

Started with MMS slowly, adding one drop a day

GF/CF/SF diet

It took her 1 1/2 months to get to full dose.

Noticed improvement in physical health & behavior

Began parasite program

Sept. 18, 2012 Atec=24

Continued with 6-8 doses/day & baths

More improvements

School discontinued IEP, because she was doing so well academically and socially

January 15, 2013 Atec=19

My daughter, who is not vaccinated, comes down with Chicken Pox

No one at school or in community had it before her. It appears to be an isolated case.

It may have been in her system and released as parasites died?

Fever of 102 degrees for two weeks was the lead up to the Chicken Pox. Seemed like her immune system woke up! After chicken pox, huge gains! That is when we noticed she was recovered!

April 25, 2013 Atec=6

Yeah!

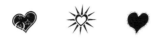

Please share your experiences!

Testimonials are one of the best ways to share your experiences with this protocol. Perhaps you learned about it by reading or watching a video testimonial?

If you don't tell us your experiences, we can't share them or take action on issues that need improving or correcting...

Send your testimonials to:

testimonials@cdautism.org

Also, let us know if we are free to publish your testimonial, with or without your name.

It's in our interest to take care of others. Self-centredness is opposed to basic human nature. In our own interest as human beings we need to pay attention to our inner values. Sometimes people think compassion is only of help to others, while we get no benefit. This is a mistake. When you concern yourself with others, you naturally develop a sense of self-confidence. To help others takes courage and inner strength.

~ *Dalai Lama*

Appendix 2

CD Autism Worldwide

Since September of 2011 over 5,000 families in 58 countries have used CD to help with an autism spectrum disorder. Here is a list of all the countries who have at least one family using CD to help heal the symptoms known as autism. This list is constantly updated at www.CDAutism.org.

- Argentina
- Australia
- Austria
- Belgium
- Bolivia
- Brazil
- Bulgaria
- Canada
- Chile
- China
- Colombia
- Costa Rica
- Cuba
- Czech Republic
- Dominican Republic
- Ecuador
- Egypt
- England
- France
- Germany
- Ghana
- Greece
- Hungary
- India
- Iraq
- Ireland
- Italy
- Japan
- Jordan
- Kenya
- Kuwait
- Malaysia
- Mexico
- Montenegro
- Morocco
- New Zealand
- Norway
- Panama
- Peru
- Philippines
- Poland
- Portugal
- Puerto Rico
- Qatar
- Russia
- Scotland
- Singapore
- Slovakia
- Slovenia
- Somalia
- South Africa
- Spain
- Swaziland
- Sweden
- Tanzania
- Turkey
- United Arab Emirates
- United States
- Venezuela

If you are using CD for autism in a country not listed above please email us so we can add you to the list... kim@cdautism.org.

Conformity is the jailer of freedom and the enemy of growth.

~ Robert F. Kennedy

Appendix 3

AutismOne on Healing Autism:
<u>Accidental Cure by Optimists</u>
by Simon Yu, MD

Accidents happen. We accept the reality of them as is and we usually move on. On the other hand, accidental discovery is another story. For some people, they ask questions like, "why me?" Or keep asking for a deeper meaning: Is this really an accident or a message to understand? An accident is a fertile ground to find out if you are a pessimist or optimist.

Tom Jacobs, story teller from Kansas City, recently told a story about a pessimist and optimist: Two sales men were assigned to Africa in the early years of the shoe industry to sell their shoes. One week later, one salesman telegrammed to his boss, "Business situation in Africa is hopeless. Nobody wears shoes". On the other side of the continent, the other salesman excitedly telegrammed to his boss, "Unlimited potential in Africa. Nobody wears shoes!"

I don't know about you but I would rather be an optimist. I always encourage my patients to look at the bright side and be cautiously optimistic no matter how grim their conditions might be. Hope is a powerful driving force to promote healing. Pessimists do not call themselves pessimists. Just realists.

Today, I saw a 77 year old patient with a history of chronic pulmonary fibrosis, bronchiectasis and rheumatoid arthritis with a recent diagnosis of stage one bladder cancer. She has been depressed and joined a cancer support group because of feeling a sense of hopelessness.

After a long discussion, I told her how lucky she is that her lung and rheumatoid conditions have been stable and she has only a relatively benign early stage of bladder cancer. I told her if you are going to have cancer, this is the kind of cancer to have and she should be thankful. All of a sudden, her doom and gloom mood was lifted with a broad smile. The rest of our session was uplifting.

The AutismOne 2013 conference was held in Chicago during Memorial Day weekend. I was invited to give a talk on parasites, allergies, and autism. Autism is not my field. I usually see adults as an Internist. However, beginning in 2012, I have been seeing autistic children with rather interesting responses. In May 2013, I wrote an article about a medical hypothesis of a relationship between parasite infection and autism in preparation for my lecture for the AutismOne conference.

I attended a full day of lectures and was awestruck by the thousands of autism parents from all over the country attending the lectures. Multiple lectures were conducted by many autism specialists at the same time covering a large variety of topics. This conference was driven by a grass roots movement of parents with a hope to help their children. Here is a short synopsis of the lectures.

Dr. Anju Usman, MD from the Chicago area covered gut-brain connection and biofilms by pathogens in the gut. Symptoms such as depression, anxiety, poor attention and focus, and obsessive compulsive behaviors may be related to the delicate balance of bugs which produce a mucous slime known as biofilm.

Andreas Ludwig Kalcker, Ph.D. Bio-Physicist from Spain, who studied under German bio-physicist Fritz Albert Popp, Ph.D., discussed parasites in depth. He demonstrated a successful treatment for more than 65 children around the world with his parasite protocol over a one year period.

Kerri Rivera, from Mexico, one of the main leaders of the group running the AutismOne conference, showed many cases of successfully treated autistic children including her child. She has been using chlorine dioxide in conjunction with diet, nutritional supplements, detox, and hyperbaric oxygen.

By the time I presented my medical hypothesis on parasite infection and autism, they had already had numerous discussions about parasites and had been saying all along how parasite infection might be one of the major underlying problems for autism that has been overlooked. I felt like I was repeating what had already been presented.

Dr. Andreas Kalcker and Kerri Rivera collaborated using chlorine dioxide for two years with prescribed parasite medications, albendazole and pyrantel pamoate, to turn around autistic children. Professionally, I have no experience using chlorine dioxide on my patients. The difference with my therapy was that I was using acupuncture meridian assessment as a guide to detect and treat parasites.

If what they are reporting is even partially true for these autistic children, it would be a major breakthrough in the autism community. Some of the audience was crying in excitement but some were skeptical and saying it sounded too good to be true. I could feel the excitement of the audience but also a sense of fear that Kerri Rivera and Andreas Ludwig Kalcker will be attacked by special interest groups. Chlorine dioxide is too inexpensive to a fault.

Is this an accidental finding leading into an accidental cure for autism? It is too early to tell but any chronic medical conditions like cancer, heart disease, diabetes, arthritis, Alzheimer's dementia, or autism seems driven by epigenetic influences from environmental toxins, parasites, hidden dental problems, and faulty diet and nutrition.

I spent several hours with Andreas Kalcker after our lectures were over. We found a common ground for treating parasites: his experience as a bio-physicist and my experience as a military medical officer. Few people truly understand and are aware of the magnitude of parasite problems. This man was very passionate to rescue these children from the scourge of autism.

Kerri Rivera just published a book called [Healing the Symptoms Known as Autism]. I just finished the book. This book is for everyone but especially for both autism parents and all medical professionals involved in the care of autistic children. The book contains much important information that is not available in the main stream autism community.

Most pediatricians might be sympathetic but they are rather pessimistic regarding the care of autistic children. Andreas Kalcker and Kerri Rivera are true optimists in the midst of skeptics and pessimists. They see unlimited potential for the cure for autism based on diet, nutrition, and parasite eradications using chlorine dioxide and parasite medications. If you want to know more about autism and what is possible, I highly recommend reading [Healing the Symptoms Known as Autism] by Kerri Rivera. The book explains in detail the Kalcker parasite protocol.

Dr. Simon Yu, M.D. is a Board Certified Internist. He practices Internal Medicine with an emphasis on Alternative Medicine to use the best each has to offer. For more articles and information about alternative medicine as well as patient success stories, and Dr. Yu's revolutionary health book Accidental Cure: Extraordinary Medicine for Extraordinary Patients, visit his web site at...

www.PreventionAndHealing.com

...or call Prevention and Healing, Inc., 314-432-7802. You can also attend a free monthly presentation and discussion by Dr. Yu on Alternative Medicine at his office on the second Tuesday each month at 6:30 pm. Call to verify the date. Seating is limited, arrive early.

Appendix 4

Autism Evaluation
Treatment Checklist (ATEC)

The next page contains a copy of the original *Autism Evaluation Treatment Checklist* (ATEC) developed by the late Dr. Bernard Rimland, the founder of the *Autism Research Institute*. We are not suggesting you use this particular copy. It is only included here for those not familiar with the evaluation so you have an idea what the ATEC involves since we mention it throughout this book.

The survey consists of a series of questions to be answered by a parent about what they are observing in their child's CURRENT behavior. It is not uncommon for both parents to take the survey separately and compare/average the scores.

The best way to take the survey is online at the *Autism Research Institute's* website. Here is the direct link to the current survey:

www.autism.com/index.php/ind_atec_survey

After completing the questions, a score is generated that can range from 0 to 180. 0 means no autism while 180 would mean that the answer to every question was in the most negative extreme.

We consider a child recovered from autism if their score is between 0 and 10.

You are encouraged to complete an ATEC before starting the Protocol, and every 3 months thereafter so you can clearly see the progress you are making.

Also, please share your results with us; we collect data on the children whose parents follow the Protocol as explained in this book. Send your name, date of the survey, general location (city, state, country) and score to:

atec@cdautism.org

If you have a history of ATEC results while on the protocol, please include them all.

NOTE: Do not send questions to this email address! You are unlikely to get any response from this address! It is just a collection point.

ARI/Form
ATEC-1/11-99

Autism Treatment Evaluation Checklist (ATEC)
Bernard Rimland, Ph.D. and Stephen M. Edelson, Ph.D.
Autism Research Institute
4182 Adams Avenue, San Diego, CA 92116
fax: (619) 563-6840; www.autism.com/ari

Project/Purpose:
Scores: I	II	III	IV	Total

This form is intended to measure the effects of treatment. Free scoring of this
form is available on the Internet at: www.autism.com/atec

Name of Child _____ _____ ☐ Male   Age _____
                        Last   First   ☐ Female   Date of Birth _____
Form completed by: _____ Relationship: _____ Today's Date _____

Please circle the letters to indicate how true each phrase is:

I. Speech/Language/Communication: *[N] Not true   [S] Somewhat true   [V] Very true*

N S V 1. Knows own name	N S V 6. Can use 3 words at a time (Want more milk)	N S V 11. Speech tends to be meaningful/relevant
N S V 2. Responds to 'No' or 'Stop'	N S V 7. Knows 10 or more words	N S V 12. Often uses several successive sentences
N S V 3. Can follow some commands	N S V 8. Can use sentences with 4 or more words	N S V 13. Carries on fairly good conversation
N S V 4. Can use one word at a time (No!, Eat, Water, etc.)	N S V 9. Explains what he/she wants	N S V 14. Has normal ability to communicate for his/her age
N S V 5. Can use 2 words at a time (Don't want, Go home)	N S V 10. Asks meaningful questions	

II. Sociability: *[N] Not descriptive   [S] Somewhat descriptive   [V] Very descriptive*

N S V 1. Seems to be in a shell – you cannot reach him/her	N S V 7. Shows no affection	N S V 14. Disagreeable/not compliant
N S V 2. Ignores other people	N S V 8. Fails to greet parents	N S V 15. Temper tantrums
N S V 3. Pays little or no attention when addressed	N S V 9. Avoids contact with others	N S V 16. Lacks friends/companions
N S V 4. Uncooperative and resistant	N S V 10. Does not imitate	N S V 17. Rarely smiles
N S V 5. No eye contact	N S V 11. Dislikes being held/cuddled	N S V 18. Insensitive to other's feelings
N S V 6. Prefers to be left alone	N S V 12. Does not share or show	N S V 19. Indifferent to being liked
	N S V 13. Does not wave 'bye bye'	N S V 20. Indifferent if parent(s) leave

III. Sensory/Cognitive Awareness: *[N] Not descriptive   [S] Somewhat descriptive   [V] Very descriptive*

N S V, 1. Responds to own name	N S V 7. Appropriate facial expression	N S V 13. Initiates activities
N S V 2. Responds to praise	N S V 8. Understands stories on T.V.	N S V 14. Dresses self
N S V 3. Looks at people and animals	N S V 9. Understands explanations	N S V 15. Curious, interested
N S V 4. Looks at pictures (and T.V.)	N S V 10. Aware of environment	N S V 16. Venturesome - explores
N S V 5. Does drawing, coloring, art	N S V 11. Aware of danger	N S V 17. "Tuned in" — Not spacey
N S V 6. Plays with toys appropriately	N S V 12. Shows imagination	N S V 18. Looks where others are looking

IV. Health/Physical/Behavior: *Use this code:* *[N] Not a Problem   [MI] Minor Problem   [MO] Moderate Problem   [S] Serious Problem*

N MI MO S 1. Bed-wetting	N MI MO S 9. Hyperactive	N MI MO S 18. Obsessive speech
N MI MO S 2. Wets pants/diapers	N MI MO S 10. Lethargic	N MI MO S 19. Rigid routines
N MI MO S 3. Soils pants/diapers	N MI MO S 11. Hits or injures self	N MI MO S 20. Shouts or screams
N MI MO S 4. Diarrhea	N MI MO S 12. Hits or injures others	N MI MO S 21. Demands sameness
N MI MO S 5. Constipation	N MI MO S 13. Destructive	N MI MO S 22. Often agitated
N MI MO S 6. Sleep problems	N MI MO S 14. Sound-sensitive	N MI MO S 23. Not sensitive to pain
N MI MO S 7. Eats too much/too little	N MI MO S 15. Anxious/fearful	N MI MO S 24. "Hooked" or fixated on certain objects/topics
N MI MO S 8. Extremely limited diet	N MI MO S 16. Unhappy/crying	N MI MO S 25. Repetitive movements (stimming, rocking, etc.)
	N MI MO S 17. Seizures	

Appendix 5

MOLECULAR MIMICRY
What It Is
&
How it Relates to
The Gluten Syndrome

by Mrs. Olive Kaiser

After reading the short answers in *The Diet* Chapter (page 64), we understand (simply) the basics of how some of these departments of the immune system function. It is easier to grasp how, through molecular mimicry, gluten can damage so many different tissues in different people, and sometimes cause other foods that *look like* gluten to also be reactive. Before we go any further, I would like to thank the following professionals for their contributions to our family's well-being and a wider understanding of the gluten syndrome and other related topics. If you would like to conduct further research into this topic, the body of work that the following professionals have contributed would be a great place to start. There is so much more to learn.

Dr. Alessio Fasano, MD, shook America awake on gluten awareness in the 1990's and in 2003 published a landmark paper[1] on one small subset of the gluten syndrome, villi damaged celiac disease. That study provided the impetus that brought gluten awareness to the table (or sadly, OFF many tables) across our nation.

Dr. Thomas O'Bryan, DC, Functional Medicine, and international gluten syndrome educator - www.thedr.com. Dr. O'Bryan is my functional medicine doctor. He taught me much of what I learned about gluten and other topics and led me to his mentor, Dr. Aristo Vojdani. Later Dr. O'Bryan's amazing research review seminars on gluten contributed hugely to my knowledge base and bolstered my confidence to manage our new lifestyle in a then difficult social era.

Dr. Aristo Vojdani, PhD., MsC, Immunologist, CEO owner of *Immunosciences Lab*, Los Angeles, CA. Dr. Vojdani is also chief scientific advisor of *Cyrex Laboratories*, Phoenix, AZ. Dr. Vojdani has published nearly 150 excellent research papers.[2,3,4] They fit the community like a glove.

Dr. Rodney Ford, MD, pediatric gastroenterologist, NZ, grasped the extent of neurological injury,[5] and "silenced nerves phenomenon."[6] This compellingly suggests why many of us do not recognize symptoms of gluten damage until we are in deep trouble. This builds on the previous work of Dr. Marios Hadjivassiliou, Professor of Neurology, Sheffield, UK.[7]

Dr. Kenneth Fine, MD, gastroenterologist, Dallas, Texas, owner of an investigative research lab, *Enterolab* (www.Enterolab.com). His lab ran the only accurate gluten antibody tests our family received back in 2004.

Without the courage of these astute researchers, we would still be wandering in the dark. Thank you all, and other individuals who thought outside the box. Kerri you are one of those thinkers. Thank you!

Lastly, special thanks to **LuEllen Giera**, my support group leader, for leading me to Dr. O'Bryan and Dr. Vojdani.

1. What is Molecular Mimicry? How does gluten damage us?

The structure of gluten resembles the structure of many of our body tissues. When the immune system attacks gluten or partly digested "pieces" of gluten it may also attack body tissues that "look like" those pieces of gluten. There may also be other processes that we do not yet understand.

What is gluten? - Gluten is a stretchy protein found in some bread grains. The problematic types are found in wheat, barley, and rye, and now early research suspects possibly rice, corn and oats (Dr. Peter Osborne, DC, CCN, www.glutenfreesociety.org).

What are proteins? - Proteins are a class of materials found in living tissues, such as hair, nerves, enzymes, etc. Molecularly, all proteins look like necklaces of beads strung into various color sequences. The different sequences make the proteins different, and the "colored beads" represent 22 separate amino acids. Our digestive system uses enzymes to cut up these necklaces into single beads so they are small enough to cross the gut wall properly and be restrung into new proteins. See image on page 452.

Unfortunately, many folks today are toxic and poorly nourished and do not have strong digestion, so the gluten "necklaces" may never completely break down. As weaker bonds between the beads break, "pieces", called "peptides," of gluten are formed. Gliadin is a well known gluten piece and there are many others.

Our immune system - has "departments" to protect us in various ways, including IgA, IgG, IgE, IgM, IgD and others. IgE can cause immediate allergic reactions to bee stings or peanuts, etc. IgA, IgG and IgM may react more slowly with less drama. They all manufacture "workers" or "soldiers", called antibodies, each custom designed to patrol our bodies, looking for the bead sequence of one particular enemy. When they find that bead sequence, they "tag or stick onto" it. Our killer white blood cells interpret the antibody tag as a condemned sign and know to surround and destroy that protein.

If an antibody test lists "Gliadin – IgA", "Gliadin – IgG", and "Gliadin – IgM" it means the test checked for gliadin antibodies in the IgA, IgG and IgM departments. If the antibodies are high it means the immune system is does not like gliadin and is working to destroy it.

Weak, leaky barriers - Our gut wall and other barrier membranes such as the skin, lung, placental, and blood brain barriers are held together with "tight junction proteins" that act like velcro. Inflammation, parasites, gluten, medications, infections, electrosmog, etc, may damage the "velcro" or open them up too much. Substances may slip through them into places they should not be and cause trouble.

Unfortunately if the gut wall does not hold together well, i.e., is "leaky", pieces of incompletely digested gluten strings (and others) may slip through and run into the immune system—our dutiful "guard dog" on the other side. Due to their too-large size "he" may raise the alarm. The invader strings are "frisked out" i.e., examined. If they are rejected, one or more of the immune departments make matching antibodies to "tag" them so the killer cells know to go after them.

It is at this point more problems may arise. A gluten antibody may "run by" a natural body tissue, for example a nerve in the heart. It may see in that innocent nerve tissue a sequence of "beads" that matches or partly matches the gluten sequence it was designed to "tag" and stick to that section of the nerve protein instead. This, unhappily, attracts killer cells to the misidentified nerve, resulting in autoimmune injury to the nerve. This is molecular mimicry.

Other foods and proteins beside gluten may also initiate molecular mimicry when they prematurely cross a leaky gut, and may prompt allergies (IgE) or intolerances (IgA, IgM, or IgG). However specialists agree that gluten's particular "bead" (amino acid) sequences are uniquely guilty in their ability to upset the immune system and instigate molecular mimicry between "their" antibodies and our tissues.

Molecular mimicry can take place between non-food proteins and body tissues also. Infectious microbe sequences such as strep, for example, are believed to partially match, (in the case of strep), heart and joint proteins and so injure the heart muscle or valves, and (rheumatic) joints. Ditto is suspected for root canal and cavitation infections that may circulate and injure specific tissues, including the heart. Flu microbe sequences can resemble gluten and may trigger or surface gluten syndrome. There are numerous other examples of mimicry between infections, foods and body tissues.

Consider the image below. An antibody may be made to seek the shorter "bead" sequence of a gluten piece that crossed the gut wall, but it might also recognize a similar sequence, a partial match, in the longer nerve protein sequence. The antibody "tags" or "sticks to", the part of the nerve tissue that matches the gluten piece that it seeks.

Gluten Peptide (and antibody) Sequence
Note: the different colors represent different amino acids.

					pink	blue	white	brown	brown	brown	red	red	green		

Nerve Sequence

orange	orange	yellow	green	red	red	blue	white	brown	brown	brown	red	orange	green	blue	yellow

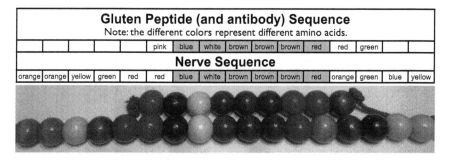

It gets more complicated, but eventually the victim tissue is attacked by killer cells on an ongoing basis. This process may be slow but stealthy. In time, the nerve may malfunction and the organ it serves may also begin to fail; for example, heart failure. This is termed autoimmunity. The body attacks its own tissue.

Molecular mimicry can occur in hundreds of places in the body since gluten can break up into numerous pieces having amino acid sequences that partly match many of our natural tissues. This may explain why gluten syndrome presents so differently in different people.[2]

Once this process starts, like elephants who never forget, the memory B cells that manufacture the antibodies never forget the sequence of the "invader" gluten pieces. If gluten is removed, antibody manufacture eventually stops, but any time the immune system sees even a tiny amount of that protein sequence, antibody production is retriggered. This is why specialists insist the gluten-free diet is strict and lifelong.

Gluten removal stops production of the initial antibody, which decreases the inflammatory process significantly. Literature shows the gluten-free diet may reverse or improve many serious conditions, but it may not always arrest an advanced autoimmune disease. Prevention is key.

Example: Once a ball is pushed down a hill, further pushing will only send it downhill faster, but it will roll on its own. To correlate, molecular mimicry between the gluten antibody and victim tissue starts the ball rolling. Removal of gluten stops pushing the process, and the sooner the better. The longer the exposure[8], and to other factors as well in a triad of autoimmunity (a. environmental stress, toxins, infections, etc.; b. a faulty blood brain barrier; and c. susceptible genetics), the higher the chance of autoimmune disease.

Dr. Vojdani comments, "If it is detected early enough and steps are taken early enough the condition may be reversed. If any condition is advanced enough you can reach a point when simple removal may not be enough. Autistic children generally have autoimmune reactivity rather than full-blown autoimmune disease, which is why they show great improvement upon the removal of gluten."

2. Does gluten always damage the villi of the small intestine as the celiac story teaches? Many other tissues such as thyroid, pancreas, blood vessels, joints, brain, nerves, liver, bone, etc. may be involved in this disorder. Does all that other damage arise due to poor nutrient absorption from injured gut villi?

No, according to published research many researchers and practitioners now believe the villi are not always damaged in an autoimmune gluten reaction.[2] Where there is no villi damage, injury to other organs cannot be due to nutrient deficiencies caused by villi damage. Molecular mimicry provides a mechanism for direct autoimmune gluten injury to many other tissues and organs when the villi are fine. It is also possible that several tissues and organs, *including villi,* may be injured and then nutrient deficiencies from poor villi absorption may affect other areas.

Dr. Vojdani's abstract in his editorial, *The Immunology of Gluten Sensitivity Beyond the Intestinal Tract,*[2] supports that the villi are not always injured. To quote his editorial abstract, "Evidence has been accumulated in literature demonstrating that gluten sensitivity or celiac disease can exist even in the absence of enteropathy" [gut/villi damage], "but affecting many organs."

3. I do not have damaged villi, and my tTG/gliadin blood tests were negative, but I feel so much better gluten-free. Why?

The tests were likely false negative. That is very, very common. As gluten is processed in the digestive system, it can break into more pieces than we have tests developed to check them, and the immune system makes an antibody for each separate piece. The test probably missed your antibodies because they were different from the one or two the test checked. Many patients have proven this because they received negative results to the standard test, and then found a number of positive gluten related antibodies when they ran a more comprehensive panel. Cyrex Laboratories (www.cyrexlabs.com), runs 28 gluten related antibodies in 3 areas of the immune system.

Your properly performed* biopsy was probably negative because likely your gut villi are fine.** Your gluten injury may have targeted other organs or tissues, not the villi.*** For instance, if gluten has damaged the heart, snipping intestinal villi will not help find the heart injury. Damage in either place is not ok.

More detail on False Negative Tests

The blood and saliva tests - Standard celiac blood and saliva tests only check tissue transglutaminase IgA, (tTG – IgA) as an initial screener. Most doctors give up if that test is negative. However, the literature shows that standard tTG-IgA tests are only elevated when the villi are completely destroyed. Dr. Vojdani finds that form of tTG is often not found in other gluten injured tissues. Therefore the standard tTG-IgA test is a poor screener for most patients, and returns many false negatives. More forms of tTG have now been discovered.

Doctors might also order a standard test for deamidated gliadin IgA and possibly IgG. Unfortunately these tests also have a miserable failure rate for picking up gluten syndrome because many patients have other

---

* If there IS villi damage it is possible for the biopsy to miss it if the damage is patchy or further down the duodenum than the villi samples are taken. Most good "gluten aware" gastroenterologists take a number of samples to try to avoid this possibility.

** It is possible that very early villi damage may slowly accumulate long before it shows up on a pathology report. An elevated IEL count, (intraepithelial lymphocyte, an early sign of inflammation) of the villi tissue indicates this process is underway. Ask the gastroenterologist to specify that the pathologist do an IEL count.

*** I am careful to specify the "villi of the gut". There may actually be gut damage, but not to the villi. There are many types of tissue in the gut, such as nerves, for instance. The villi may be fine, but it is still possible that some other gut tissue may be damaged by molecular mimicry or other processes we do not yet understand. For instance, if the nerves that control peristalsis (wave like gut motion) are injured, it could result in chronic constipation.

antibodies beside those two. The gluten "string" can break up into many other pieces, plus other "departments" of the immune system may react.

Villi biopsy vs. positive antibodies for diagnosis? - To add insult to injury, even if antibodies are discovered, many celiac, villi focused specialists may still insist that the villi biopsy is the final word for "celiac" diagnosis and they trust a negative villi biopsy over positive antibodies. Many folks have positive antibodies and suspicious symptoms, including improvement upon gluten removal, but no apparent villi damage. Their doctors assure them they can eat gluten! This is a serious mistake for many patients.

More on the villi biopsy – By now it is easy to understand why even properly performed* villi biopsies are only useful for the relatively small subset of patients in which the villi of the duodenum are injured. Most patients do not happen to have damaged villi. Their damage is somewhere else in their body, other organs, nerves, etc., or some enzyme or functional item has been damaged by gluten antibodies. Scientists such as Dr. Aristo Vojdani[2,3,4,] do NOT recommend villi biopsies for gluten syndrome diagnosis (there may be other reasons to scope the gut, such as tumors, etc). Dr. Vojdani explains that if there are elevated antibodies to gluten, the immune system is screaming "I do NOT want this substance! I am manufacturing antibodies to tag and destroy it." That is sufficient reason to remove gluten from the diet. It is less expensive to check an extensive array of gluten antibodies than undergo an endoscopy anyway, and is much less invasive.

4. Why do many gluten syndrome patients not only react to wheat, barley, and rye but also sometimes to other foods, particularly oats, milk, corn, soy, egg, coffee, sesame, yeast, chocolate and others.

These foods have similar amino acid sequences to gluten. Now that we grasp molecular mimicry, this is logical. The immune system may misrecognize them for gluten, causing cross reactions which may keep the gluten antibodies running high even on a gluten-free diet. Happily, this does not always occur. Cyrex labs, Array # 4, checks a list of cross reactive and gluten substitute foods, IgA and IgG.

5. The diet seems excessively strict? Why does it take so little gluten to start a reaction?

We understand that miniscule amounts of bee venom, or peanut, can trigger emergency allergic reactions, and very tiny medication pills can cause major effects on our bodies. This is also true of gluten reactions, both immediate allergic IgE, and delayed IgA, IgG, and IgM.[3] "Crumbs matter." The difference is that delayed reactions are not as obvious as the allergic reaction. They may go unnoticed for hours to decades, but may be a long, slow, serious process. Their lack of drama robs these reactions of the compliance respect they deserve.

6. The silent syndrome - Why do many people react to gluten, proven by antibody tests, but they have few or no warning signs, or seemingly unrelated symptoms they do not recognize or connect with their diet for a long time. Then they crash with something serious, often or usually autoimmune?

Gluten is famous for slowly injuring nerves[5] by molecular mimicry, and in many cases the nerves are silenced by that injury.[6] The patient does not realize there is a problem until the tissue or organ that those nerves supply begins to fail. Furthermore some areas of the body do not contain many pain nerves, so we may not feel the damage. Slow silent damage is understood in other diseases. Heart damage, cancer, and aortal aneurysms are examples of conditions that develop silently and then suddenly flare. Prevention is best.

For years, celiac literature recognized 2 neurological conditions, peripheral neuropathy and gluten ataxia. In the wider perspective of gluten syndrome, nerve damage may be one of the most important areas of injury.[5]

Dr. Rodney Ford, MD, suggests in his book, *The Gluten Syndrome: Is Wheat Causing You Harm,*[6] that this is primarily a neurological disease[5], injuring and in some cases silencing nerves, compromising the health and function of the tissues they serve. This idea was reinforced by an astute observation made by Dr. Ford of one of his patients, an elementary school child who had not achieved bowel control. After she went gluten-free, the problem resolved. Dr. Ford realized the child now recognized the signal to visit the toilet, and accidents were avoided. The nerves in the lower bowel apparently "woke up" once the antibodies that injured them disappeared. This is an interesting and logical theory to explain "silent gluten injury", and it fits the community. Here is an abstract of Dr. Ford's published paper which discusses a possible widespread neurological focus:[5]

The Gluten Syndrome: A Neurological Disease, by R.P. Ford

Hypothesis: gluten causes symptoms, in both celiac disease and non-celiac gluten-sensitivity, by its adverse actions on the nervous system. Many celiac patients experience neurological symptoms, frequently associated with malfunction of the autonomic nervous system. These neurological symptoms can present in celiac patients who are well nourished. The crucial point, however, is that gluten-sensitivity can also be associated with neurological symptoms in patients who do not have any mucosal gut damage (that is, without celiac disease). Gluten can cause neurological harm through a combination of cross reacting antibodies, immune complex disease and direct toxicity. These nervous system affects include: dysregulation of the autonomic nervous system, cerebella ataxia, hypotonia, developmental delay, learning disorders, depression, migraine, and headache. If gluten is the putative harmful agent, then there is no requirement to invoke gut damage and nutritional deficiency to explain the myriad of the symptoms experienced by sufferers of celiac disease and gluten-sensitivity. This is called "The Gluten Syndrome."[5]

7. Why do so many of us react now, when for centuries most people appeared to be fine with wheat? After all, wheat is spoken of positively in the Bible and many other historical documents.

There may or may not be a conclusive answer to this question, but a few factors may play a role.

a. Many folks have higher toxin levels now, their nutritional status is worse, and digestive strength is weaker.

b. Today's wheat is different. Gluten grains have been subjected to a lot of changes, some genetically violent, according to Nina Federoff, a pro GMO scientist. She asserts in her book, *Mendel in the Kitchen*, that gluten grains were altered with nuclear radiation and chemical mutation by the 1950's – 1960's.[9] Recently a stash of old blood samples from that era, stored in a freezer by the military, were checked with standard celiac antibody tests. The incidence of positive antibodies was much less in those samples than is typically found in the general public today.

c. Wheat seed is sometimes treated with mercury. Might this play into unintended results?

8. Why do specialists and researchers insist that the gluten-free diet must be life long? Can't we heal the gut and go back to our beloved wheat bagels, croissants, and brownies?

Our scientists insist that gluten-free is a strict lifelong commitment. The memory B cells in the immune system never forget what the enemy "looks like." Today's gluten is a violently altered substance according to the very scientists who defend genetic alterations.[9] It is not worth playing with today's wheat. There is something strange and unpredictable about it. Even if a leaky gut has healed, future circumstances, toxins and stress might injure it and retrigger the syndrome, perhaps silently. Researchers say gluten creates leaky gut for a few hours in everyone.

Particularly since gluten appears to be the "bad boy" that predisposes to other intolerances, I prefer to walk away for life and concentrate on other nutrient dense foods. However, it is wise to consume whole foods rich in B vitamins, (ex., liver or bee pollen), and silica (the herb horsetail, "equisetum hymale" species, is a source,) as gluten grains contain those nutrients.

9. Traditional peoples soaked and/or sprouted their wheat berries and then made sourdough bread with it. Does that process alter the gluten sufficiently for gluten syndrome patients to safely consume it today, particularly organic spelt and einkorn?

No. These methods make bread more digestible, but the fermented products and ancient gluten grains still contain gluten and can trigger reactions in research trials. Even if there are no visible reactions, silent injury cannot be ruled out without long term research. Additionally, the preparation process before fermentation is completed is definitely gluten based, so significant cross contamination issues come into play in the kitchen. Healing the gut is a challenge. Other areas crop up that need cleanup too, such as the parasite issues. Gluten specialists advise us to go gluten-free, stay that way, and move on.

10. What are gluten withdrawals?

Rarely, a few days to a few weeks after going gluten-free, or after being glutened, a patient may experience a few hours to a couple of weeks of a parade of varied and unusual symptoms including dizziness, black pit depression, crying, physical or emotional exhaustion, even as in difficulty getting up to use the rest room, and other odd symptoms. In severe cases they may experience an inability to socialize, make eye contact, make decisions or hold a normal conversation. Children or teens may act out in extreme ways during this situation. Often patients cannot bring themselves to discuss this experience afterward. However, a patient reluctantly described her experience 2 years later as "encountering an empty white board with nothing on it." The rest of life around her seemed to be "across the Grand Canyon." This appears to be a temporary crisis that resolves anywhere from a few hours to a couple of weeks or so according to folks who contact me about them. It is assumed that this phenomenon is due to particular pieces of gluten strings called gluteomorphins with amino acid sequences which resemble opiate drugs. When these gluten pieces disappear from the blood stream the patient may experience "withdrawal," very much like a drug withdrawal. Another theory for why this may happen involves changes in blood flow to the brain that may create a temporary neurological crisis. Autistic children may suffer these withdrawals and may take longer to stabilize, but they usually make nice gains after the crisis passes. Happily, once withdrawal is over the patients are usually much better, and they are VERY vigilant with their diet.

In the rare event that this type of reaction might occur, family and friends of the person do well to understand that the person may (or may not) be able to prepare their own food, for instance, but not be able to verbally communicate much, make eye contact, hold a conversation, answer questions, and may be uncharacteristically snappy particularly if others attempt to communicate with them. Family members may wish to be quietly and unobtrusively nearby until the person passes through this stage. If the patient has children to care for, help may be needed, and also solitude, rest, and simply prepared "real" nourishing food that is gluten-free and easy to digest such as bone broth. Probiotics or old fashioned fermented raw veggies or sauerkraut from the refrigerated section of the health food store may be helpful. Family and friends should not take the person's temporarily withdrawn personality personally.

For details on these unstudied rare reactions, or if you need support during a crisis, see...

www.theglutensyndrome.net /Adverse_reactions.htm

...or contact me at *jka8168@sbcglobal.net*. I collect testimonials, so feel free to contribute if you have experienced this type of reaction. We hope these reactions will eventually be studied.

11. Should I replace all the gluten foods I routinely eat with gluten-free substitutes?

No, most gluten-free substitutes are still mainly expensive processed food (aka junk food). For the first few weeks it is normal for newbies to look for substitutes to replace their "old gluten friends" and it helps them make the very real emotional transition, but there are better, more nutrient dense food choices. The substitutes are still high carb, (potato, corn, tapioca, rice), and most contain sugar, processed gums, GMOs and ingredients that do not help us get well. We may actually eat more of them BECAUSE they are gluten-free. Additionally they are expensive and not always easy to prepare at home.

Many experienced gluten-free folks gradually wean themselves off a constant diet of the rather junky substitutes in favor of other real unprocessed foods, such as meat, eggs, veggies, fruits, nuts, fermented vegetables, bone broths, and so on according to their digestive abilities. The gluten-free substitutes become the occasional treat, such as pizza crust. Gluten free families are wise to find the healthiest GF versions of just the items they miss the most, and skip the rest. For example, at our house, I had served gluten spaghetti for years, but when I dropped that habit, no one noticed. However, my husband wanted his breakfast toast, so we found a gluten free brand he liked and continued that tradition. Each family works out these adjustments for themselves.

Lettuce wraps are crunchy and yummy instead of sandwiches. Hamburger patties without the bun but with onion for the onion lovers, are still tasty and they feel better afterward. In our family we now use watermelon or a watermelon basket for birthday "cake", complete with candles and a bow in the summer. Fruit pizza with a nut flour or nut/date crust, avocado chocolate or other dairy-free or fruit based pudding for the sauce, and an artistic fruit/coconut topping works for parties. There are lots of ways to celebrate happy healthy gluten-free, junk free birthdays.

12. Warning! Formal gluten challenges for testing purposes – risky!

A word of caution. Antibody tests must be performed while the patient is still consuming gluten or shortly after going gluten-free. Sometimes doctors advise patients who are already gluten-free to go back on gluten, 4 slices a day for 4-6 weeks to restart the antibodies for testing purposes. Patient experience has shown that once the system is fairly clean of gluten, going back to perform a formal gluten challenge for testing purposes may be risky. The secondary reactions for some individuals can be significant, particularly neurologically. Challenges have been known anecdotally to trigger psychological black pit crashes, fibromyalgia, and other organ injury. Autistic children may have a hard time when they just go gluten-free initially or consume gluten accidentally. A planned challenge for them may be very unwise.

13. Intermittent infractions (aka cheats) are seriously unwise and may increase injury.[10]

This is not a fad, or cheater's diet. The gluten-free diet is a medical diet to treat or control serious autoimmune, inflammatory, and often neurological diseases. There is no room for casual infractions. Research suggests that repeated, intermittent cheats, even every few weeks, over time may actually influence mortality rates.[10] This is not a reason to avoid the diet, but to take it seriously. Once the strictness of the diet is embraced the patient or family adjusts and discovers that it is doable. Gluten-free food bars, nuts, a packet of gluten-free soy sauce, and GlutenEase™ or other brands of DPP IV enzymes are good to keep in the glove compartment or backpack to handle emergencies. NOTE: DPP IV (pronounced DPP 4) digestive enzymes help break down gluten but they do not stop a reaction and are NOT a reason to cheat. However if there is a possibility of exposure it makes sense to take them for whatever help they might afford. In the case of a confirmed gluten exposure, take the enzymes, keep the bowels moving, stay calm and deal with it. Worry and drama makes everything worse.

14. Discrepancy –The celiac focus uses villi biopsy for diagnosis. The wider perspective relies on positive antibodies or improvement on the diet. Question? How did villi damage become the gold standard?

The first place the medical profession found conclusive damage by gluten in the 1950's – 60's was to the villi of the gut. After the endoscopy tool was developed, villi damage and subsequent healing upon gluten removal could be observed. They concluded that gluten damaged the villi. This was true. The particular subset of cases they scoped had villi damage, but their conclusion that the villi were the only target of damage for everyone with gluten syndrome was too narrow according to research today.[2] In most patients the target damage was NOT the villi, but the bones, joint lining, heart, thyroid, pancreas, liver, brain, almost any organ, blood vessel walls, nerves almost anywhere in the body, and so on. The patients might even have injury to multiple tissues, BUT NOT NECESSARILY ALWAYS TO THE VILLI. When the villi biopsy was declared the gold standard for gluten syndrome diagnosis, it cut out most of the patients who were reacting to gluten. Snipping villi does no good if the damage is in the thyroid or brain. For the next 60 years very few patients were prescribed a gluten-free diet because most of them did not have damaged villi, (or the doctor never thought to look at all). Their gluten-induced injury was somewhere else in their body, so they were never diagnosed.

15. Discrepancy - The villi damaged celiac disease story teaches that celiac disease is autoimmune and much worse than "non autoimmune" non-celiac gluten syndrome (NCGS). The wider gluten syndrome perspective teaches that both are autoimmune and serious.[2,3,4]

A significant disagreement exists over the autoimmunity of non-celiac gluten syndrome (NCGS). In the beginning, antibodies to gluten could not be found in NCGS patients, therefore it was assumed that NCGS was not autoimmune. However, Dr. Vojdani insists NCGS IS autoimmune. The NCGS patients have plenty of antibodies, just different ones than the standard tests check. His tests, which check and find more antibodies,[****] the illnesses these patients develop, and recoveries or improvements on the diet all prove his point. He also asserts that NCGS can indicate a gut wall in worse shape than the celiac villi damaged subset.[2,3,4] The damage is simply somewhere else, not to the villi. See the link below for diagrams of these reactions, and compare the condition of the gut wall in the celiac diagram with the gut wall in the gluten intolerance diagram.

www.TheGlutenSyndrome.net/ VojdaniDiagrams.htm

[****] Dr. Vojdani's research found several more forms of both tTG, and gliadin antibodies, (alpha, gamma, omega), gluteomorphins, glutinins, and others. His saliva and blood panels check 12 separate antibodies in 3 different immune departments and 2 mediums, totaling 28 gluten related antibodies. The two panels, run together, nearly always find antibodies if they are present in the patient, translating to far fewer false negatives.

This disagreement fosters confusion among NCGS patients that villi damaged celiac disease is the "big bad boy" to avoid (true, it is bad), but that NCGS is less severe, not autoimmune. This translates in real life to gluten birthday cake for the Friday night party and then back on the gluten-free bandwagon Saturday morning, "so I won't eventually develop villi damaged celiac disease." Yes, that could happen also, particularly if the person seesaws on the diet, but the notion that NCGS is not as bad as villi damaged celiac disease is a misunderstanding according to Dr. Vojdani.[2,3,4] To repeatedly seesaw off and on gluten indiscriminately is unwise according to medical literature,[10] and community experience. Gluten exposure needs to be an accident, which happens occasionally even to the most vigilant. Casual cheats are a more risky mindset, usually meaning "more frequent."[10] Take it seriously, nerves, blood vessels, and organs are precious.

Gluten Tests with a Good Track Record

Some families cannot afford to test or good tests are not available. In the case of autism this protocol and most others require gluten-free and that is the end of the matter. Kerri takes this position partly due to cost and the miserable record of false negatives that standard tests return. The protocol does not work without the diet. Period.

Some adults are also willing to go gluten-free without a test. Their bodies tell them what they need, they listen, and are happy to find answers. Social pressure does not sway their decision or ability to comply.

In many other situations, a positive test is very meaningful. It gives patients confirmation that gluten-free is right for them, silences critics, and helps them comply with the diet. In the case of children it provides proof to the other parent, grandparents, therapists, doctor, etc. It may also come in handy if the child turns into an invincible teen who doubts he ever needed the diet in the face of pizza and beer, ditto for his future spouse and in-laws. The catch is that the test must be adequate. A false negative misvalidates the skeptics. These are decisions every individual or family must evaluate for themselves. Thankfully there are test panels with good track records now.

Absolutely, regardless of any test result, if the body is able to communicate a reaction to gluten or its removal, then that is the final answer. Be grateful and go gluten-free.

This testing section is for those who wish to test for their own confirmation or social support.

NOTE: If a patient has been ill for a very long time it is possible for the immune system to be so worn out that few antibodies are manufactured. Lower antibody counts might show a false negative but not prevent injury to innocent tissues. Also, due to the wide variety of antibodies a patient may happen to make, it is possible to run any antibody panel and miss those particular antibodies. The more antibodies that are checked the less likely this may occur, but should be considered in the event of a negative test that the patient or practitioner questions. In this case a gene test may be helpful.

Enterolab - Stool and 1 part gene tests

For 10 years Enterolab's mail in home collection research stool test stood in the gap for thousands of patients who received false negative standard tTG and gliadin blood tests. It has saved many lives, and gave our family the social confirmation we needed. This unpublished research test checks stool for tTG-IgA and gliadin-IgA only. The use of stool as the testing medium appears to pick up those antibodies most of the time, much much more often than standard tTG or gliadin IgA blood tests. However, since only two antibodies are checked, it may miss in some cases.

Dr. Fine's lab also offers a one part gene test which he believes is adequate for a reasonable price. Dr. Fine finds if a gene is present, nearly always so are the antibodies, and two genes are worse. Villi damaged celiac specialists recognize only HLA DQ 2 and 8 as gluten related, but Dr. Fine includes 1 and 3 and their subsets 5, 6, 7 and 9. In fact according to Enterolab, HLA DQ 4 is the only DQ gene that does NOT correlate with gluten syndrome. According to him, a patient needs 2 copies of the HLA DQ 4 gene to miss the predisposition. This translates to 81% of the Caucasian population with a predisposition to trigger gluten syndrome at some point in their lifetime, including before they are born.

Cyrex Labs - Better blood and saliva tests

Cyrex Labs (www.CyrexLabs.com) opened their doors in 2010 in Phoenix, Arizona. They run much more complete antibody panels designed by Dr. Aristo Vojdani, PhD., their scientific advisor, an immunologist, and researcher. Dr. Vojdani found a wider variety of gliadin antibodies, (alpha, gamma, omega) and variations of tTG in other tissues, plus gluteomorphins, and several others. He also checks an IgM antibody due to possible malfunctions in that system. Cyrex blood and saliva panels, Array #1 and #3, combined, test for 28 gluten related antibodies between 3 immune departments, 2 mediums, plus IgA insufficiency. They rarely miss a diagnosis because they look for so many antibodies. (Note: Vojdani believes stress, toxins and infections, i.e. environment, can trigger a gluten reaction without the genes.)

Gluten Free Society - Two Part Gene Test

A third approach espoused by Dr. Peter Osborne, *The Gluten Free Society*, Sugarland, Texas, (www.glutenfreesociety.org), is to run only the gene test, since any antibody panel may theoretically miss the particular ones the patient may have. He uses a 2 part test, the most complete method, and looks for both celiac and gluten sensitivity genes. A positive gene test does not prove a current immune response as do antibodies, but predisposition to it. Presence of 2 genes indicates a more severe case. Gene tests have an advantage in that they can be run anytime, gluten consumption is unnecessary, and depending on the results, useful information can be gleaned for immediate and extended family members.

Elimination Diet

The elimination diet is inexpensive. Often/usually it demonstrates improvement upon removal of gluten, or worsening upon reintroduction. Many "heads up" practitioners accept this as reason enough to go gluten-free.

There are occasional complications or interpretation issues for the elimination diet as follows:

a.   Reintroduction of gluten (gluten challenge) can trigger stronger, sometimes risky reactions.[10] Stop a challenge upon negative symptoms, including depression and emotional instability, or best, don't challenge. An accidental infraction may come up that provides insight.

b.   Occasionally it takes several months to see the difference, or a silent reaction may mask symptoms.[6]

c.   If the patient later decides to test and is already "clean" on the gluten-free diet, blood tests will not work unless gluten is reintroduced for many weeks.[10] No! Stool/gene tests are safer.

d.   There is no lab confirmation to silence naysayers.

Other Related Tests

Cyrex Labs Array # 2 - Intestinal Permeability Panel focuses on specific causes of leaky gut. This helps strategize treatment, and is an improvement over the old lactulose/mannitol test.

Cyrex Labs Cross Reactive Foods and Gluten Substitutes, Array # 4. - This specific list checks foods that commonly cross react with gluten and also foods commonly used to replace gluten. It helps customize an anti-inflammatory diet.

Cyrex Labs Predictive Antibody panels determine if or which tissues are currently under antibody attack. This predicts autoimmunity years ahead of time and gives the patient advance notice in order to address trouble spots.

Enterolab (www.Enterolab.com) offers several stool based food antibody panels and gut related stool tests.

What are the lab instructions?
Do I need to consume gluten for testing?

Antibody tests, (blood, saliva, stool), prove a reaction and require recent gluten consumption. Ideally, test first, then go gluten-free. If the patient is off gluten, call the lab for advice on the time window before the test will not work.

Cyrex Labs (www.CyrexLabs.com) tests require prescriptions and a saliva specimen and/or blood draw. If a doctor is needed to write the script, check www.thedr.com for a partial list of practitioners who are familiar with Cyrex Labs. Results are sent to the prescribing doctor.

Enterolab stool specimens are ordered online, kits are sent, home collected and mailed. No prescription is required. Results arrive on email. Enterolab's test works for several months after going gluten-free.

Gene tests do not require gluten consumption or a script and can be run at any time. Genes prove a predisposition to gluten reaction.

Enterolab's gene test is a relatively inexpensive "one part" test. It is a mail in cheek swab and reports the patient's actual genes.

Gluten Free Society (www.Glutenfreesociety.org) gene test is a "two part" (more complete) mail in cheek swab and reports yes or no for both celiac and gluten sensitivity genes.

For information on testing (I have no financial interests) see:

www.TheGlutenSyndrome.net

The latest version of this article and a complete list of references is available at:

www.TheGlutenSyndrome.net /Molecular_Mimicry.pdf

Author's note: While the information Olive has provided can be extremely helpful for adults or children who are not on the spectrum or who are suffering from other ailments, a gluten-free diet is non-negotiable for healing autism. We need to remove foods that cause inflammation and mucous, and which can produce gluteomorphin in the body. I have seen many families waste time and money doing testing only to get confused by false negatives—time and money they could have spent on recovering their child.

Online Gluten Summit – A Chance to Support CDAutism

Recently, in November 2013, Dr. Thomas O'Bryan, an internationally recognized gluten educator, put together an amazing online Gluten Summit. Twenty nine iconic experts on Celiac Disease and its wider perspective, Gluten Sensitivity, also called Gluten Syndrome, covered every possible aspect before 115,000 appreciative viewers. This set of interviews plus extra materials is available for purchase at only $3.30 per speaker and is a priceless addition to all our libraries. It also is a great gift and a good way to inform friends and family. Often our closest loved ones accept new information better from a respected professional rather than from us.

Arrangements are in place to contribute half of your purchase price of The Gluten Summit interviews to the CDAutism project. Go to the link below to order and also credit CDAutism with your contribution.

gg110.infusionsoft.com/go/tgso/Kerri

Appendix 6

Measuring the Strength
of Your CD, CDS & CDH

by Charlotte Lackney

CD, CDS, and CDH work because all of them contain chlorine dioxide (ClO_2). ClO_2 is made when a 22.4% solution of sodium chlorite ($NaClO_2$) is activated with an acid, usually 4% hydrochloric acid (HCl) for CD and CDH; and 10% HCl for CDS.

Sometimes it might be useful to measure the amount of ClO_2 in those solutions, although that has not been done in the past when using CD. And, it may only be necessary to know the amount of chlorine dioxide if you are not getting the expected results. There could be a problem with the ingredients or process and knowing the amount of ClO_2 in the solution could be helpful in determining what might be wrong.

The amount of ClO_2 in a solution is measured in *parts per million* (ppm). It is always necessary to specify the volume of solution when talking about ClO_2 ppm because the ppm will vary depending on the dilution of the solution.

If using CDH or CDS with the protocol in this book, it is assumed that you are preparing them at 3000ppm. If using CDS, please keep in mind that the relative strength of one milliliter of CDS is approximately 60% of one drop of CD.

However, if the ingredients are of good quality and the CD or CDH protocol is closely followed, there is usually no need to know or measure the ClO_2 concentration.

Both CD and CDH may continue to activate inside the body from whatever sodium chlorite has not been activated outside the body. That is not the case with CDS, as it has no sodium chlorite to continue activating inside the body. Some believe that this is why many people can tolerate a higher dose of CDS than an equivalent dose of CD.

Measuring the concentration of ClO_2 can easily be done at home. You will need to purchase ClO2 test strips made by *LaMotte* or others. I have only used LaMotte Insta-Test® High-Range Test Strips, 0 to 500ppm (code #3002). The container's label has a chart showing seven colors on it wih each color indicating a ClO_2 concentration in ppm. Note: LaMotte recently changed the appearance of their labels, as shown on the right. Both are the same product. For more information, see their website:

www.lamotte.com/ en/water-wastewater/test-strips/3002.html

Directions for how to use the LaMotte test strips are printed on the side of the container and need to be followed in order to get an accurate ClO_2 concentration reading.

The numbers below each of the seven colors represent 0, 10, 25, 50, 100, 250 and 500ppm. Many people who use the test strips think the 50ppm color is the best one to use for color matching, because they can see the difference in color below and above that color more easily than the others.

If the ClO_2 solution you want to measure is suspected to be 3000ppm, how do you measure that if the test strips highest ClO_2 concentration color is 500ppm? Recall that I had said that it is always necessary to specify the volume of solution when talking about ClO_2 ppm, because the ppm will vary depending on the dilution of the solution.

So if we dilute the suspected 3000ppm ClO_2 stock solution with more water, the same amount of ClO_2 will now be evenly spread out in the larger amount of solution if stirred. There will be less ClO_2 in any one spot than before dilution, because the ClO_2 is now dispersed into a larger volume of water. Visualize what happens when a drop of red food coloring falls into a glass of water. It disperses throughout the water if stirred, and that dark red color is now much lighter because it is diluted in the water.

In order to read 3000ppm with a test strip, and have it match the 50ppm color on the container, we will need to dilute a small sample of the stock solution.

Stock solution (1ml)	÷	Desired dilution in ppm	=	Volume of water for dilution.
3000ppm		50ppm		60ml

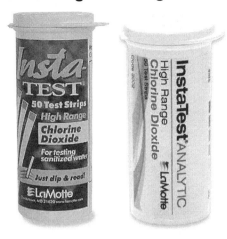

The chlorine dioxide test strips (code #3002) made by LaMotte are available on the market with two different labels, although both are the same product. Both labels show the same measuring color chart on the outside of the container.

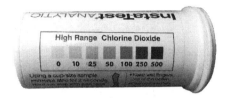

So, if we take a 1ml sample of the stock solution and add it to 60ml of water, then the stock solution is diluted 60 times its original volume. Technically, one should add the 1ml of stock solution to 59ml of water, for a total of 60ml, but using 60ml is easier to measure and you would not see the difference in ClO_2 readings if 59ml of water was used.

To measure, pour 60ml of distilled water into a small glass and then add 1ml of stock solution. Stir well to evenly distribute the ClO_2 sample in the water. Then take one of the test strips—taking care not to touch the pad of chemicals on the end of the strip—and dip it in the solution for two seconds. Keep the strip in one place in the solution and do not move it around during the two-second period.

Without flicking any of the solution off the strip, remove the strip from the test solution with the pad facing up and wait ten seconds. Now compare the color of the test strip pad to the color chart on the side of the test strips container (as shown above).

If the stock solution is 3000ppm, then the color on the test strip will match the 50ppm color on the container. Multiply 50 times 60 (the amount of dilution) and you get 3000ppm.

If the color on the test strip does not match the 50ppm color on the container, try to estimate the ppm number between container colors and multiply that number by 60 to get the ClO_2 concentration.

Tip: You can cut the strips lengthwise to get 100 strips instead of 50; just be sure not to touch the strip's pad with your fingers or your readings may not be accurate. Also it is important to keep the container tightly capped to keep moisture out which can affect the readings.

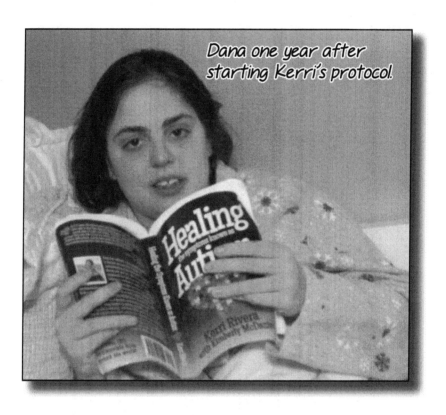

Dana one year after starting Kerri's protocol.

Appendix 7

Diluting HCl Concentration

The protocols in this book use two different concentrations of hydrochloric acid (HCl): 10% & 4%. Some suppliers sell both concentrations, while others only one. You may also find a source with a different concentration and wish to dilute it to 4 or 10%. The math to determine how much to dilute your stock solution is rather simple. You should have no problem if you know how to multiply, divide, add and subtract. Note: The same calculation works for citric acid if you have 50% and need to go down to 35%.

What you will need is:

- Bottle of concentrated HCl (10% or higher)
- Receiving bottle to store the resulting diluted HCl
- Graduated cylinder or other measuring cup

On the next page is a graphical representation of the dilution equation. It may look intimidating at first glance, but it is actually quite simple and is made up of three simple mini-calculations. Each box is labeled with a letter which refers to the graphic. Just fill in the numbers with a pencil and follow the directions.

We'll go over one example here: Let's say you have 10% HCl and want to make 1 liter of 4% HCl. Here's what you would have to calculate:

Desired Volume	×	Desired HCl %	=	Temporary Number
1000ml		4%		4000

Temporary Number	÷	Stock HCl %	=	Amount of 10% HCl
4000		10%		400ml

Desired Volume	−	Amount of 10% HCl	=	Amount of water
1000ml		400ml		600ml

So, in this example, you would need 400ml of 10% HCl and 600ml of water to make 1 liter of 4% HCl. If you add them together, you should have 1000ml (1 liter).

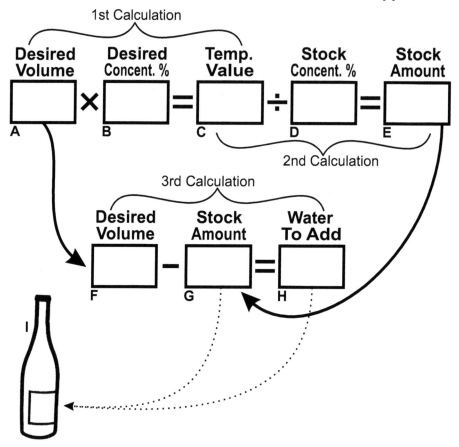

A	Determine the volume of the receiving bottle in milliliters. For example, if you have a 1 liter bottle, you would enter the number "1,000" for 1,000ml.
B	This is where you enter the % of the final solution. If you are making 4%, then enter "4" in this box.
C	Multiple **A** and **B** and enter the result into box **C**. This is a temporary value you will need for the next calculation.
D	This is where you enter the percentage of your concentrated stock solution–the HCl you want to dilute. If you have 10%, then enter a "10" in this box.
E	Now divide the temporary value in **C** by D and enter the result in **E**. This is the amount of concentrated stock HCl (in milliliters) you will need.
F	Copy what you entered in **A** to F for the next calculation.
G	Copy the result from **E** to **G**.
H	Do the subtraction of **F** − **G** and enter he value in **H**. This is the number of milliliters of distilled or filtered water you will need.
I	Measure the resulting volume of water calculated in **H** and pour it into the receiving bottle **I**. Finally, measure out the value in **G** and pour it into the receiving bottle **I**.

Appendix 8

Other Uses of Chlorine Dioxide

Bladder Infection Protocol (for Adults)
The protocol for bladder infection is three oral drops of CD eight times a day with a douche of 10 drops CD three times the first day, and then once every day thereafter, for 30 days (for females).

Ear, Eye, Nose Protocol
Make a mixture that contains one ounce of water for every one drop of CD. Use one drop of that mixture in the affected orifice every hour until symptoms disappear. If the issue is acute you can use one drop every 15 minutes. This method can be used in the ears for infections, in the nose for congestion/infection, and the eye for infection or conjunctivitis.

General Fever Protocol
If the person has a fever, or if you want clarification of any kind, email Kerri, but in the meantime, this will hopefully get you started:

1. Give baths interspersed with enemas, approximately eight hours apart (e.g. bath in the evening and enema in the morning or vice versa).

2. Give oral CD doses (using the person's usual number of drops) 12 to 16 times or more a day (essentially every hour); unless they stop eating, in which case, stop oral dosing. Enemas and baths can continue.

3. Have them drink lots of water.

4. Cool clothes on forehead and neck.

Please see Chapter 14, page 335 for more information on fever therapy.

Teeth
Ten activated drops of CD per one ounce of water. Put this in a spray bottle and spray on the toothbrush.

Throat Spray
Ten activated drops of CD (chlorine dioxide) in one ounce of water. Spray on throat once/hour. Recommended in the case of a sore throat.

Vaginal Douching for Yeast Infections:

Put six activated drops of CD in 60 ml of water. Hold this in for two minutes every day for a few weeks or between periods. Six drops MAX in the vagina.

CD Skin Spray

Use ten drops of activated CD per one ounce of water in a spray bottle.

CD spray is great for a variety of ailments.

- Skin
- Dandruff
- Scrapes
- Cuts
- Rashes
- Toe Fungus

Burns

Any burn should be sprayed with full strength sodium chlorite solution (no acid added) directly from a small spray bottle. Do not add citric acid or HCl at all! If you don't have a spray bottle available drip sodium chlorite solution directly onto the burn, making sure the area is soaked with it.

Wait up to five minutes, but no longer before rinsing off with room temperature water. If you fail to rinse off the sodium chlorite solution, the burn will continue to hurt and get worse.

This technique will cause the burn to heal in 1/4 the time normally required. The pain should stop almost immediately or reduce to almost zero within several minutes.

Sunburns should be treated the same way. Spray the red area, wait 1 to 5 minutes, and rinse off. If the area is still sore, in about an hour spray the area again and wait 5 minutes before rinsing off. Remember, DO NOT allow the sodium chlorite to remain in place. It must be rinsed off! The pain should be gone in a couple of minutes. Generally two doses will overcome most sunburns, but on rare occasions if the discomfort is not all gone you can use a third dose. Be sure to rinse it off.

Note that sodium chlorite is alkaline and burns are acidic. Therefore the sodium chlorite neutralizes the acidity that resides in the burned areas. This is part of the reason why burns heal rapidly after sodium chlorite applications.

Appendix 9

Blank Kalcker Parasite Protocol Chart

The next page contains a blank Kalcker Parasite Protocol Daily Chart identical to those found on pages 199 through 217. You are encouraged to copy this chart for use in your parasite protocol planning. Setting the copy machine to enlarge at 125% should fill a standard letter-sized page.

Time	Meal Time	CD / CDS / CDH	CD / CDS / CDH Bath	CD / CDS / CDH Enema	Ocean Water	Diatomaceous Earth	Lepidium Latifolium Extract (Rompepiedras / RP)	Pyrantel Pamoate (Combantrin®)	Mebendazole	Castor Oil	Neem	Probiotic
6:00 AM												
6:30 AM												
7:00 AM												
7:30 AM												
8:00 AM												
8:30 AM												
9:00 AM												
9:30 AM												
10:00 AM												
10:30 AM												
11:00 AM												
11:30 AM												
12:00 PM												
12:30 PM												
1:00 PM												
1:30 PM												
2:00 PM												
2:30 PM												
3:00 PM												
3:30 PM												
4:00 PM												
4:30 PM												
5:00 PM												
5:30 PM												
6:00 PM												
6:30 PM												
7:00 PM												
7:30 PM												
8:00 PM												
8:30 PM												
9:00 PM												
9:30 PM												

Appendix 10

Lunar Phase Calendar
for Kalcker Parasite Protocol

As covered in Chapter 8, the Kalcker Parasite Protocol is administered over a period of 19 days and scheduled according to the lunar cycle. We have included an easy to follow calendar starting on the next page for the years 2014 through 2016.

Each chart page shows 6 months with each month broken up into 3 columns: Column 1 is the day of the month; column 2 indicates the lunar phase; and column 3 shows the corresponding Parasite Protocol day.

The full moon is identified with an "F" in the second column and the new moon is identified by an "N" in each month section, which usually occurs towards the end of each protocol cycle.

We have used New York as our center point since it is roughly the center of the majority of those using this book in the US and Europe. The moon phase may occur 1 day before or after the dates shown if you are in another part of the world, but the difference is not great, so feel free to use the dates shown. However, you are welcome to be precise for your particular location. The Farmer's Almanac is a great source and provides an online calendar that can be adjusted to your location:

www.almanac.com/moon

You may also wish to install a moon phase app into your smart phone. Many free options exist.

2014 - Lunar Phases for New York, NY

Jan			Feb			Mar			Apr			May			Jun		
1	N	18	1			1	N	18	1			1	N		1		
2			2			2			2			2			2		
3			3			3			3			3			3		
4			4			4			4			4			4		
5			5			5			5			5			5		
6			6			6			6			6			6		
7			7			7			7			7			7		
8			8			8			8			8			8		
9			9			9			9			9			9		
10			10			10			10			10			10		0
11			11		0	11			11			11			11		1
12		0	12		1	12			12		0	12			12		2
13		1	13		2	13		0	13		1	13		0	13	F	3
14		2	14	F	3	14		1	14		2	14		1	14		4
15	F	3	15		4	15		2	15	F	3	15		2	15		5
16		4	16		5	16	F	3	16		4	16	F	3	16		6
17		5	17		6	17		4	17		5	17		4	17		7
18		6	18		7	18		5	18		6	18		5	18		8
19		7	19		8	19		6	19		7	19		6	19		9
20		8	20		9	20		7	20		8	20		7	20		10
21		9	21		10	21		8	21		9	21		8	21		11
22		10	22		11	22		9	22		10	22		9	22		12
23		11	23		12	23		10	23		11	23		10	23		13
24		12	24		13	24		11	24		12	24		11	24		14
25		13	25		14	25		12	25		13	25		12	25		15
26		14	26		15	26		13	26		14	26		13	26		16
27		15	27		16	27		14	27		15	27		14	27	N	17
28		16	28		17	28		15	28		16	28		15	28		18
29		17				29		16	29	N	17	29		16	29		
30	N	18				30	N	17	30		18	30	N	17	30		
31						31		18				31		18			

2014 - Lunar Phases for New York, NY

Day	Jul		Aug		Sep		Oct		Nov		Dec	
1												
2												
3										0		0
4										1		1
5						0		0		2		2
6						1		1	F	3	F	3
7				0		2		2		4		4
8				1	F	3	F	3		5		5
9		0		2		4		4		6		6
10		1	F	3		5		5		7		7
11		2		4		6		6		8		8
12	F	3		5		7		7		9		9
13		4		6		8		8		10		10
14		5		7		9		9		11		11
15		6		8		10		10		12		12
16		7		9		11		11		13		13
17		8		10		12		12		14		14
18		9		11		13		13		15		15
19		10		12		14		14		16		16
20		11		13		15		15		17		17
21		12		14		16		16		18	N	18
22		13		15		17		17	N			
23		14		16		18	N	18				
24		15		17	N							
25		16	N	18								
26	N	17										
27		18										
28												
29												
30												
31												

2015 - Lunar Phases for New York, NY

Jan			Feb			Mar			Apr			May			Jun		
1		0	1		1	1			1		0	1		1	1		2
2		1	2		2	2		0	2		1	2		2	2	F	3
3		2	3	F	3	3		1	3		2	3	F	3	3		4
4	F	3	4		4	4		2	4	F	3	4		4	4		5
5		4	5		5	5	F	3	5		4	5		5	5		6
6		5	6		6	6		4	6		5	6		6	6		7
7		6	7		7	7		5	7		6	7		7	7		8
8		7	8		8	8		6	8		7	8		8	8		9
9		8	9		9	9		7	9		8	9		9	9		10
10		9	10		10	10		8	10		9	10		10	10		11
11		10	11		11	11		9	11		10	11		11	11		12
12		11	12		12	12		10	12		11	12		12	12		13
13		12	13		13	13		11	13		12	13		13	13		14
14		13	14		14	14		12	14		13	14		14	14		15
15		14	15		15	15		13	15		14	15		15	15		16
16		15	16		16	16		14	16		15	16		16	16	N	17
17		16	17		17	17		15	17		16	17		17	17		18
18		17	18	N	18	18		16	18	N	17	18	N	18	18		
19		18	19			19		17	19		18	19			19		
20	N		20			20	N	18	20			20			20		
21			21			21			21			21			21		
22			22			22			22			22			22		
23			23			23			23			23			23		
24			24			24			24			24			24		
25			25			25			25			25			25		
26			26			26			26			26			26		
27			27			27			27			27			27		
28			28			28			28			28			28		0
29						29			29			29			29		1
30						30			30		0	30		0	30		2
31		0				31						31		1			

2015 - Lunar Phases for New York, NY

Jul			Aug			Sep			Oct			Nov			Dec		
1	F	3	1		4	1		6	1		7	1		8	1		9
2		4	2		5	2		7	2		8	2		9	2		10
3		5	3		6	3		8	3		9	3		10	3		11
4		6	4		7	4		9	4		10	4		11	4		12
5		7	5		8	5		10	5		11	5		12	5		13
6		8	6		9	6		11	6		12	6		13	6		14
7		9	7		10	7		12	7		13	7		14	7		15
8		10	8		11	8		13	8		14	8		15	8		16
9		11	9		12	9		14	9		15	9		16	9		17
10		12	10		13	10		15	10		16	10		17	10		18
11		13	11		14	11		16	11		17	11	N	18	11	N	
12		14	12		15	12		17	12	N	18	12			12		
13		15	13		16	13	N	18	13			13			13		
14		16	14	N	17	14			14			14			14		
15	N	17	15		18	15			15			15			15		
16		18	16			16			16			16			16		
17			17			17			17			17			17		
18			18			18			18			18			18		
19			19			19			19			19			19		
20			20			20			20			20			20		
21			21			21			21			21			21		
22			22			22			22			22		0	22		0
23			23			23			23			23		1	23		1
24			24			24		0	24		0	24		2	24		2
25			25			25		1	25		1	25	F	3	25	F	3
26			26		0	26		2	26		2	26		4	26		4
27			27		1	27	F	3	27	F	3	27		5	27		5
28		0	28		2	28		4	28		4	28		6	28		6
29		1	29	F	3	29		5	29		5	29		7	29		7
30		2	30		4	30		6	30		6	30		8	30		8
31	F	3	31		5				31		7				31		9

2016 - Lunar Phases for New York, NY

Jan			Feb			Mar			Apr			May			Jun		
1		10	1		12	1		11	1		12	1		12	1		14
2		11	2		13	2		12	2		13	2		13	2		15
3		12	3		14	3		13	3		14	3		14	3		16
4		13	4		15	4		14	4		15	4		15	4	N	17
5		14	5		16	5		15	5		16	5		16	5		18
6		15	6		17	6		16	6		17	6	N	17	6		
7		16	7		18	7		17	7	N	18	7		18	7		
8		17	8	N		8	N	18	8			8			8		
9	N	18	9			9			9			9			9		
10			10			10			10			10			10		
11			11			11			11			11			11		
12			12			12			12			12			12		
13			13			13			13			13			13		
14			14			14			14			14			14		
15			15			15			15			15			15		
16			16			16			16			16			16		
17			17			17			17			17			17		0
18			18			18			18			18		0	18		1
19			19		0	19			19		0	19		1	19		2
20		0	20		1	20		0	20		1	20		2	20	F	3
21		1	21		2	21		1	21		2	21	F	3	21		4
22		2	22	F	3	22		2	22	F	3	22		4	22		5
23	F	3	23		4	23	F	3	23		4	23		5	23		6
24		4	24		5	24		4	24		5	24		6	24		7
25		5	25		6	25		5	25		6	25		7	25		8
26		6	26		7	26		6	26		7	26		8	26		9
27		7	27		8	27		7	27		8	27		9	27		10
28		8	28		9	28		8	28		9	28		10	28		11
29		9	29		10	29		9	29		10	29		11	29		12
30		10				30		10	30		11	30		12	30		13
31		11				31		11				31		13			

2016 - Lunar Phases for New York, NY

Jul			Aug			Sep			Oct			Nov			Dec		
1		14	1		16	1	N	17	1		18	1		18	1		
2		15	2	N	17	2		18	2			2			2		
3		16	3		18	3			3			3			3		
4	N	17	4			4			4			4			4		
5		18	5			5			5			5			5		
6			6			6			6			6			6		
7			7			7			7			7			7		
8			8			8			8			8			8		
9			9			9			9			9			9		
10			10			10			10			10			10		0
11			11			11			11			11		0	11		1
12			12			12			12			12		1	12		2
13			13			13		0	13		0	13		2	13	F	3
14			14			14		1	14		1	14	F	3	14		4
15			15		0	15		2	15		2	15		4	15		5
16		0	16		1	16	F	3	16	F	3	16		5	16		6
17		1	17		2	17		4	17		4	17		6	17		7
18		2	18	F	3	18		5	18		5	18		7	18		8
19	F	3	19		4	19		6	19		6	19		8	19		9
20		4	20		5	20		7	20		7	20		9	20		10
21		5	21		6	21		8	21		8	21		10	21		11
22		6	22		7	22		9	22		9	22		11	22		12
23		7	23		8	23		10	23		10	23		12	23		13
24		8	24		9	24		11	24		11	24		13	24		14
25		9	25		10	25		12	25		12	25		14	25		15
26		10	26		11	26		13	26		13	26		15	26		16
27		11	27		12	27		14	27		14	27		16	27		17
28		12	28		13	28		15	28		15	28		17	28		18
29		13	29		14	29		16	29		16	29	N	18	29	N	
30		14	30		15	30	N	17	30	N	17	30			30		
31		15	31		16				31						31		

Three things cannot be long hidden:
the sun, the moon, and the truth.

~ Buddha

Appendix 11

Health Benefits of
Diatomaceous Earth

by Dee McCaffrey, CDC

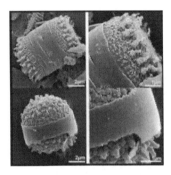

You've probably never heard of one of the best and most economical supplements to improve your health and cleanse your body. In fact, this supplement is perhaps one of the best kept secrets ever. This relatively unknown "food" supplement is called Diatomaceous Earth, also known as DE. It is a completely natural substance that is rich in naturally occurring silica, a mineral whose list of documented health benefits continues to grow as more research is being conducted.

Some of the most recent studies show that it can strengthen bones and joints, prevent osteoporosis and restore bone health if you already have osteoporosis, boost the immune system, ward off Alzheimer's, prevent premature aging and wrinkling of the skin, and strengthens the arterial walls to maintain good heart health. Another of the benefits of silica is that it helps to destroy bad fats in the body. Used as a daily treatment, diatomaceous earth can alleviate the potentially deadly risks of high cholesterol, high blood pressure, and obesity.

Additionally, because of its physical structure, diatomaceous earth is a highly effective anti-inflammatory and internal cleansing agent for the body. It can remove intestinal bacteria, parasites, e-coli, viruses, pesticides, heavy metals, and other toxins. It has also been known to assist with vertigo, headaches, tinnitus, and insomnia.

Sound too good to be true? Read on to learn more about this overlooked multi-purpose supplement and how it can improve many aspects of your health at a fraction of the cost of other supplements.

What is Diatomaceous Earth?

Diatomaceous earth is the fossilized shells of microscopic water-dwelling organisms known as diatoms. Diatoms are one-celled plants (algae or phytoplankton) that are the primary food source for marine life. These plants have been part of the earth's ecology since prehistoric times, yet their species still exists today in both salty and fresh waters all over the world.

Diatoms use soluble silica (sand) from their environment to make their shells, or exoskeletons. As diatoms die, their shells fall to the bottom of the bodies of water in which they live. It is believed that 30 million years ago the diatoms piled up to form thick beds of chalky fossilized sediment. These beds, known as diatomite or diatomaceous earth, were discovered after the waters receded.

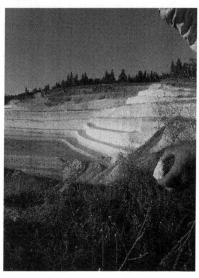

Today, hundreds of large deposits of diatomaceous earth occur all over the world. Some are still underwater and some are found in ancient dried lake bottoms. It has been estimated that one cubic inch of diatomaceous earth may contain as many as 400 million shells, that's how small diatoms are!

Diatomite is mined and ground into a powder that looks and feels like talcum powder. This all natural powder is called Diatomaceous Earth (DE) or fossil shell flour. It is made up of approximately 33% silicon, 19% calcium, 5% sodium, 3% magnesium 2% iron and many other trace minerals such as titanium, boron, manganese, copper and zirconium.

What Do Fossilized Shells Have to Do With Improving Your Health?

It's all about the silica.

As I mentioned earlier, the shells of diatoms are made up mostly of silica (known by chemists as silicon dioxide). Silica is one of the most abundant minerals on the planet, but most of it is in a form that is unabsorbable by humans, and there are limited numbers of foods that contain an adequate amount of the absorbable form to supply the quantity our body needs. Silica is the most important trace mineral for human health. It plays an important role in many body functions and has a direct relationship to mineral absorption. For optimal health, the average human body needs to hold approximately seven grams of silica, a quantity far exceeding the figures for other important minerals such as iron and calcium.

Silica can be found in such foods as alfalfa, beets, brown rice and oats. Bell peppers and leafy green vegetables also provide silica, while asparagus, Jerusalem artichokes, parsley, sunflower seeds and grain husks, such as barley, millet and wheat contain smaller amounts.

Years ago, the silica found in our foods was adequate, but with today's depleted soils, only about one-third of the silica needed by our body is supplied in our food.

In our youth, our tissues absorb and maintain high levels of silica— enabling our bodies to remain flexible, resilient, and energetic—but as we age, and as our dietary sources of silica are not meeting our needs, our silica levels steadily decline until they become almost non-existent. In fact, 80% of all of our body's silica is used up by the time we become adults.

Our bodies need silica regardless of our age and even when diet is not the primary factor in cases of deficiencies, we often become deficient in this essential trace element simply thorough the aging process. The effect of this steady decrease in silica levels is a progressive decline in health, increasing fatigue and acceleration of the aging process.

Diatomaceous earth, which is very high in the absorbable form of silica, can replenish silica levels in the body, which can vastly improve your health and reverse many chronic problems. Studies show that high levels of silica can:

Improve Bone Health and Stop Osteoporosis: Calcium and vitamin D alone are not sufficient for bone growth, density, strength, and flexibility. In fact, the body cannot absorb and use calcium without the presence of silica. Recent data suggests that instead of promoting healing, calcium supplements actually speed up the leeching away of bone calcium and accelerate the degenerative process of osteoporosis and similar diseases that affect the connective tissues in the human body!

To re-mineralize and repair damaged bones, it is now advised that a sufficient silica supplement be taken daily because bones are composed of mainly of the minerals phosphorus, magnesium and calcium; however, these minerals need the presence of silica to be deposited into the bones, especially calcium. Silica hastens the healing of fractures and also diminishes scarring at the location of a fracture. A great deal of research evidence indicates that silica has the ability to "morph" itself into calcium through a transmutation process. Yes, silica actually has the ability to be turned into calcium when there is a calcium deficiency and the body needs it!

That fact alone should be reason enough to supplement with DE!!

Ward Off Alzheimer's: Scientists and researchers have long hypothesized that Alzheimer's disease is linked to a build up of aluminum in the brain, and links between aluminum in drinking water supplies and Alzheimer's have now been ascertained. A factor that had been overlooked is that silica reduces the accumulation of aluminum. When researchers added silica to aluminum-laced water supplies, it inhibited the aluminum from being absorbed. It also caused a proliferation in the excretion of aluminum in urine and lowered aluminum concentrations in the brain, liver, bone, spleen and kidneys. Silica, therefore, may be important in supporting neurological health.

Improve Heart and Lung Health: Silica can hinder the effects of coronary disease by fortifying blood vessels. Studies confirm that with age, silica disappears from the aorta, the heart's key blood vessel—thus weakening its critical connective tissue, and resulting in a greater cardiac risk. Studies have shown diatomaceous earth to significantly lower cholesterol by removing plaque and keeping arteries and veins supple. It also helps to regulate blood pressure. Silica also aids in the repair and maintenance of vital lung tissues and defending them from pollution.

Stop Premature Wrinkling and Sagging Skin: Silica is excellent for supporting bones and connective tissue. Your body needs healthy connective tissue for internal organs and the largest organ which is your skin. And you probably know that degrading connective tissue, with age is why wrinkles appear and skin begins to sag. Perhaps it is not age, but rather not enough silica that makes this happen.

Collagen, which is mostly made up of silica, is the glue that holds us together. Collagen accounts for up to 75% of the weight of the dermis and is responsible for the resilience and elasticity of the skin. Our connective tissues consist of collagen, elastin, mucopolysaccharides and mucous carbohydrates which aid in moisture retention. Their capacity to hold on to moisture keeps the connective tissue resilient and has apparent importance in the prevention of premature aging. All these valuable molecules house large quantities of silica. Also, many people with advanced arthritis suffer from bone deformation when tendons and ligaments in the joints lose flexibility due to loss of collagen. Tendons and ligaments need silica for health and flexibility.

Boost the Immune System: Silica may play an important role in the immune system and its biological response to harmful stimuli. Silica is necessary for the body to produce antibodies that fight off viruses, bacteria, allergens and other invaders that the body views as foreign.

Other Ways Diatomaceous Earth Can Improve Your Health

One of the most sought after benefits of diatomaceous earth is to cleanse the digestive tract. Many people consume a variety of processed foods, which contain various harmful chemicals and toxins. Plus, as air quality has decreased, we are constantly putting more toxins in our body that need to be removed.

Diatomaceous earth can purge any parasite, virus, bacteria, or toxin that is clinging to our digestive tract. While diatomaceous earth feels like a soft powder, the truth is that diatomaceous earth is actually a small cylinder with extremely sharp edges. As we consume diatomaceous earth, these sharp edges scrape away parasites, toxins, and viruses clinging to the lining of our digestive tract. Plus, any toxins or bacteria floating in our digestive tract are absorbed and trapped by diatomaceous earth. It has also been shown to cling to bad fats in the body, effectively reducing bad cholesterol. Diatomaceous earth is then expelled through our bowel movements and these harmful materials are removed.

Our skin and organs are strong and thick enough not to be affected by these sharp edges, which is why we feel no pain taking diatomaceous earth. After a few days, the body's digestive system can be thoroughly cleansed and can operate much more efficiently.

Are All Forms of Diatomaceous Earth the Same?

No! There are two types of DE—Food Grade and Pool Grade.

Most deposits of diatomaceous earth are from salt water sources, while only a few are from fresh water sources. Of the hundreds of DE deposits that exist worldwide, only 4 of them can be called food grade. The DE sourced from fresh water beds are of extremely high purity—so pure that it is called Food Grade Diatomaceous Earth, or also known as fossil shell flour. Food grade diatomaceous earth, the only form safe for human consumption, is a white powder, while other forms of diatomaceous earth may have a brown/reddish tint.

Also, there are two types of naturally occurring silica—crystalline silica and non-crystalline (amorphous) silica. Crystalline silica can be very dangerous, especially to our lungs if inhaled, while non-crystalline silica is completely safe, even for human and animal consumption. The fresh water diatoms contain mainly non-crystalline silica, while salt water diatoms can contain both types, with higher amounts of the crystalline form.

PERMA-GUARD™ is the trade name known worldwide for using a grade and quality of Diatomaceous Earth (DE) that is extremely pure. Brands that use Perma-Guard™ food grade Diatomaceous Earth contains less than 0 .5% crystalline silica. It is important to have a consistent shape diatom and no unwanted sediment. The shape of the diatom must be tubular with holes on the walls. It must be from fresh water because the fresh water diatoms form a harder shell and are less fragile that those from salt water. Salt water deposits contain a mix of diatom species. These deposits shapes and sediments are inconsistent making them unusable for safe human consumption.

Other types of diatomaceous earth have other industrial uses. It is heated to a very high temperature (about 1000°C or 1800°F). This type of DE is called "calcined." It is used for pool filters and other types of filtering but it is also used as a filler and can end up in paints, cosmetics, drugs, chemical insecticides, and other things. Food grade DE is never heated.

Bottom Line: ONLY use Food Grade Diatomaceous Earth for health purposes!!! Food grade diatomaceous earth is the purest form of diatomaceous earth and can be consumed and used by humans. Food grade diatomaceous earth is heavily regulated and must contain less than a certain amount of specific minerals.

Pool grade DE is calcinated and is a stronger, more potent form of DE. It is not to be used by humans and pool grade DE must be handled with gloves and a mask to ensure no throat irritations occur.

All DE should have a label that tells you if it has been calcined and how much crystalline silica it contains.

How Much to Take—How Safe Is It?

Food grade diatomaceous earth is a very fine powder and is very light due to its high porosity. It mixes easily into liquids and foods. Most people take a teaspoon or a tablespoon two or three times a day (up to a total of one quarter cup per day) for best results. Mix it into water, juice, smoothies or other foods.

It sort of resembles putting a spoonful of baking soda in water and drinking it!

Silica is water soluble; hence, once you get it into your body it easily absorbed via the intestinal wall and is also rapidly excreted. It does not accumulate in the body, so consistent daily supplementation is important. Studies have not found any negative side effects from too much silica. Its safety and extensive range of uses makes silica one of the most important minerals used in complementary therapy and alternative medicine. Regular supplementation could make a significant difference in your health.

Being approved by the FDA, Diatomaceous Earth has absolutely no dangerous side effects. It can be used by anyone, as long as the person doesn't suffer from a serious illness. As with any other health supplement, talk to a doctor before using DE. You might have some intolerance to it, so it's advisable to not risk your health. Pregnant and breastfeeding mothers can use it as long as their doctor has agreed.

What Other Uses Does DE Have?

One of the most commonly known uses for diatomaceous earth is as a non-toxic bug killer. DE is almost pure silica (with some beneficial trace minerals); under a microscope, it looks like shards of glass (glass is made from silica). On any beetle-type insect that has a carapace, like ants, fleas and cockroaches, the DE works under the shell and punctures the body, which then dehydrates their innards and the insect dies. DE is totally nontoxic. There is no buildup of tolerance like there is to poisons because the method of killing is PHYSICAL, not chemical. But rest assured, food grade DE doesn't hurt people or animals. In fact, it makes a great flea killer for your pets, and can also be added to their food as de-wormer. Many farmers use it to keep farm animals healthy, both inside and out. Food grade DE is also added to grains in storage because it keeps bugs from eating the grain. So if you eat any grains, you're probably already eating a little bit of DE!

Where to Get It!

You can buy food grade diatomaceous earth online. Processed-Free America sells it through its online store.

Written by Dee McCaffrey, CDC, who lost 100 pounds and has kept it off for over 20 years. For more info, go to: www.processedfreeamerica.org

Appendix 12

Summary of Protocols

The purpose of this list is to have all the protocols in one place, so you don't have to be hunting and flipping pages to find something. This information is also available on our website www.cdautism.org if you would like to print anything full size.

Diet

Permitted Foods List:

Note: Organic products are better but not required.

Proteins

- ☐ Beef
- ☐ Chicken
- ☐ Eggs
- ☐ Fish (small not large size)
- ☐ Pork
- ☐ Turkey

Fruit

- ☐ Most fresh fruits are permitted (except citrus, mango, pineapple, kiwi, and limit berries).
- ☐ Frozen fruit without added cream or sugar.
- ! NO canned fruit (nothing canned ever).
- ! Be careful of dried fruit as it may contain sugar.

Vegetables

- ☐ All vegetables are fine!!!
- ☐ Including French fries, however, not frozen fries or fries from fast food chains; these are often coated in flour.

Nuts

- ☐ Almonds
- ☐ Cashews
- ☐ Coconut
- ☐ Hazelnuts
- ☐ Walnuts

Grains

- ☐ Amaranth
- ☐ Buckwheat
- ☐ Corn
- ☐ Millet
- ☐ Quinoa
- ☐ Rice
- ☐ Sorghum
- ☐ Tapioca
- ☐ Xanthan gum

Beans

- ☐ All beans—EXCEPT soy
- ☐ Split Pea
- ☐ Garbanzo
- ☐ Lentils
- ☐ Navy
- ☐ Peanuts

Sweeteners

- ☐ Stevia (Best choice of all sweeteners)
- ☐ Agave syrup
- ☐ Honey
- ☐ Maple syrup (without added sugar)
- ☐ Xylitol

Prohibited Foods List

- ⊘ Acetic acid (E260)
- ⊘ Artificial flavoring
- ⊘ Artificial sweeteners
- ⊘ Bouillon cubes
- ⊘ Bread
- ⊘ Candy
- ⊘ Cane sugar
- ⊘ Carrageenan
- ⊘ Catsup
- ⊘ Chocolate milk
- ⊘ Coloring
- ⊘ Corn flakes
- ⊘ Corn syrup
- ⊘ Cow's milk in any form (even lactose-free milk products)
- ⊘ Flour tortillas
- ⊘ Gelatin
- ⊘ Malt
- ⊘ Margarine
- ⊘ Mayonnaise
- ⊘ Microwave popcorn
- ⊘ MSG
- ⊘ Natural flavoring
- ⊘ Noodle soup
- ⊘ Oatmeal (except for Bob's Red Mill GF oats)
- ⊘ Pasta
- ⊘ Piloncillo (unrefined sugar)
- ⊘ Children's nutritional shakes
- ⊘ Play-Doh™
- ⊘ Preservatives
- ⊘ Processed meats (hotdogs, ham, sausage, bologna, cold cuts)
- ⊘ Shellfish (full of toxins)
- ⊘ Sodas
- ⊘ Soy/fruit beverages
- ⊘ Soy milk
- ⊘ Soy sauce
- ⊘ Sports drinks
- ⊘ Sugar
- ⊘ Yeast

1.	Start by filling the baby bottle with 8 fl. oz. (237ml) of water (distilled or reverse osmosis). NO alkaline water!	
2.	Place 1 drop of sodium chlorite solution into the CLEAN and DRY shot glass.	
3.	Add 1 drop of acidic activator (hydrochloric acid or citric acid) to the shot glass containing the drop of sodium chlorite. The number of drops may be higher if you are using a weaker activator. See chart on page 94.	
4.	Now wait the appropriate time for the mixture to react (see chart on page 94). You should see the color change from clear to slightly yellow. If there were more drops in the shot glass, the color change is more noticeable. You are also likely to notice the chlorine-like smell coming from the shot glass. Remember, this is NOT chlorine, but rather chlorine dioxide.	
5.	After the activation time has passed, pour a little water from the baby bottle into the shot glass and let it mix. This mostly stops the chemical reaction and insures you get most of the mixture out in the next step.	
6.	Lastly, pour all of the watered down mixture in the shot glass back into the baby bottle, and seal it tightly with the cap—don't leave it sitting open for any length of time. Think partially used soda pop and how you would want to keep that closed.	

Estimated Full Oral CD Doses by Weight

Use these numbers as a guide only. You may need to go up by as much as 50% or more over the indicated drops. Read chart as: **POUNDS / KILOGRAMS → DROPS OF CD (per 8 fl. oz. water)**

25/11→8	62/28→17	99/45→24	136/62→29	173/78→33	210/95→37
26/12→8	63/29→17	100/45→24	137/62→29	174/79→33	211/96→37
27/12→9	64/29→17	101/46→24	138/63→29	175/79→34	212/96→37
28/13→9	65/29→18	102/46→24	139/63→30	176/80→34	213/97→37
29/13→9	66/30→18	103/47→24	140/64→30	177/80→34	214/97→37
30/14→9	67/30→18	104/47→25	141/64→30	178/81→34	215/98→37
31/14→10	68/31→18	105/48→25	142/64→30	179/81→34	216/98→37
32/15→10	69/31→18	106/48→25	143/65→30	180/82→34	217/98→37
33/15→10	70/32→19	107/49→25	144/65→30	181/82→34	218/99→38
34/15→10	71/32→19	108/49→25	145/66→30	182/83→34	219/99→38
35/16→11	72/33→19	109/49→25	146/66→30	183/83→34	220/100→38
36/16→11	73/33→19	110/50→26	147/67→31	184/83→35	221/100→38
37/17→11	74/34→19	111/50→26	148/67→31	185/84→35	222/101→38
38/17→11	75/34→20	112/51→26	149/68→31	186/84→35	223/101→38
39/18→12	76/34→20	113/51→26	150/68→31	187/85→35	224/102→38
40/18→12	77/35→20	114/52→26	151/68→31	188/85→35	225/102→38
41/19→12	78/35→20	115/52→26	152/69→31	189/86→35	226/103→38
42/19→12	79/36→20	116/53→26	153/69→31	190/86→35	227/103→38
43/20→13	80/36→21	117/53→27	154/70→31	191/87→35	228/103→38
44/20→13	81/37→21	118/54→27	155/70→31	192/87→35	229/104→38
45/20→13	82/37→21	119/54→27	156/71→32	193/88→35	230/104→39
46/21→13	83/38→21	120/54→27	157/71→32	194/88→35	231/105→39
47/21→14	84/38→21	121/55→27	158/72→32	195/88→36	232/105→39
48/22→14	85/39→21	122/55→27	159/72→32	196/89→36	233/106→39
49/22→14	86/39→22	123/56→27	160/73→32	197/89→36	234/106→39
50/23→14	87/39→22	124/56→28	161/73→32	198/90→36	235/107→39
51/23→15	88/40→22	125/57→28	162/73→32	199/90→36	236/107→39
52/24→15	89/40→22	126/57→28	163/74→32	200/91→36	237/108→39
53/24→15	90/41→22	127/58→28	164/74→32	201/91→36	238/108→39
54/24→15	91/41→23	128/58→28	165/75→33	202/92→36	239/108→39
55/25→16	92/42→23	129/59→28	166/75→33	203/92→36	240/109→39
56/25→16	93/42→23	130/59→28	167/76→33	204/93→36	241/109→39
57/26→16	94/43→23	131/59→28	168/76→33	205/93→36	242/110→39
58/26→16	95/43→23	132/60→29	169/77→33	206/93→37	243/110→39
59/27→16	96/44→23	133/60→29	170/77→33	207/94→37	244/111→40
60/27→17	97/44→24	134/61→29	171/78→33	208/94→37	245/111→40
61/28→17	98/44→24	135/61→29	172/78→33	209/95→37	246/112→40

CD Enemas:

I recommend enemas no less frequently than every other day. You can do them more often particularly if you see parasites coming out. The ratio is 1-2 drops chlorine dioxide per 100 ml of filtered warm water. Work your way up to 500 mL – 1.5 L of water per enema, depending on the size of your child. You have the following options for methods of administering the enemas: a catheter and syringes, a multipurpose enema/douche bag, empty out a fleet enema, or a gravity bag. (note, if your child suffers from constipation you can add enemas and baths in before you get to full dose, alternating them on opposite days or opposite ends of the day).

Enemas should be started when the child reaches full oral dose. However, if your child suffers from constipation you can add enemas and baths on day one (see page 113), before you get to the full oral dose. However, alternate them on opposite days or opposite ends of the day. The following chart is an approximate amount of water based on the size of the person, and calculated the maximum of 2 drops of CD per 100mL of water.

Age/Size	Water Volume	Drops of CD
Child	1/2 Liter (500ml)	10
Adolescent	1 Liter (1,000ml)	20
Teen/Adult	up to 2 Liters (2,000ml)	40

CD Baths:

10-100 Activated drops of CD in a hot (to tolerance) bath with enough water to cover the child's body. Soak for 20 minutes. Apply on alternate enema days, unless you are doing daily enemas, in which case apply on opposite ends of the day.

The CD baths can go from as low as 10 drops to as high as 80 to 100 drops; it just depends on the person, and the size of your tub. With younger/smaller children we start with ten drops. Since we're doing baths every other day, start with ten drops on Monday, 11 drops on Wednesday, and 12 drops on Friday. Just keep going up until you get to 20 drops. The bigger and older the person is, the more drops they can tolerate. Fill the tub to a level that maximizes skin contact.

72/2 Protocol

Give one dose of CD every 2 hours for 72 hours straight, including the middle of the night. Apply every possible weekend.

This involves giving one dose of CD every two hours for 72 hours straight—including the middle of the night. Here are some additional thoughts and guidelines:

- Start protocol when you pick up your child from school on Friday.
- Give them the last 72/2 dose when you drop them off at school on Monday.
- Avoid giving CD enemas or CD baths during this protocol, UNLESS they are dumping parasites, in which case you might need to reduce the amount of CD on both the oral and enema dose to insure the child doesn't have a Herxheimer reaction.
- Why not give hourly doses during the day at the usual dose? It's simply too much if you are doing it all night as well.
- Watch for improvements on Tuesday or Wednesday each week.
- Ideally, get your spouse or significant other to help with every other nightly dose.

Supplement Dosing Overview

Supplement	Dose	Time of Day	Empty Stomach (ES) or With Food (WF)
Probiotics	1 cap	Before Bed	ES
Omega-3/ Omega-6	1 Tbsp	With any meal 1-3x / day	WF
L-Carnitine	250-1000mg/day	With any meal 1-3x / day	WF
GABA	Up to 2,500mg 2x/day	Upon waking & at bedtime	ES
5-HTP	50-200mg	Morning & Evening	WF
L-Theanine	Work up to 200-250mg/day	Mornings or Mornings & Nights	ES
Pycnogenol	25-40mg a day/as needed	Morning	WF
L-Carnosine	200-400mg 2x / day	Morning & Evening	WF
Taurine	500-1500mg/day	Morning, Noon & Night	ES
DMG	900mg/day	Morning	ES
TMG	500mg/day	Morning	ES
Enzymes	1 cap w/meals	Morning, Noon & Night	WF

Parasite Protocol

Please see the complete explanation of the parasite protocol starting on page 187. Day-to-day protocol charts can be found on page 198.

Chelation:

I suggest that when you decide to add clay baths into your child's protocol that you do so on the off days of the CD baths.

Follow the instructions on the package, and follow septic tank precautions if you have one.

Three days or so later, you can add in the Bio-Chelat. Again, follow the instructions on the package, and you can always start slowly and work your way up. Since Bio-Chelat™ doesn't alter the CD, the drops can be added to a single dose of CD. In addition, since the drops have no flavor, it is suitable to add them to water or any other drink your child might consume throughout the day.

Hyperbarics:

Option #1:

Two sessions of 60 minutes each for 20 days for a total of 40 sessions at 1.75 ATA.

Option #2:

One 90-minute session a day for twenty days at 1.75 ATA.

Instead of thinking outside of the box, get rid of the box.

~ Deepak Chopra

Appendix 13

Body Burden
The Pollution in Newborns

W̶hen I came across the following investigation I knew it was the perfect precursor to the incredible "Avoiding Autism" by Dr. Anju Usman and Beth Hynes. Babies are exposed to toxins in the womb and this study by the Environmental Working Group demonstrates so perfectly why the advice in the "Avoiding Autism" article is so very crucial to health of our children and for our species as a whole.

Body Burden — The Pollution in Newborns
A benchmark investigation of industrial chemicals, pollutants and pesticides in umbilical cord blood.

Environmental Working Group, July 14, 2005

Summary. In the month leading up to a baby's birth, the umbilical cord pulses with the equivalent of at least 300 quarts of blood each day, pumped back and forth from the nutrient- and oxygen-rich placenta to the rapidly growing child cradled in a sac of amniotic fluid. This cord is a lifeline between mother and baby, bearing nutrients that sustain life and propel growth.

Not long ago scientists thought that the placenta shielded cord blood — and the developing baby — from most chemicals and pollutants in the environment. But now we know that at this critical time when organs, vessels, membranes and systems are knit together from single cells to finished form in a span of weeks, the umbilical cord carries not only the building blocks of life, but also a steady stream of industrial chemicals, pollutants and pesticides that cross the placenta as readily as residues from cigarettes and alcohol. This is the human "body burden" — the pollution in people that permeates everyone in the world, including babies in the womb.

In a study spearheaded by the Environmental Working Group (EWG) in collaboration with Commonweal, researchers at two major laboratories found an average of 200 industrial chemicals and pollutants in umbilical cord blood from 10 babies born in August and September of 2004 in U.S. hospitals. Tests revealed a total of 287 chemicals in the group. The umbilical cord blood of these 10 children, collected by Red Cross after the cord was cut, harbored pesticides, consumer product ingredients, and wastes from burning coal, gasoline, and garbage.

This study represents the first reported cord blood tests for 261 of the targeted chemicals and the first reported detections in cord blood for 209 compounds. Among them are eight perfluorochemicals used as stain and oil repellants in fast food packaging, clothes and textiles — including the Teflon chemical PFOA, recently characterized as a likely human carcinogen by the EPA's Science Advisory Board — dozens of

Chemicals and pollutants detected in human umbilical cord blood

Hg

Mercury (Hg) - tested for 1, found 1
Pollutant from coal-fired power plants, mercury-containing products, and certain industrial processes. Accumulates in seafood. Harms brain development and function.

PAH

Polyaromatic hydrocarbons (PAHs) - tested for 18, found 9
Pollutants from burning gasoline and garbage. Linked to cancer. Accumulates in food chain.

BD/F

Polybrominated dibenzodioxins and furans (PBDD/F) - tested for 12, found 7
Contaminants in brominated flame retardants. Pollutants and byproducts from plastic production and incineration. Accumulate in food chain. Toxic to developing endocrine (hormone) system

PFC

Perfluorinated chemicals (PFCs) - tested for 12, found 9
Active ingredients or breakdown products of Teflon, Scotchgard, fabric and carpet protectors, food wrap coatings. Global contaminants. Accumulate in the environment and the food chain. Linked to cancer, birth defects, and more.

D/F

Polychlorinated dibenzodioxins and furans (PCDD/F) - tested for 17, found 11
Pollutants, by-products of PVC production, industrial bleaching, and incineration. Cause cancer in humans. Persist for decades in the environment. Very toxic to developing endocrine (hormone) system.

OC

Organochlorine pesticides (OCs) - tested for 28, found 21
DDT, chlordane and other pesticides. Largely banned in the U.S. Persist for decades in the environment. Accumulate up the food chain, to man. Cause cancer and numerous reproductive effects.

PBDE

Polybrominated diphenyl ethers (PBDEs) - tested for 46, found 32
Flame retardant in furniture foam, computers, and televisions. Accumulates in the food chain and human tissues. Adversely affects brain development and the thyroid.

CN

Polychlorinated Naphthalenes (PCNs) - tested for 70, found 50
Wood preservatives, varnishes, machine lubricating oils, waste incineration. Common PCB contaminant. Contaminate the food chain. Cause liver and kidney damage.

PCB

Polychlorinated biphenyls (PCBs) - tested for 209, found 147
Industrial insulators and lubricants. Banned in the U.S. in 1976. Persist for decades in the environment. Accumulate up the food chain, to man. Cause cancer and nervous system problems.

Source: Chemical analyses of 10 umbilical cord blood samples were conducted by AXYS Analytical Services (Sydney, BC) and Flett Research Ltd. (Winnipeg, MB).

widely used brominated flame retardants and their toxic by-products; and numerous pesticides.

Of the 287 chemicals we detected in umbilical cord blood, we know that 180 cause cancer in humans or animals, 217 are toxic to the brain and nervous system, and 208 cause birth defects or abnormal development in animal tests. The dangers of pre- or post-natal exposure to this complex mixture of carcinogens, developmental toxins and neurotoxins have never been studied.

Chemical exposures in the womb or during infancy can be dramatically more harmful than exposures later in life. Substantial scientific evidence demonstrates that children face amplified risks from their body burden of pollution; the findings are particularly strong for many of the chemicals found in this study, including mercury, PCBs and dioxins. Children's vulnerability derives from both rapid development and incomplete defense systems:

- A developing child's chemical exposures are greater pound-for-pound than those of adults.

- An immature, porous blood-brain barrier allows greater chemical exposures to the developing brain.

- Children have lower levels of some chemical-binding proteins, allowing more of a chemical to reach "target organs."

- A baby's organs and systems are rapidly developing, and thus are often more vulnerable to damage from chemical exposure.

- Systems that detoxify and excrete industrial chemicals are not fully developed.

- The longer future life span of a child compared to an adult allows more time for adverse effects to arise.

The 10 children in this study were chosen randomly, from among 2004's summer season of live births from mothers in Red Cross' volunteer, national cord blood collection program. They were not chosen because their parents work in the chemical industry or because they were known to bear problems from chemical exposures in the womb. Nevertheless, each baby was born polluted with a broad array of contaminants.

U.S. industries manufacture and import approximately 75,000 chemicals, 3,000 of them at over a million pounds per year. Health officials do not know how many of these chemicals pollute fetal blood and what the health consequences of in utero exposures may be.

Had we tested for a broader array of chemicals, we would almost certainly have detected far more than 287. But testing umbilical cord blood for industrial chemicals is technically challenging. Chemical manufacturers are not required to divulge to the public or government health officials methods to detect their chemicals in humans. Few labs are equipped with the machines and expertise to run the tests or the funding to develop the methods. Laboratories have yet to develop methods to test human tissues for the vast majority of chemicals on the market, and the few tests that labs are able to conduct are expensive. Laboratory costs for the cord blood analyses reported here were $10,000 per sample.

A developing baby depends on adults for protection, nutrition, and, ultimately, survival. As a society we have a responsibility to ensure that babies do not enter this world pre-polluted, with 200 industrial chemicals in their blood. Decades-old bans on a handful of chemicals like PCBs, lead gas additives, DDT and other pesticides have led to significant declines in people's blood levels of these pollutants. But good news like this is hard to find for other chemicals.

The Toxic Substances Control Act, the 1976 federal law meant to ensure the safety of commercial chemicals, essentially deemed 63,000 existing chemicals "safe as used" the day the law was passed, through mandated, en masse approval for use with no safety scrutiny. It forces the government to approve new chemicals within 90 days of a company's application at an average pace of seven per day. It has not been improved for nearly 30 years—longer than any other major environmental or public health statute—and does nothing to reduce or ensure the safety of exposure to pollution in the womb.

Because the Toxic Substances Control Act fails to mandate safety studies, the government has initiated a number of voluntary programs to gather more information about chemicals, most notably the high production volume (HPV) chemical screening program. But these efforts have been largely ineffective at reducing human exposures to chemicals. They are no substitute for a clear statutory requirement to protect children from the toxic effects of chemical exposure.

In light of the findings in this study and a substantial body of supporting science on the toxicity of early life exposures to industrial chemicals, we strongly urge that federal laws and policies be reformed to ensure that children are protected from chemicals, and that to the maximum extent possible, exposures to industrial chemicals before birth be eliminated. The sooner society takes action, the sooner we can reduce or end pollution in the womb.

Tests show 287 industrial chemicals in 10 newborn babies

Pollutants include consumer product ingredients, banned industrial chemicals and pesticides, and waste byproducts

Sources and uses of chemicals in newborn blood	Chemical family name	Total number of chemicals found in 10 newborns (range in individual babies)
Common consumer product chemicals (and their breakdown products)		47 chemicals (23 - 38)
Pesticides, actively used in U.S.	Organochlorine pesticides (OCs)	7 chemicals (2 - 6)
Stain and grease resistant coatings for food wrap, carpet, furniture (Teflon, Scotchgard, Stainmaster...)	Perfluorochemicals (PFCs)	8 chemicals (4 - 8)
Fire retardants in TVs, computers, furniture	Polybrominated diphenyl ethers (PBDEs)	32 chemicals (13 - 29)
Chemicals banned or severely restricted in the U.S. (and their breakdown products)		212 chemicals (111 - 185)
Pesticides, phased out of use in U.S.	Organochlorine pesticides (OCs)	14 chemicals (7 - 14)
Stain and grease resistant coatings for food wrap, carpet, furniture (pre-2000 Scotchgard)	Perfluorochemicals (PFCs)	1 chemicals (1 - 1)
Electrical insulators	Polychlorinated biphenyls (PCBs)	147 chemicals (65 - 134)
Broad use industrial chemicals - flame retardants, pesticides, electrical insultators	Polychlorinated naphthalenes (PCNs)	50 chemicals (22 - 40)
Waste byproducts		28 chemicals (6 - 21)
Garbage incineration and plastic production wastes	Polychlorinated and Polybrominated dibenzo dioxins and furans (PCDD/F and PBDD/F)	18 chemicals (5 - 13)
Car emissions and other fossil fuel combustion	Polynuclear aromatic hydrocarbons (PAHs)	10 chemicals (1 - 10)
Power plants (coal burning)	Methylmercury	1 chemicals (1 - 1)
All chemicals found		287 chemicals (154 - 231)

Source: Environmental Working Group analysis of tests of 10 umbilical cord blood samples conducted by AXYS Analytical Services (Sydney, BC) and Flett Research Ltd. (Winnipeg, MB).

The ultimate ignorance is the rejection of something you know nothing about and refuse to investigate.

~ Dr. Wayne Dyer

Appendix 14

Avoiding Autism

By Anju Usman, MD and Beth C. Hynes JD, MBA

Whether or not you are the parent of a special needs child, please pay special attention to this article, we do believe autism is totally preventable and that starts with pregnancy. Here's to your health!

Every parent's dream is to have a healthy baby. Over the past ten years of working with families devastated by the diagnosis of autism, we, along with our patients' parents, have realized one key fact: if we knew then what we know now, the diagnosis of the disease called autism could very well have been prevented. Considering that the cause(s) of the current epidemic of autism spectrum disorders (ASD) are unknown (and scant research dollars are being dedicated to finding the most likely culprits), there is no surefire method to avoid having your infant regress into this devastating state. That sad fact, however, does not mean that there are no proactive steps parents can take to try to mitigate the chances of this disease overtaking their baby and stealing their hopes and dreams for that child's life.

Having reviewed the medical and laboratory test results of thousands of children afflicted with ASD, clinicians using a biomedical approach to treating autism see repeating patterns in these children—impaired methylation and detoxification, mitochondrial dysfunction, gastrointestinal distress, and immune dysregulation compounded by chronic viral, fungal and bacterial infections and a burden of heavy metals and other toxins. From this perspective, we have come to view autism as a multifactorial medical disease that can be treated and overcome and, therefore, possibly avoided. Coming straight from the heart, this advice is for thinking, active parents and prospective parents who want to know what they can do to reduce the risk that their infant will regress into autism. In our practice, we have helped many parents go on to have healthy children even though they already have a child with autism. Considering that the information provided here is not harmful but, to the contrary, is helpful in promoting improved maternal and fetal health, there is little downside to pursuing these strategies while simultaneously minimizing the risk of having your child slip away into the autism epidemic. According to the latest statistics out of California, that epidemic continues to grow from the already shocking 1 out of 150 children. The aim here is to provide an analytical construct that will guide parents in making choices for both their own health and that of their baby before, during, and after pregnancy.

Think of the analogy of the straw that broke the camel's back. Human beings start life as infants with some "straws" in their saddle – these are predispositions to be harmed by certain chemicals, to be susceptible to certain diseases, or to have a less robust detoxification capacity. The goal of gestating and parenting an infant in today's toxic world is to not accumulate additional straws during your baby's gestation and infancy, thereby avoiding adding the straw that breaks the camel's back. Autism seems to occur when the infant's body is so overwhelmed by toxins, viruses and/or pathogenic elements that typical development is arrested and/or derailed.

Children diagnosed with autism have a variety of medical problems, the underpinnings of which can be ameliorated and/or healed. The symptoms associated with autism occur through malfunctioning of the infant immune, gastrointestinal, and central nervous systems ("Infant Body Systems") – all of which, when functioning properly, contribute to the healthy development of the brain. Viruses, heavy metals, toxins, fungi, and bacteria together form a weapon that disrupts the development of, and harms the functioning of, these critical Infant Body Systems. As researchers have recently found, "a single toxicant may promote different immune-associated diseases that are dependent upon the specific window of early life exposure, the gender of the exposed offspring, and the genetic background of the offspring." Our construct will consist of actions you can take to promote the healthy development of these Infant Body Systems as well as steps you can take to avoid upsetting the healthy development of those systems.

Due to the symbiotic relationship between a mother and her developing fetus, care must be taken by the mom before, during, and after pregnancy (if nursing) to both avoid exposure to harmful elements and to promote optimal maternal detoxification processes so that the host body remains as clean an environment as possible within which vigorous infant development can unfold.

Only recently have researchers begun closely linking environmental factors with developmental delays in our children. A host of studies show how environmental factors including diet, nutrition, air quality, clean water, heavy metals (e.g., mercury, lead, arsenic, and aluminum), xenobiotics (e.g., chemicals, pesticides, plasticizers, and perchlorates), pharmaceuticals, and vaccinations can change your child's inborn risk.

This area of study is called epigenetics – the molecular changes in our DNA caused by environmental factors. In 2003, researchers at Duke University found that rats carrying a gene for obesity, cancer, and diabetes, when fed a diet high in B-12, folic acid, choline, and methyl-rich foods, had babies that were born healthy and with a reduced risk of developing disease; this research revealed that these genetic changes persisted across four generations. Thus, when you eat a healthy diet, you are affecting not only the health of your own kids but also your grandchildren, great-grandchildren, and great-great-grandchildren. Researchers are finding hundreds of unwanted and potentially toxic chemicals in the placenta and cord blood of newborns as well as in mothers' breast milk. That means that today's children are born with a toxic burden their infant bodies must contend with from day one. Studies out of China, Texas, and San Francisco show that if pregnant mothers can decrease their exposure to pollutants during gestation, they can improve health outcomes for their children – especially brain development. Compounds such as mercury, cadmium, nickel, trichloroethylene, and vinyl chloride in the air around the birth residence caused a 50% increase in the risk of autism.

Numerous studies document the neurotoxic effects of heavy metals – especially dangerous to the developing brain is mercury. Yet, many of our children are actually injected with the mercury-containing preservative thimerosal in their infant vaccines. Although thimerosal has been removed from, or perhaps phased out of, many childhood vaccines, it still remains in the flu vaccine, which is recommended by health authorities to pregnant woman as well as to children under age 2. Mercury exposure is such a concern that pregnant women are advised by health authorities not to eat fish because of potential mercury contamination – yet injecting thimerosal is much more damaging than the exposure suffered through eating it in food such as fish. Vaccines also contain aluminum, formaldehyde, and other toxic elements as well as live viruses that, in a subset of infant bodies, can trigger harmful impacts. Heavy metals have also been identified as factors affecting human fertility. Diagnosing and reducing the heavy metal burden of women improved the spontaneous conception chances of infertile women. Women with many dental amalgams had a higher incidence of miscarriages and a higher excretion of mercury when given the chelating agent DMPS (2,3-Dimercapto-1-propanesulfonic acid). It has been found that DMPS was a useful and complementary method to increase fertility compared to hormone therapy in infertile women.

With all this evidence mounting against various environmental toxins affecting human development, an international assembly of scientists, doctors, toxicologists, and researchers sponsored by the

World Health Organization (WHO), the European Environmental Agency, the Centers for Disease Control (CDC), and the National Institutes of Health (NIH) gathered in the Faroe Islands in May 2006. Their consensus statement was clear: "it is time to take action, now." As expected, the declaration highlighted the results of hundreds of studies that showed early fetal exposures to toxic substances, even at low concentrations, can cause health problems later in life. There are a growing number of chemicals that affect the developing embryo, fetus, and infant, including the pesticides DDT, atrazine, methoxychlor, and vinclozolin. Also suspect are plastics and the epoxy resin bisphenol A, plasticizing agents called phthalates, mercury, lead, arsenic, organotoxins, polychlorinated biphenols (PCBs), carbon monoxide, smog, tobacco smoke, and alcohol. The health problems caused by exposure to these substances comprise a dizzying array of maladies including cancer, diabetes, obesity, asthma, and allergies as well as reproductive, cardiovascular, neurological, cognitive, endocrine, psychological, immune, and respiratory troubles.

Other troubling chemicals include parabens (found in various creams and lotions) and triclosan, an antibacterial agent (found in toothpaste, soaps, and cleaning products). Although parabens and triclosan are not ingested, absorbing chemicals through the skin can be far more dangerous than swallowing because transdermal applications are transported directly to the bloodstream. Most women absorb 51 pounds of chemicals every year from their cosmetics alone! Additional exposures emanate from daily lifestyle, profession, and locale. For those elements for which we have the flexibility to make choices, we must choose wisely. After all, it is not just our health that is being affected by our choices but the health of our children and progeny as well.

Basic principles to guide you in decision making surrounding pregnancy are as follows:

1. You are what you eat (and drink); therefore, make healthy choices in what you consume.
2. Skin is the largest organ in the body, so be very careful of what you rub into yours and your baby's.
3. Think beyond "green": What is "green" for the environment is not always what is healthiest for the body, but what is healthiest for the body is always "green."

Suggestions to promote these principles are below and are cumulative, so keep following each set of suggestions as this journey into and through parenthood progresses.

Pre-Pregnancy

While planning a pregnancy, we recommend that you clean up any toxicity in your body and begin to follow a more organic, healthy lifestyle. Remember, the less toxic you are, the better for you and your future baby. Undertake a sequential detoxification program that targets the liver and colon; this type of program can take six months or more and should not be done while pregnant. In a careful manner, with an experienced dentist, remove amalgams from your teeth, which also can take six months or more. Take the time now to find organic, nontoxic makeup, hair, and body products that you like and start integrating them into your daily life. Ask your doctor to run some tests to determine any additional specific supplementation you may need to optimize levels within your body; a good place to start is your copper-zinc ratio (1:1 is the ideal ratio), thyroid function (TSH, free t3, free t4), Vitamin D 25 OH, vitamin A levels, and total cholesterol (low cholesterol is associated with preterm births).

Next, clean up your living and working environment. Remove all harmful chemical cleaning agents from your cleaning routine at home and at the office, and instead use cleaning products labeled level 1 by the EPA. Do not forget to include products for dishwashing and clothing detergent in your cleanup, and avoid toxic dry cleaning as much as possible. Finally, improve your nutrition with a targeted vitamin supplementation program to include omega-3 essential fatty acids, sublingual methyl B-12, folinic acid, vitamin D3, zinc, and antioxidants.

DO	DON'T
• Eat organic, hormone-free food	• Consume fish or foods w/MSG or food dyes
• Drink organic green tea, filtered water, and antioxidant rich organic juices	• Drink soda, carbonated beverages, or alcohol
• Use stevia, raw organic honey, and xylitol as sweeteners	• Consume artificial sweeteners
• Go for walks and get some sunshine daily	• Be exposed to lawn chemicals or second-hand smoke
• Use aluminum-free natural deodorant in them	• Use moisturizers or makeup with chemicals or parabens
• Use natural hennas to color your hair	• Use chemical dyes, perms, or other such hair treatments
• Use cast iron, glass, or stainless steel cookware	• Cook with pans that are non-stick, Teflon coated, or made from aluminum
• Use chemical-free cleaning products in your home	

During Pregnancy

We would suggest that you find a holistic health practice to guide you during pregnancy and delivery as there are many decisions to make during this time. In general, we suggest avoiding medications to the extent possible as well as acetaminophen because it hinders normal detoxification. Add zinc, calcium, essential fatty acids, and prenatal vitamins to your daily supplement intake. Discontinue use of nail polish and any makeup (including lipstick) products that contain parabens and other toxins. Use fluoride-free toothpaste as fluoride interferes with iodine metabolism, which is an issue implicated in mental retardation worldwide.

DO	DON'T
• Yoga and engage in stress management techniques, such as massages and listening to soothing music	• Start a rigorous exercise program, sit in a sauna, or get dental work (not even cleanings)
• Eat fermented foods, cook with organic coconut oil, use organic raw apple cider as salad dressing, and consume healthy fats, and cold pressed oil	• Wait until labor arrives to discuss NOT subjecting your baby to vaccines
• Use natural remedies for pain, like homeopathic arnica	• Talk on a cell phone without a headset or work with a laptop computer on your lap
• Drink kombucha and take probiotics	• Undertake a major home renovation (concern is for lead and other toxins in the process)
• Run an air filter in your bedroom while you sleep	

Infancy

Healthy babies grow and develop perfectly when nature's biochemical processes are allowed to unfold uninterrupted. The sequence of events that leads an infant to begin to focus, develop gross and fine motor skills, begin to speak and to walk is based on a delicate but deliberate series of biochemical processes and chemical interactions. A primary goal of raising a healthy infant is to avoid disruption or interference with this sequence. Babies look fragile and, indeed, they are. An infant's immune system, which guards the rest of the body from harm, is immature and requires time and peace to mature maximally. Thus, help your infant progress uninterrupted by avoiding the introduction of toxins, viruses, allergens, and heavy metals into their bodies. In light of this, parents should consider an alternate, gradual vaccine schedule of carefully thought through vaccines for infants being raised in the domestic United States.

If you have amalgams and plan to nurse, you should send a sample of your breast milk to a specialty lab for heavy metal testing. If you plan to use formula, use those containing DHA (docosahexanenoic acid), an essential fatty acid critical to the healthy development of the central nervous system. In terms of food introduction, organic baby food is recommended. Start feeding with organic rice cereal. Avoid the introduction of soy, gluten, or dairy until after the baby turns two years of age. After one year, supplement your baby with a quarter teaspoon of mercury-free cod liver oil – again this is to increase the supply of omega-3 essential fatty acids.

In terms of coping with baby colds and other minor illnesses, unless symptoms are severe, less is more when it comes to treatment. For fevers over 101°F, treat with a tepid bath or dye-free ibuprofen. Fevers, while nerve-wracking for new parents, are the response of a healthy immune system reacting to kill off an invading virus through heat. Antibiotics should be used sparingly and only for confirmed bacterial infections (they do not alleviate viral infections). Remember, antibiotic use disrupts the normal gut flora and promotes the overgrowth of yeast and resistant organisms that, in turn, harms the optimal functioning of the immune system. Bear in mind that most ear infections are viral and are thus not treatable with antibiotics. Use homeopathic ear drops to help ease the symptoms associated with ear infections and colds.

DO	DON'T
• Invest in an organic baby matress, bedding and pillows and hypo allergenic encasements	• Clothe the baby in pajamas soaked in flame retardant chemicals
• Bathe your baby daily in warm filtered water — enjoy the experience with your baby!	• Use soaps, moisturizers, or other "baby products" on the skin as such items are unnecessary and contain harmful chemicals
• Feed with all organic and hormone-free products	• Introduce dairy, gluten, or soy until after age two
• Feed baby using glass bottles	• Feed baby from plastic bottles or cups or microwave formula or breast milk
• Wearing a hat, walk outside with baby to get 10 to 15 minutes of sunshine daily	• Take your infant into polluted and heavily populated locations
• Run an air filter in baby's bedroom	

Source: http://www.autismfile.com/what-is-autism-facts/autism-symptoms/avoiding-autism

Reprinted with permission.

When a truth is not given complete freedom,
freedom is not complete.

~ Vaclav Havel

Appendix 15

RECIPES
Cooking with Ana

Since 2001 Ana Bobadilla has been a chef to Kerri Rivera and family, including her son Patrick, who has a diagnosis of regressive autism. Over the years she has mastered gluten-free/casein-free to vegan to Atkins and back again. Her dishes always impress and nourish guests and family members alike.

One of the most important pieces to the autism recovery puzzle is diet. As Kerri always says, if your goal is to heal autism, you must do *The Diet*. However, that is easier said than done for many families whose children have self-limited to grilled cheese sandwiches and pizza.

A book is in the works containing dozens of delicious recipes using natural ingredients that can be found in almost any country. Ana has found unique ways to make foods that children on the spectrum can enjoy, without breaking the bank. The ingredients that she uses can be found all over the world, not just the US. They are presented here in a very approachable way so even if you are not a whiz in the kitchen your child will be able to enjoy what you serve.

The following is a sneak peek from *Cooking with Ana*:

Almond Milk

Amount: 1 L of milk

- 1 cup of peeled almonds
- 1 L of filtered water
- Stevia and vanilla to taste

Preparation:

To a saucepot of boiling water, add the almonds. Remove immediately from the fire. Allow almonds to soak for 20 minutes, remove them from water, rinse, dry and blend in a liter of filtered water. Strain the liquid through a piece of cheesecloth until all the water is drained. Add agave syrup and vanilla to taste.

Vegetable Fries

3 Servings

Ingredients:

- 3 Carrots
- 1 cup oil
- Salt to taste

Preparation:

Peel the carrots and then form very thin slices using the same peeler. Pat dry with a piece of cloth to remove any excess water. Heat oil in a frying pan and fry carrots. When frying be very careful because they can quickly burn, be sure to have a slotted spoon ready to remove from the oil as soon as they are crisp. After frying carrots remove excess oil with a paper towel and sprinkle some salt on top of them.

You can also do this recipe with banana, potato, sweet potato or jackfruit. This is a great alternative to French fries or if you want to eat something crunchy.

Beef or Chicken Tostadas

4 Servings

Ingredients:

- 5 ground chicken breasts or beef filets
- 1 cup of rice or coconut flour
- 1 cup of oil
- Salt and pepper to taste

Preparation:

In a mixing bowl, combine the ground chicken, flour, salt, pepper and a ½ cup of oil. Mix thoroughly until a uniform dough results. Take approximately 2 tablespoons of the dough and form small tortillas/flat circles with it. They should be approximately ¼ inch think and 4 inches wide. Fry in a layer of oil until cooked through, and a thin outer crust forms, or bake in a 350 degree oven, after pouring a dollop of oil on top of each tostada.

Coconut Bars

15-18 bars

Ingredients:

- 3 cups of vegan butter (or coconut oil)
- 1 cup of honey
- 1 cup of raisins
- 1 cup of grated of coconut
- 1 cup of walnuts
- 1 tablespoon of salt

Preparation:

In a saucepan over medium heat combine honey and butter, stirring constantly for a few minutes until thoroughly combined. Remove from heat and mix with all other ingredients. Spread in a 9x13 casserole pan without oil, and bake in an 350°F (180°C) over for 25 minutes until it sets. Allow to cool, and cut into small rectangles.

*Get people back into the kitchen
and combat the trend toward
processed food and fast food.*

~ Andrew Weil

Appendix 16

Websites We Like

General:

♥ Our website containing the latest information about our research, videos, forums, etc.
www.cdautism.org

♥ The Spanish version of our website.
www.autismo2.com

♥ *Curando el Autismo* is a Puerto Rican organization created by three mothers of children recovered from autism who have an interest in helping the community learn about their options.
www.curandoelautismo.com

♥ Defeating Autism - Non-Profit Organization in Venezuela that utilizes Kerri's Protocols.
www.fundacionvenciendoelautismo.blogspot.mx

♥ Autism Research Institute originally founded by Dr. Bernard Rimland. Home of the ATEC survey.
www.autism.com

♥ Our public Facebook page.
www.facebook.com/groups/AutismCD

♥ *CD Health*: Facebook group dedicated to using the protocol for non-autism related issues.
www.facebook.com/groups/mojoother

Diet:

♥ **Website forcused on the *Specific Carbohydrate Diet*™ (SCD) in English.**
www.pecanbread.com

♥ **Top 10 FAQs about the *Specific Carbohydrate Diet* (SCD) in Spanish.**
www.pecanbread.com/pandenuez/10preguntas.html

♥ **Autism Network for Dietary Intervention**
www.autismndi.com

♥ **Gluten Free/Casein Free Diet Intervention website.**
www.gfcfdiet.com

♥ **Intestinal health through diet with the Specific Carbohydrate Diet™**
www.breakingtheviciouscycle.info

♥ **Resource for naturally healing digestive disease, reducing stress and living a long, healthy life.**
www.scdlifestyle.com

♥ ***The Feingold® Association* is a non-profit organization helping provide dietary management and generate public awareness of the role food and synthetic additives play in behavior, learning and health problems.**
www.feingold.org

Chlorine Dioxide (CD):

♥ **Jim Humble's MMS (CD) website.**
www.jimhumble.org

♥ **Another popular site about MMS (CD).**
www.mmswiki.org

♥ **Spanish site selling various books about MMS (CD)**
www.voedia.com

♥ **Andreas Kalcker's website (in English)**
www.andreaskalcker.com

♥ **CD research site by Andreas Kalcker (in Spanish)**
www.medicasalud.com

♥ **A huge public health forum with thousands of discussions about every imaginable health topic. Also includes surveys about various topics.**
www.curezone.com

♥ **Good sources of CD and other related supplies.**
www.wps4sale.com
www.mightyguts.com

♥ **The latest information on CDH.**
http://www.mmsinfo.org/infosheets/infosheet_cdh.pdf

Hyperbarics:

♥ **Good source of information about Hyperbaric Oxygen Therapy.**
www.hyperbaric-oxygen-info.com

Other Valuable Source of Information:

♥ **PubMed comprises of more than 23 million citations for biomedical literature from MEDLINE, life science journals, and online books.**
www.ncbi.nlm.nih.gov/pubmed

♥ **Parents Helping Parents - P.A.N.D.A.S. Network: A Resource Library of Medical Studies and Case Histories**
www.pandasnetwork.org

♥ **International OCD Foundation**
www.ocfoundation.org/PANDAS/

Videos / Audio of Interest:

💜 **Video Testimonials. This link contains various health testimonials related to MMS, many are about autism.**
www.youtube.com/mmstestimonials

💜 **AutismOne 2012: 38 Children Recovered in 20 months with MMS by Kerri Rivera**
www.autismone.org/content/38-children-recovered-20-months-mms-0

💜 **Video about Kerri, produced by Daniel Bender in 2012.**
www.youtube.com/watch?v=HnCiX5bll-Y

💜 **Kerri speaks in Bulgaria, 2013 (Voice in English, slides in Bulgarian)**
www.youtube.com/watch?v=4OxNGIEWzds

💜 **Kerri on the Robert Scott Bell Show**
http://www.youtube.com/watch?v=-1zJhr5VhxE

💜 **MMS Autism Webinars**
http://www.ustream.tv/channel/mms-autism-webinar%20

💜 **Patrick Timpone interviews Kerri Rivera (8/15/2013)**
http://oneradionetwork.com/health/kerri-rivera-healing-the-symptoms-known-as-autism-children-are-not-born-with-autism-so-they-should-not-die-with-it-august-15-2013/

💜 **Patrick Timpone interviews Kerri Rivera (11/18/2013)**
http://oneradionetwork.com/health/kerri-rivera-encore-interview-healing-the-symptoms-known-as-autism-using-parasite-protocols-and-chlorine-dioxide-november-18-2013/

💜 **Bulletproof Executive Radio with Dave Asprey (11/27/2013)**
http://www.youtube.com/watch?v=R7s7IYj2SCs

Appendix 17

<u>Direct Help from Kerri Rivera</u>

Consults

Since the release of the first edition of the book, we have found that when families decide to implement The Protocol some do not need further assistance beyond reading the information in this book, using our online support groups, YouTube videos, and attending conferences. However, there are some of us who need a more personalized approach and support to navigate the information, or would like ideas on dosing or timing.

For those of us who need or want that additional support, consults are perfect. We can work together to map out a plan for the parent/family and child, brainstorm through challenges, or just know that you will never walk alone. Whatever the case may be I am available if you need me. I am fluent in English and Spanish, and we can use a translator for other languages. We can speak over the phone or on Skype.

As time goes on, more and more practitioners will be able to support families while using this protocol. In the meantime, If you would like to set up a consult with me, please click on the "Consult Kerri" button on...

www.CDAutism.org

...and follow the instructions there.

> Kerri Rivera's undivided attention + discussing your child + $100 = priceless. Tonight, instead of living it up in Mexico, Kerri spent her Friday evening on the phone doing a consult with me. Not only was the consult informative but also highly enjoyable. Kerri's energy is contagious, her vision boundless and her sense of humor edgy (just the way I like it). Kerri thank you for rocking our world! You are an amazing lady and my family is eternally grateful for your love of our children. Peeps, if you are new, stuck, confused or you want a better understanding of the protocol PLEASE, PLEASE, PLEASE take advantage of this opportunity. I've done a million consults over the years but this was by far my favorite.

Note: A consult with Kerri does not constitute medical advice, nor is it a substitute for a consult with your doctor or healthcare provider. As always, you are responsible for your health, and for the health of your children.

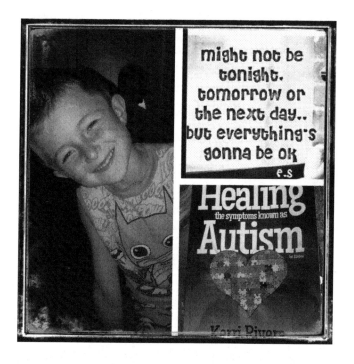

References

Chapter 3 - Diet

1. Siri, Ken, and Tony Lyons. Cutting-Edge Therapies for Autism 2011-2012. New York: Skyhorse, 2011. Print.

2. Knivsberg, A.M., K.L. Reichelt, T. Høien, and M. Nødland. "A randomized, controlled study of dietary intervention in autistic syndromes. Nutritional Neuroscience 5.4 (2002) : 251-261. Print.

3. "Frequently Asked Questions." The GFCF Diet Intervention – Autism Diet. TheGFCDiet.com, n.d. Web. 19 Mar. 2013.

4. Reichelt, Karl L., Dag Tveiten, Anne-Mari Mari Knivsberg, and Gunnar Brønstad. "Peptides´ role in autism with emphasis on exorphins." Microbial Ecology in Health & Disease 23 (2012). Web. 11 May 2013.

5. Shattock, Paul, and Paul Whiteley. "Biochemical aspects in autism spectrum disorders: updating the opioid-excess theory and presenting new opportunities for biomedical internvention. Expert Opinions on Therapeutic Targets 6 (2002) : 175–183. Print.

6. Fasano, A. "Dr. Fasano on Leaky Gut Syndrome and Gluten Sensitivity. " Gluten Free Society, n.d. Web. 11 May 2013.

7. "How does gluten and casein relate to the problem of autism?" University of Florida. Department of Pediatrics Division of Genetics and Metabolism, n.d. Web. 11 May 2013.

8. Appleton, Nancy, and G.N. Jacobs. Suicide by Sugar A Startling Look at Our #1 National Addiction, New York: Square One, 2009. Print.

9. Tobacman, J.K. "Review of harmful gastrointestinal effects of carrageenan in animal experiments." Environmental Health Perspectives 109.10 (2001) : 983-994. Print.

10. McMillan, Tricia. "Does Splenda sugar substitute have chlorine in it?" Livestrong.com, Demand Media. 11 June 2011. Web. 11 May 2013.

11. "Food and Drugs." 21 CFR 102.22. 2012. Web. 11 May 2013.

12. Wallinga, David, Janelle Sorensen, Pooja Mottl, and Brian Yablon. Institute for Agriculture and Trade Policy. "Not So Sweet: Missing Mercury and High Fructose Corn Syrup." 2009. Web. 11 May 2013.

13. Gottschall, Elaine. "About the Diet." Breaking the Vicious Cycle, n.d. Web. 11 May 2013.

14. Gottschall, Elaine. "Autism & GI Problems." Breaking the Vicious Cycle. n.d. Web. 11 May 2013.

15. Reasoner, Jordan. "Phenols and Salicylates: What They Are and Why it Matters." SFK. Web. 2010. 11 May 2013.

16. Campbell-McBride, Natasha. Gut and Psychology Syndrome: Natural Treatment for Autism, Dyspraxia, A.D.D., Dyslexia, A.D.H.D., Depression, Schizophrenia. 2nd ed. Cambridge UK: Medinform. 2010. Print.

17. Sarah. "Don't Waste Your Time: Why the Candida Diet Doesn´t Work." The Healthy Home Economist. Austus Foods. 15 Nov. 2012. Web. 11 May 2013.

Chapter 4 - An Introduction to Chlorine Dioxide

1. Port, Tami. "Gram Negative (Gram-) Bacteria." Suite101. 27 July 2007. Web. 11 May 2013.

2. Toxicological Profile for Chlorine Dioxide and Chlorite. U.S. Department of Health and Human Services. Public Health Service. Agency for Toxic Substances and Disease Registry. September 2004. Pg 25. 3.2.2 Oral Exposure. 3.2.2.1 Death. Web. 11 May 2013.

Chapter 5 - Chlorine Dioxide (CD)

1. Lubbers, Judith R., Sudha Chauan, and Joseph R. Bianchine. "Controlled Clinical Evaluation of Chlorine Dioxide, Chlorite and Chlorate in Man." Environmental Health Perspectives 46 (1982) : 57-62. Print.

2. Ballantyne, Coco. "Strange but True: Drinking Too Much Water Can Kill You." Scientific American. 21 June 2007. Web. 11 May 2013.

3. "Woman died from too much water´." BBC News. 12 Dec. 2008. Web. 11 May 2013.

4. Humble, Jim. The Master Mineral Solution of the Third Millennium. 5th ed. Jim V. Humble 2011. Print.

5. Harman, D. "Aging: a theory based on free radical and radiation chemistry." Journal of Gerontology 11.3 (1956) : 298-300. Print.

6. Harman, D. "The biologic clock: the mitochondria?" Journal of the American Geriatrics Society 20 (1973) : 145–147. Print.

7. Watson, J. "Oxidants, antioxidants and the current incurability of metastatic cancers." Open Biology. 12 April 2013. Web. 11 May 2013.

8. Tarr, Peter. "Nobel laureate James Watson publishes novel hypothesis on curing late-stage cancers." Cold Spring Harbor Laboratory. 7 January 2013. Web. 11 May 2013.

9. Kilic, Eser, Süleyman Yazar, Recep Saraymen, and Hatice Ozbilge. "Serum malondialdehyde level in patients infected with Ascaris lumbricoides." World Journal of Gastroenterology 9 (2003) : 2332-2334. Print.

10. Kosenko, Elena, Yuri Kaminski, Oksana Lopata, Nikolay Muravyov, and Vicente Felipo. "Blocking NMDA receptors prevents the oxidative stress induced by acute ammonia intoxication." Free Radical Biology & Medicine 26 (1999) : 1369-1374. Print.

11. Lee, J.K., E.H. Choi, K.G. Lee, and H.S. Chun. "Alleviation of aflatoxin B1-induced oxidative stress in HepG2 cells by volatile extract from Allii Fistulosi Bulbus." Life Science 77 (2005) : 2896-2910. Print.

12. Nielsen, F., B.B. Mikkelsen, J.B. Nielsen, H.R. Andersen, and P. Grandjean. "Plasma malondialdehyde as biomarker for oxidative stress: reference interval and effects of life-style factors." Clinical Chemistry 43 (1997) : 1209-1214. Print.

13. Anwar, H., M.K. Dasgupta, and J.W. Costerton. "Testing the susceptibility of bacteria in biofilms to antibacterial agents." Antimicrobial Agents and Chemotherapy 34.11. (1990) : 2043-2046. Print.

14. Usman, Anju. AutismPedia. 12 May 2010. Web. 11 May 2013.

15. Budinger, Mary. "Lyme-Induced Autism Conference Focuses on Biofilm and Toxicity." Public Health Alert. 4.8. Publichealthalert.org. Aug. 2009. Web. 11 May 2013.

16. "Children With Autism Have Mitochondrial Dysfunction, Study Finds." Science News. 30 November 2010. Web. 11 May 2013.

17. MMS Autism Webinar - May 10, 2012, Andreas Kalcker & Kerri Rivera.

Chapter 8 - The Kalcker Parasite Protocol

1. Volinsky, Alex, A., Nikolai V. Gubarev, Galina M. Orlovskaya, and Elena V. Marchenko. "Developmental stages of the rope´ human intestinal parasite" Submitted to arxiv.org 13 Jan. 2013. Web. 11 May 2013.

2. United States. Department of Health and Human Services, Food and Drug Administration, Centre for Food Safety and Applied Nutrition. Fish and Fishery Products Hazards and Controls Guidance 4th Edition. Florida: Government Printing Office, 2011. Web. 11 May 2013.

3. Zam, S.G., Martin, W.E., and Thomas Jr., L.J. "In Vitro uptake of Co^{60} –vitamin B_{12} by Ascarias suum." The Journal of Parasitology 49 (1963): 190-196. Print.

4. Vasudevan D.M., Sreekumari, S., and Vaidyanathan, K. "Textbook of BIOCHEMISTRY for Medical Students. 6th ed." Section D: Nutrition. New Delhi, 2011. 404. Print.

5. "Water related diseases; Ascariasis." Water Sanitation Health. WHO. 2013. Web. 11 May 2013.

6. "Mebendazole Dosage." Drugs.com. n.d. Web. 11 May 2013.

7. Wina, Peter. "Clay Uses – Parasite Removal – Yes, You Do Have Worms!" aboutclay.com. n.d. Web. May 13 2013.

8. "Parasites – Cysticercosis." Centers for Disease Control and Prevention. n.d. Web. 11 May 2013.

9. Nielsen, Flemming, Mikkelsen, Bo Borg, Nielsen, Jesper Bo, Andersen, Helle Raun, and Grandjean, Philippe. "Plasma malondialdehyde as biomarker for oxidative stress: reference interval and effects of life-style factors." Clinical Chemistry 43 (1997) : 1209-1214. Print.

Chapter 9 - Other Supplements

1. "What are probiotics?" Theralac. Master Supplements. n.d. Web. 11 May 2013.

2. "Frequently Asked Questions About Theralac." Purest Colloids. 2013. Web. 11 May 2013.

3. "Autism." The Probiotic Revolution. Freedom. n.d. Web. 11 May 2013.

4. Messaoudi, Michaël, Robert Lalonde, Nicolas Violle, Hervé Javelot, Didier Desor, Amine Nejdi, Jean-François Bisson, Catherine Rougeot, Matthieu Pichelin, Murielle Cazaubiel, and Jean-Marc Cazaubiel. "Assessment of psychotropic-like properties of a probiotic formulation (Lactobacillus helveticus R0052 and Bifidobacterium longum R0175) in rats and human subjects." British Journal of Nutrition 105 (2011) : 755–764. Print.

5. Silk, D. B. A., A. Davis, J. Vulevic, G. Tzortzis, and G.R. Gibson. "Clinical trial: the effects of a trans-galactooligosaccharide prebiotic on faecal microbiota and symptoms in irritable bowel syndrome." Alimentary Pharmacology & Therapeutics 29 (2009) : 508–518. Print

6. "Omega-3 fatty acids." University of Maryland Medical Center. A.D.A.M. 2011. Web. 11 May 2013.

7. "Omega-6 fatty acids." University of Maryland Medical Center. A.D.A.M. 2011. Web. 11 May 2013.

8. Bell, J.G., E.E. MacKinlay, J.R. Dick, D.J. MacDonald, R.M. Boyle, and A.C.A. Glen. "Essential Fatty Acids and Phospholipase A2 in Autistic Spectrum Disorders." Prostaglandins Leukotrienes and Essential Fatty Acids 71.4 (2004) : 201-204. Print.

9. Richardson, A.J., and P. Montgomery. "The Oxford-Durham Study: A Randomized, Controlled Trial of Dietary Supplementation with Fatty Acids in Children with Developmental Coordination Disorder." Pediatrics 115.5 (2005) : 1360-1366. Print.

10. "GABA." Healing Autism & ADHD. n.p. n.d. Web. 11 May 2013.

11. English, Jim. "Saving Eli: One Family's Struggle with Autism." Jim English. 2012. Web. 11 May 2013.

12. "L-Theanine Information." L-Theanine. n.d. Web. 11 May 2013.

13. "Pycnogenol." Horphag. n.d. Web. 11 May 2013.

14. "1 in 50 US. Kids Have Autism." Autism Coach. n.d. Web. 11 May 2013.

15. Chez, Michael G., Cathleen P Buchanan, Mary C. Aimonovitch, Marina Becker, Karla Schaefer, Carter Black, and Jamie Komen. "Double-Blind, Placebo-Controlled Study of L-Carnosine Supplementation in Children With Autistic Spectrum Disorders." Journal of Child Neurology 17 (2002) : 833-837. Print.

16. Smith, Leonard. "Are You Dangerously Deficient in Taurine?" drlwilson. n.d. Web. 11 May 2013.

17. "DMG supplement." Healthcare Information Directory. iHealth Directory. n.d. Web. 11 May 2013.

18. "Dimethylglycine (DMG) for Autism." Autism Research Institute. n.d. Web. 11 May 2013.

19. "Find a Vitamin or Supplement Betaine Anyhydrous." WebMD. Therapuetic Research Faculty. 2009. Web. 11 May 2013.

20. "Nutritional DMG/TMG Treatment Overview." Autism Canada Foundation. 2011. Web. 11 May 2013.

Chapter 10 - Chelation

1. "Why Cleanse Metals." Baseline of Health Foundation. n.d. Web. 11 May 2013.

2. Klinghardt, Dietrich. "D: Amalgam/mercury detox as a treatment for chronic viral, bacterial and fungal illnesses." Explore 8 (1997) : 13-16. Print.

3. Price, Weston A. Nutrition and Physical Degeneration. 8th ed. Lemon Grove, CA: Price Pottenger Nutrition, 2008. Print.

4. "Bentonite clay for internal healing." Healing Daily. 2005. Web. 11 May 2013.

5. Clinical Evaluation of Bio-Chelate™." Bio-Chelat™. 09 Dec. 1987. Web. May 11, 2013.

Chapter 11 - Hyperbarics

1. University of Pennsylvania School of Medicine. "Penn Study Finds Hyperbaric Oxygen Treatments Mobilize Stem Cells." ScienceDaily. 28 Dec. 2005. Web. 11 May 2013.

Chapter 12 - GcMAF & Autism

1. Bradstreet, James Jeffrey, Vogelaar Emar, and Thyer Lynda. "Initial Observations of Elevated Alpha-N-Acetylgalactosaminidase Activity Associated with Autism and Observed Reductions from GC Protein—Macrophage Activating Factor Injections." Original Research. "Autism Insights 4 (2012): 31-38. Print.

Chapter 14 - Miscellaneous Information You Should Know

1. Garcia, H.H, and M. Modi. Helminthic parasites and seizures. Epilepsia 49 Suppl 6. (2008) : 25-32. Print.

2. "Self-Injurious Behavior." Autism Research Institute. n.d. Web. 11 May 2013.

3. PANDAS-PITAND Awareness & Research Support. 2011. Web. May 11 2013.

4. Jenike, Michael, and Susan Dailey. International OCD Foundation. 2012. Web. May 11 2013.

5. Jenike, Michael, and Susan Dailey. "Sudden and Severe Onset OCD – Practical Advice for Practitioners and Parents." Beyond OCD. 2013. Web. 11 May 2013.

6. Bock, Kenneth and Nellie Sabin. The road to Immunity: How to Survive in a Toxic World. New York: Pocket Books, 1997. Print.

7. "Fever." AskDrSears. 2013. Web. 11 May 2013.

8. "NINDS Febrile Seizures Information Page." National Institute of Neurological Disorders and Stroke. 2013. Web. 11 May 2013.

9. Gilbère, Gloria. "Skin & Intestinal Disorders." Leaky Gut Syndrome. Dawn
    Mellowship. 2005. Web. 11 May 2013.

10. Edward, F. "14 Common Symptoms of Parasites." Parasite Cleanse Resource
    Center. 10 June 2009. Web. 11 May 2013.

11. "Body Burden: The Pollution in Newborns. A Benchmark Investigation of
    Industrial Chemicals, Pollutants and Pesticides in Umbilical Cord Blood."
    Environmental Working Group. 14 July 2005. Web. 11 May 2013.

Appendix 5 - Molecular Mimicry

1. Fasano A, Berti I, Gerarduzzi T, Not T, Colletti RB, Drago S, Elitzur Y, Green PH,
    Guandalini S, Hill ID, Pietzak M, Ventura A, Thorpe M, Kryszak D, Fornaroli F,
    Wasserman SS, Murray JA, Horvath K. "Prevalence of celiac disease in at-risk
    and not-at-risk groups in the United States: a large multicentre study." Arch
    Intern Med. 163.3 (2003): 286-292. Print.

2. Vojdani A, O'Bryan T, Kellermann GH. "The immunology of gluten sensitivity
    beyond the intestinal tract." European Journal of Inflammation." 6.2 (2008) : 0-0.

3. Vojdani A., O'Bryan T, Kellermann GH. "The Immunology of Immediate and
    Delayed Hypersensitivity Reaction to gluten." European Journal of Inflammation
    Vol 6.1, (2008) :1-10

4. Vojdani A, O'Bryan T, Green JA, McCandless J, Woeller KN, Vojdani E, Nourian
    AA, Cooper EL. "Immune Response to Dietary Proteins, Gliadin and Cerebellar
    Peptides in Children with Autism." Nutr Neurosci. 7.3 (2004) : 151-161. Print.

5. Ford RP. "The gluten syndrome: a neurological disease. Med Hypotheses." 73.3
    (2009) : 438-440. Print.

6. Ford, RP. The Gluten Syndrome: Is Wheat Causing You Harm. Dr. Rodney Ford
    MD MBBS FRACP Smashwords 2011 ebook

7. Hadjivassiliou M, Sanders DS, Grunewald RA, Woodroofe N, Boscolo S,
    Aeschlimann D., "Gluten sensitivity: from gut to brain." Lancet Neurol.
    9.3(2010):318-30.

8. Solaymani-Dodaran M, West J. Logan RF. Long-term mortality in people with
    celiac disease diagnosed in childhood compared with adulthood: a population-
    based cohort study. Am J Gastroenterol. 102.4 (2007): 864-870. Print.

9. Fedoroff, Nina V, and Nancy Marie Brown. Mendel in the Kitchen: A Scientist's
    View of Genetically Modified Food. Washington, DC: Joseph Henry Press, 2006.
    Print.

10. Corrao G, Corazza GR, Bagnardi V, Brusco G, Ciacci C, Cottone M, Guidetti CS,
    Usai P, Cesari P, Pelli MA, Loperfido S, Volta U, Calabró A, Certo M. "Mortality
    in patients with coeliac disease and their relatives: a cohort study." Lancet.
    358.9279 (2001) : 356-361. Print

Index

C

G

H

Z

About the Author

Kerri Rivera is a native of Chicago, but has lived the last 19 years of her life in Puerto Vallarta, Mexico with her husband. Both of her sons were born there, and 13-year-old Patrick is currently in autism recovery. Kerri is the founder of AutismO2, a non-profit autism clinic based on what is formerly known as the *Defeat Autism Now!* approach. Located in Puerto Vallarta, the clinic opened in 2006. Kerri is the clinic's biomedical consultant as well as a consultant for Curando El Autismo (Latin America), and Venciendo el Autismo (Venezuela).

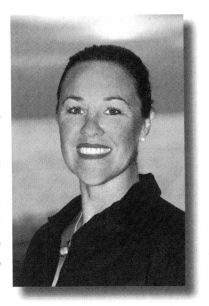

At the request of Dr. Bernard Rimland, she was responsible for translating the *Defeat Autism Now!* protocol to Spanish and donating it to the Autism Research Institute, so it could be applied throughout Latin America. Since then she has helped over 3,500 families in over 58 countries to improve the lives of their children on the autism spectrum. She has become the foremost expert on the use of CD (chlorine dioxide) for spectrum disorders. Since the addition of CD to the biomedical protocol she has seen 115 children recover from autism in the past 2.5 years.

Since 2007 Kerri has lectured internationally on the Biomedical Protocol for autism and CD for autism. She has been featured on *One Radio Network* with Patrick Timpone, *The Bulletproof Executive* with Dave Asprey, *The Mother Cub Show, Thought for Food, Enlightened Health Radio* with Justin Elledge, *Voice America*, and *The Robert Scott Bell Show*. She is the Mexican Liaison for AutismOne. Kerri graduated as a Certified Homeopath in June of 2013.

Our greatest weakness lies in giving up.

The most certain way to succeed is always to try just one more time.

~ Thomas Edison

Made in the USA
Lexington, KY
22 May 2017